Atlas of Computerized Perimetry

Atlas of Computerized Perimetry

Dr. med Jörg Weber
Büchheimer Str. 64
51063 Köln
Germany

Joseph Caprioli, M.D.
Frances and Ray Stark Professor of Ophthalmology
Chief, Glaucoma Division
Jules Stein Eye Institute
UCLA School of Medicine
Los Angeles, California

W.B. SAUNDERS COMPANY
A Division of Harcourt Brace & Company
Philadelphia London Toronto Montreal Sydney Tokyo

W.B. Saunders Company

A Division of Harcourt Brace & Company

The Curtis Center
Independence Square West
Philadelphia, Pennsylvania 19106

Library of Congress Cataloging in Publication Data

Weber, Jörg.
[Atlas der computerperimetrie. English]
Atlas of computerized perimetry / Jörg Weber, Joseph Caprioli.
p. cm.
ISBN 0–7216–6737–6
1. Perimetry Atlases. I. Caprioli, Joseph. II. Title.
RE79.P4V43 2000
617.7'15—dc21 99–16763

ATLAS OF COMPUTERIZED PERIMETRY ISBN 0–7216–6737–6

Printed in the United States of America

Last digit is the print number: 9 8 7 6 5 4 3 2 1

DEDICATION

To Dr. George L. Spaeth

Physician, Surgeon, Teacher, and Philosopher

NOTICE

Computerized Perimetry is an ever-changing field. Standard safety precautions must be followed, but as new research and clinical experience broaden our knowledge, changes in treatment and drug therapy become necessary or appropriate. Readers are advised to check the product information currently provided by the manufacturer of each drug to be administered to verify the recommended dose, the method and duration of administration, and the contraindications. It is the responsibility of the treatment physician, relying on experience and knowledge of the patient, to determine dosages and the best treatment for the patient. Neither the publisher nor the editor assumes any responsibility for any injury and/or damage to persons or property.

The Publisher

Foreword

The significance of ophthalmic disease is the deterioration of health it may cause. This is also true for the treatments used to treat ophthalmic disease. The value of these treatments is measured in terms of their ability to heal or their potential for harm. One way in which both diseases and treatments can harm is by causing loss of visual function.

There are, of course, different components of visual function, including the ability to resolve an image (visual acuity), to perceive motion, to note change of light intensity, to distinguish colors, and to locate an object in the space around the eye, that is, to appreciate the field of vision. All of these components play important roles in our ability to function. While visual acuity (the ability to resolve images) is necessary for many activities, the capacity of locating oneself in space is essential for ambulation, and the capacity to locate images in space (as occurs when reading or performing most tasks) is essential for most daily functions. Understanding the biologic basis of the visual field and how to measure the visual field provides fundamental information about how we function and how health can be enhanced or preserved. It is not surprising, then, that the study and function of the visual field have long been at the heart of the study of many types of ophthalmic and neurologic diseases. This applies to conditions as different as congenital pits of the optic nerve, drusen of the optic disc, acoustic neuromas, multiple sclerosis, retinal vein occlusions, cerebrovascular accidents, and the glaucomas. Evaluation of the visual field has been used both to understand what disease process might be present, that is to say, in diagnosis, and also to monitor the course of the disease, that is, management.

There are two essential aspects of testing the visual field: (1) the instrumentation used to define the nature of that field (hardware), and manipulation of the hardware, and (2) the interpretation of what is found (software). Modern computerized perimetry has concerned itself with both the hardware and the software.

Regarding instrumentation, there are two major ways of studying the visual field. The two methods address slightly different questions. One asks if an object can be seen when it moves; the other asks if the object can be seen when it is still. Confrontation field can be done in ways that utilize both of these methods. More sophisticated techniques for evaluating the fields can also use both these methods in different forms. Some types of abnormalities, such as those with precipitous sharp edges or those in the far periphery of the field, can best be noted by some type of motion perimetry. Arc perimetry, using moving objects, has long been used to quantitate this kinetic component of the field, and for many years was the "gold standard." Other diseases, such as glaucoma, are best studied by defining the nature of the visual field on a point-to-point basis to determine the sensitivity of receptors in a particular area, so-called static perimetry. The initial static perimeters, such as those developed in Tübingen, however, were too cumbersome to use easily in a clinical setting. Some of the newer machines provide magnificent equipment with which to detect the nature of the visual field, making static perimetry accessible, affordable, and reliable.

The present text is clear, thorough, and current in the discussion of instrumentation and how the hardware operates.

The second aspect of the visual field examination deals with the interpretation of the findings plotted by the machine or by the examiner. These interpretive aspects of perimetry are far more complex than the measurement of the field itself. They are also far more important. After all, how can one tell whether the representation of the field on the printout is an accurate, valid representation of the actual visual field? Are the changes merely artifact? Are they real, that is, representations of an abnormality in the visual field, but not representations of diseases or of what is trying to be understood? For example, is an apparent superior nasal field loss due to mispositioning of the head, the edge of the lens correcting the patient, a drooping lid, an asymmetrical cataract, normal aging, the patient fixating below the expected point of fixation, moderate glaucomatous nerve damage, or minimal glaucomatous nerve damage made apparently worse by a tiny pupil?

Interpretation requires knowing, for example, the anatomic cause of a particular type of visual field defect, which types of defects lead to particular diagnoses, which normal fluctuations occur due to chance, short- or long-term normal physiological changes, and other variabilities in the testing process. For example: When does the absence of an apparent change *really* mean that there is no change? When does the presence of an apparent change *really* mean that there has been a change? What do these changes *really* mean in terms of the health or disease of the patient?

The authors have juxtaposed anatomic considerations, clinical characteristics, and visual field results in a way that is original, clear, helpful, and in a word, brilliant. I know of no other text in which this has been done so effectively. By using numerous cases, which include a graphic depiction of the anatomical considerations, the clinical aspects (as shown, for example, in an MRI or fundus photograph), and the actual visual field plots, the clinicopathologic correlations become understandable and memorable.

The penultimate chapter provides remarkably helpful algorithms and simplifications of patterns to assist in diagnosis and differential diagnosis.

The extraordinarily beautiful Air on the G String by Johann Sebastian Bach exists in different formats: musical notation on paper, digital encoding on a compact disc, or sound waves perceived by a listener. For the overwhelming majority of people the only way the music is meaningful is in the analog form as the sound waves reach the brain and are consciously perceived. Trained musicians, however, can actually "hear" the music by scanning the musical notation. But, even though the desired information is right there on the CD, *nobody* can hear the Air on the G String by looking at the CD. The problem, however, is *not* that the information is not there, but rather that we cannot understand what is there. Testing and evaluating the visual field are like performing music. Skill both in instrumentation and interpretation is required. The real meaning, moreover, is only there for the person who knows what the "notes" mean and how they fit together to make "music."

In an elegant, artistic, and scientifically accurate way, *Atlas of Computerized Perimetry* provides readers with what they need to know about visual fields to understand the theory, the instrumentation, and the interpretation, so that they can be the most helpful in enhancing or maintaining the health of patients entrusted to their care.

George L. Spaeth, M.D.
Professor of Ophthalmology
Thomas Jefferson University
Director, Glaucoma Service
Wills Eye Hospital

Preface

It has been more than 20 years since the introduction of an automated perimetry. Since then, the field has expanded enormously, to the extent that a complete manual of computerized perimetry is not possible in a short textbook. *Atlas of Computerized Perimetry* is conceived to graphically display principles and methods and to provide an overview of findings with printouts that the practitioner will encounter. This is essentially an atlas with juxtaposition of text and figures to represent the findings clearly, and to make the complexity of the methodological details more easily understood.

In Chapter 1, though many interesting sensory phenomena are not described, the reader is confronted with some essential information, which is often provided with nongraphical definitions. The going becomes a bit easier in Chapter 2, where representations are graphical by nature. The findings in Chapter 3 represent the largest part of the book and provide information about the most frequent and perimetrically most important diseases and findings. Artifacts are also summarized in this chapter.

Interpretation and differential diagnosis is the most difficult task in perimetry. We made an effort to disassemble this process into several logical steps, which are provided in Chapter 4. Chapter 5 discusses the identification of change as it relates to the study of chronic progressive disease, especially glaucoma. Trend analysis based on sound statistical precepts provides an objective and reasonable tool to make informed judgements concerning progression or stability of visual field loss.

Finally, no text is perfect. Some parts of this text are simplified for didactic purposes, and we may later learn that some other parts contain true errors. Please forgive these transgressions. We would be very grateful if readers would communicate with us about any errors or ambiguities if they are found.

Jörg Weber, M.D.
Joseph Caprioli, M.D.

Contents

Atlas of Computerized Perimetry

1 Fundamentals and Technique

1.1 THE QUALITATIVE VISUAL FIELD

Definition

The visual field consists of all the visual space that is perceived by the eye at one time. The basic element of spatial perception is visual direction, a vector quantity. All objects which lie on the same line as this vector are projected onto a single point of the retina, regardless of their distance from the eye (Fig. 1.1A). Each point on the retina transforms light energy into electrical stimuli, which are transmitted by a series of nerve cells to a particular location in the visual cortex. Here they evoke a visual perception. Disturbances of perception involve all objects in a given visual direction. In clinical medicine, which deals mainly with disturbances of perception, the visual field is defined as the sum of all visual directions that are seen simultaneously.

Documentation

Visual directions are usually specified with a polar coordinate system which uses the dimensions of angle and eccentricity. The point of visual fixation is represented by the origin. Similar to the way in which a starry sky can be projected onto a celestial globe, the visual field can be projected onto a perimetric hemisphere. Flat maps, however, are more convenient for routine documentation and evaluation (Fig. 1.1B). The transfer of hemispheric data to a flat map causes distortions similar to those found in terrestrial and celestial maps. The most common cartographic projection is a true center-distanced, polar azimuthal projection in which the hemisphere is flattened. Meridional distances and angles from the pole are shown correctly, but the circular distances are stretched. The amount of stretching is about 5% at 30° from the center and about 30% at 60° from the center. Using this flat map, points in the visual field can be described by a rectangular (Cartesian) coordinate system in which points are located with respect to the x- and y-coordinates; distortion is still present in this type of representation. The "internal" coordinates of the corresponding retinal locations are not identical to their visual field coordinates because the optical nodal point and the anatomical center of the eye do not coincide.

Figure 1.1A. All points along the same visual direction are projected to a single location in the retina and, from there, to a particular location in the visual cortex. The visual field is represented by the sum of all directions from which light is perceived.

Figure 1.1B. The visual directions are represented by a polar coordinate system. The projection from the visual field hemisphere to a flat map causes distortion.

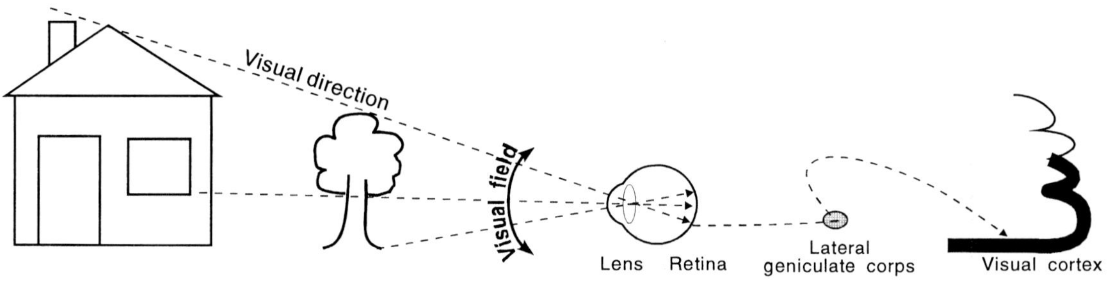
Visual direction
Visual field
Lens
Retina
Lateral
geniculate corps
Visual cortex

1.1A

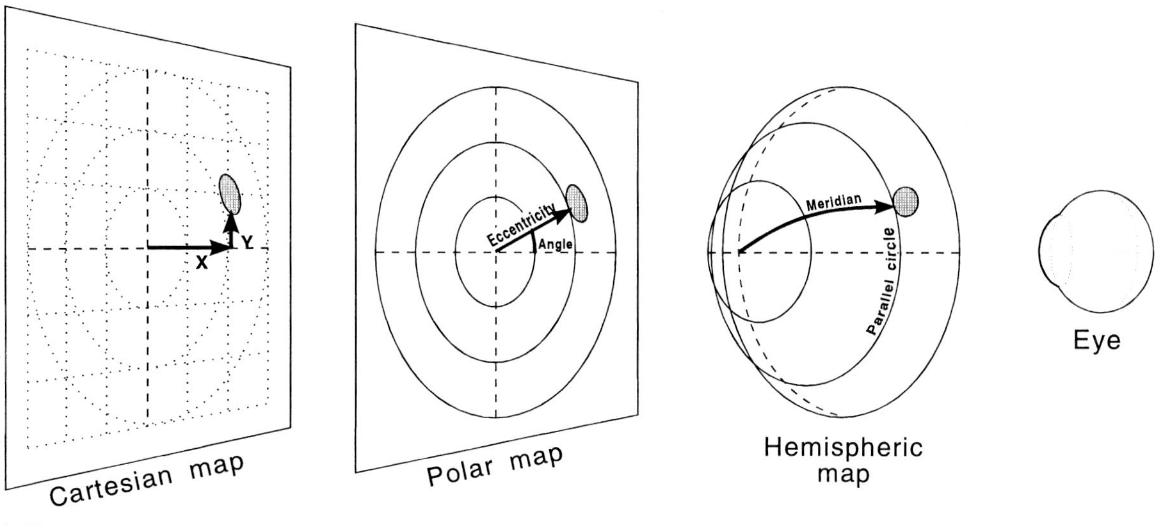
X
Y
Cartesian map
Eccentricity
Angle
Polar map
Meridian
Parallel circle
Hemispheric
map
Eye

1.1B

Normal Visual Field

The normal visual field extends up to 60° nasally and superiorly, up to 70° inferiorly, and almost 100° temporally. These upper limits are narrowed slightly with age (Fig. 1.1C).

Terminology

In the common practice of perimetry, the visual field is defined in a flat, two-dimensional way. Visual directions are called *visual field locations* or *visual field points.* The sum of all the visual directions is called the *visual field area.* The boundary between what is seen and what is not seen is called the *border.* If the visual field border is located more centrally than normal, the visual field has become constricted (Fig. 1.1D). Any area inside the outer borders which is not seen and which is surrounded by an area which is seen is called a *scotoma.* The physiological blind spot is a normal scotoma which is present in every visual field. It is caused by the interruption of the retina by the optic nerve head. This scotoma is located approximately 15° temporally and 1° below the horizontal axis. It measures about 5° horizontally and 7° vertically.

Figure 1.1C. The border of the normal visual field (right eye).

Figure 1.1D. The qualitative visual field. The solid line represents the measured outer visual field borders, and the dashed line shows the normal field border. Constrictions are central displacements of the outer field border, and scotomas are areas within these borders which are not seen. BS = physiological blind spot.

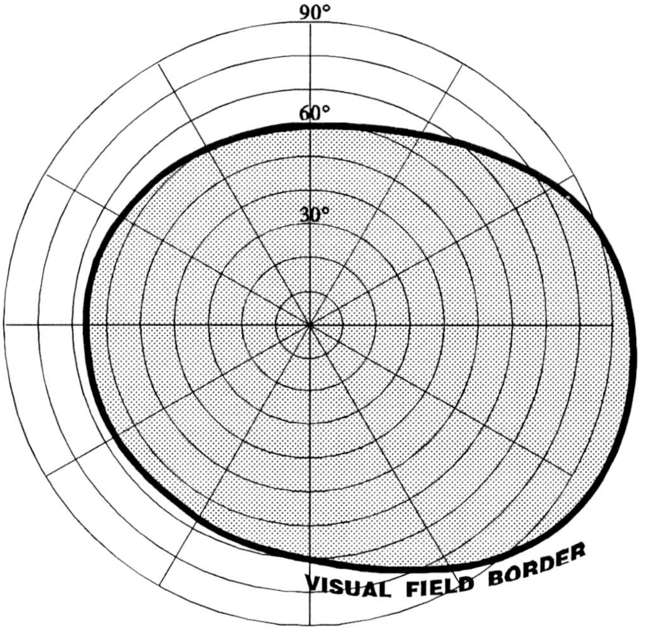
90°
60°
30°
VISUAL FIELD BORDER

1.1C

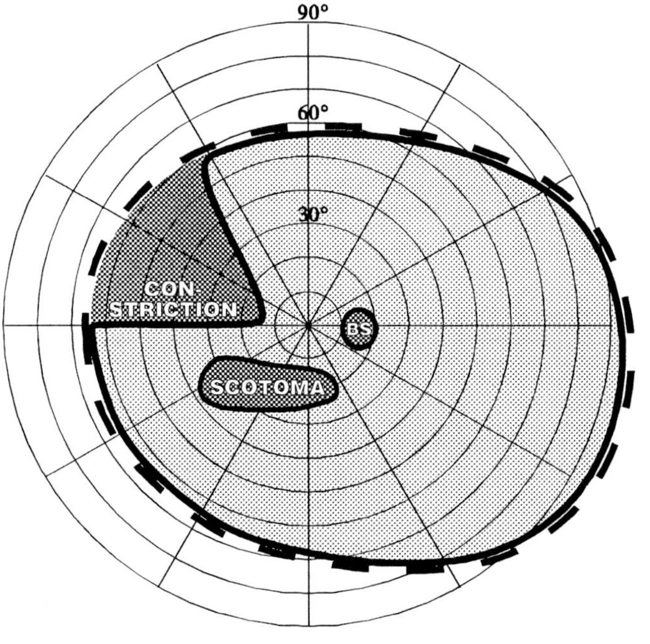
90°
60°
30°
CON-
STRICTION
BS
SCOTOMA

1.1D

1.2 THE QUANTITATIVE VISUAL FIELD

Definitions

Visual sensitivity can be measured in every visual direction (at every point in the visual field) with light stimuli of varying sizes and intensities. The field directions not only have the qualitative property of being seen or not seen, but also quantitative properties. This distinction was introduced by Bjerrum at the end of the nineteenth century when he created a scaled system of stimulus intensities. The definition of the visual field can now be extended: *the visual field is the sum of all visual directions and the visual sensitivity in these directions that are seen simultaneously.*

Documentation

Visual sensitivity may be thought of as a third dimension, although it is not a true dimension in space. The quantitative visual field can thus be thought of as a "hill" of vision, with the height of the hill representing visual sensitivity (Fig. 1.2A). The height of the hill of vision can be depicted on a flat chart by colors or shades of gray (grayscale, Fig. 1.2B).

Normal Visual Field

Visual sensitivity decreases continuously from the center toward the periphery (Fig. 1.2A–C). On the temporal side, the slope is less steep and the absolute minimum (outer border) is arrived at more peripherally than in other areas of the field. When comparing the visual fields of different individuals, age is important: at all locations of the visual field, sensitivity decreases with age. The rate at which visual sensitivity decreases with age depends on the location of the visual field; the rate of decrease with age is greater peripherally than centrally.

Figure 1.2A. The normal hill of vision: the *z*-axis represents visual sensitivity.

Figure 1.2B. grayscale display: the different shades of gray are equivalent to the color codes of a topographical map.

Figure 1.2C. Isopters: the isopters are equivalent to the lines on a topographical map which connect all points of equal altitude.

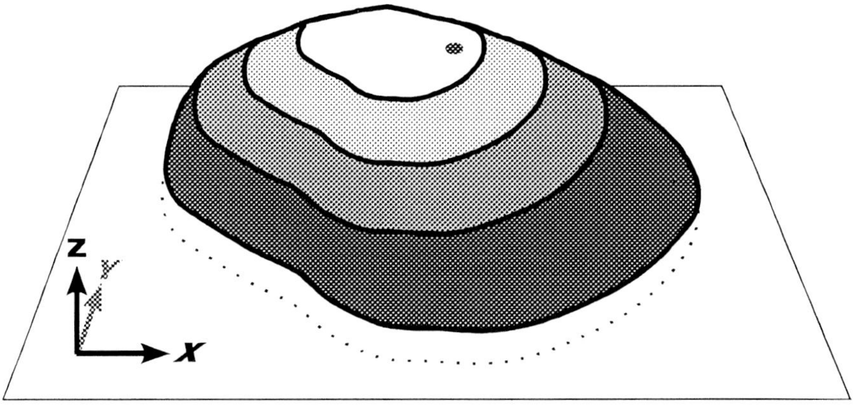

1.2A

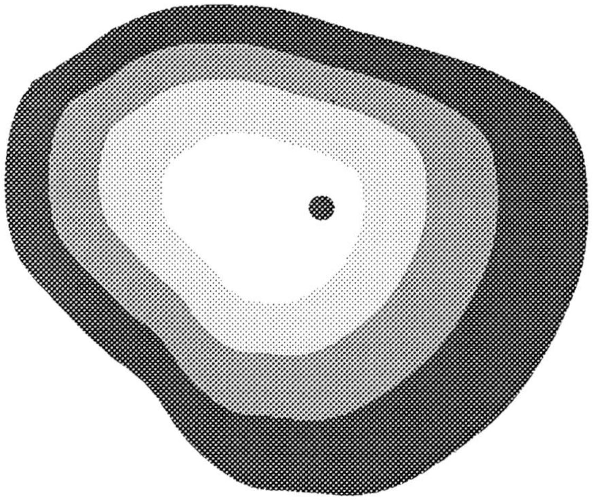

1.2B

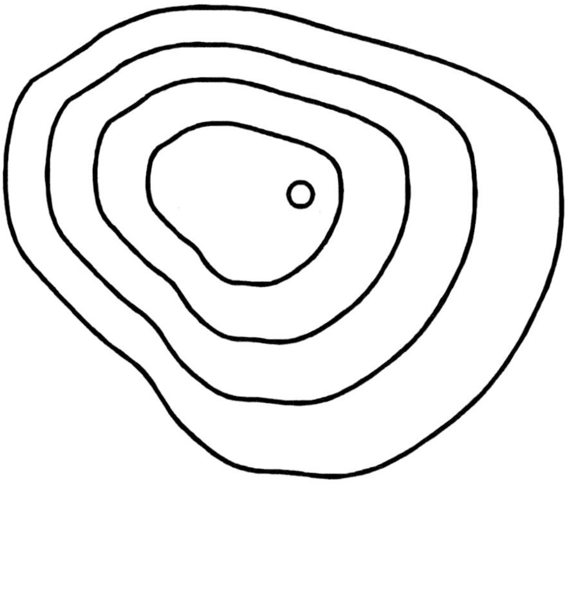

1.2C

Terminology

Pathological alterations of the visual field can be measured as reductions in visual sensitivity compared to the normal visual field. Such reductions are called *visual field defects.* The amount of reduction is the *defect depth.* In a grayscale representation, a defect is represented by a darkening of the affected area. In an isopter representation, the areas between the isopter lines are equivalent to a single shade of gray in a grayscale representation. When a defect is present, the isopters shift such that the defect lies between isopters of lower sensitivity.

Alternatively, changes in the shape of the isopter are described in terms of qualitative perimetry, such as relative constriction of an isopter or relative scotoma. To derive a realistic image of the visual hill, linear changes must be converted to spatial changes: scotomas are circumscribed defects (Fig. 1.2D); constrictions are wedge-shaped defects contiguous with the outer border (Fig. 1.2E); and concentric constrictions are generalized reductions, which may be either diffuse (Fig. 1.2F) or peripheral (Fig. 1.2G), depending on the position on the isopters.

Figure 1.2D–G. Equivalents of spatial grayscale representation and linear isopter representation.

Figure 1.2D. Scotoma.

Figure 1.2E. Peripheral constriction.

Figure 1.2F. Concentric constriction.

Figure 1.2G. Concentric constriction, especially in the periphery.

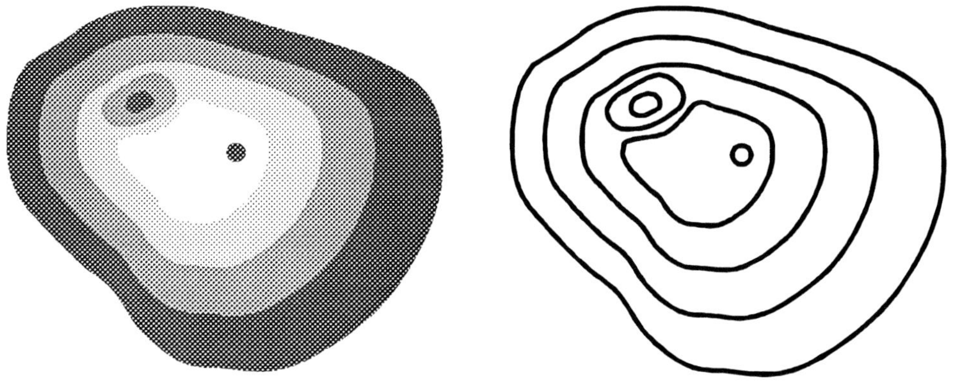

1.2D

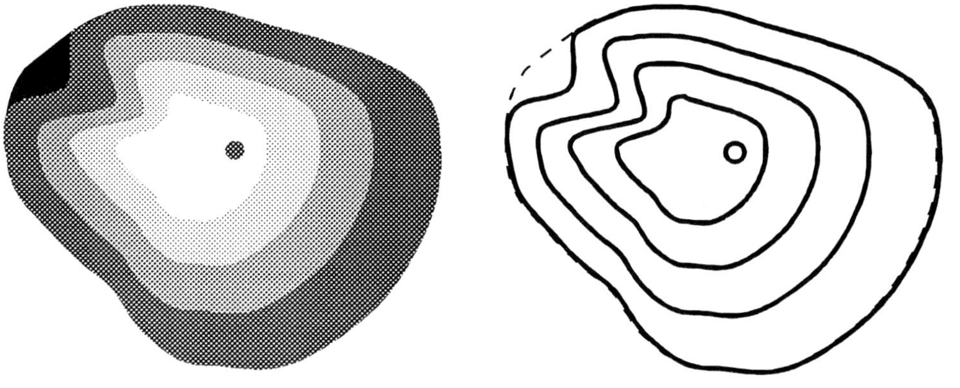

1.2E

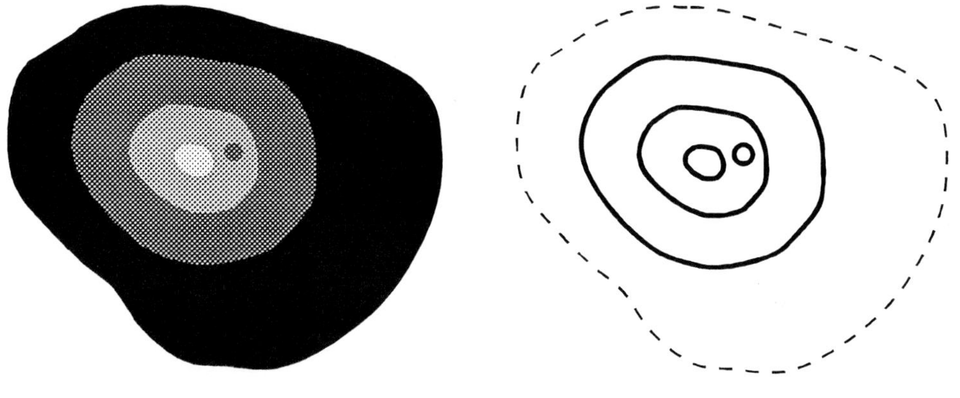

1.2F

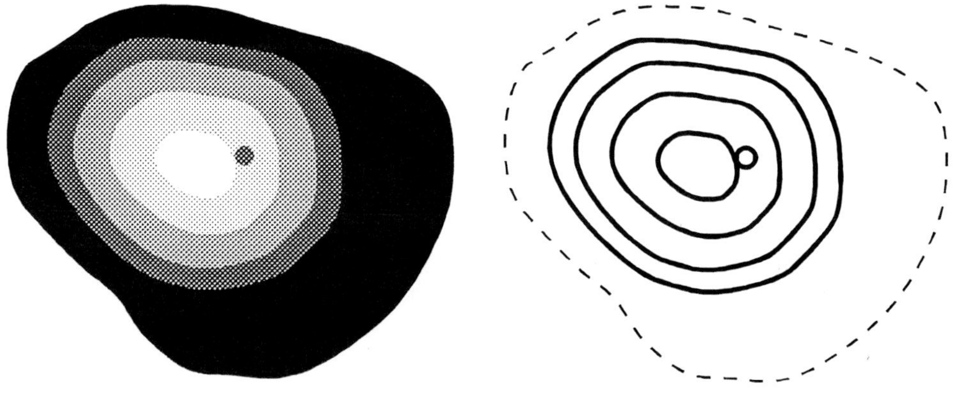

1.2G

1.3 TECHNIQUES OF COMPUTERIZED PERIMETRY

The instrument used to measure the visual field is called a *perimeter*. It consists of an optical or optomechanical unit which produces the stimulus and a control unit. In automated perimeters the control unit is a microprocessor. There are differences in the way stimuli are generated.

In conventional perimetry, visual sensitivity is measured with illuminated spots of different luminance on a background of reduced luminance. There are different ways to create such a stimulus. At present, four types of perimeters are in use: projection perimeter, retroillumination perimeter, microprojection perimeter, and cathode ray tube perimeter.

Projection Perimeter

The background is an evenly illuminated hemisphere. The stimulus is projected into the bowl with movable, often motorized, mirrors (Fig. 1.3A).

Retroillumination Perimeter

The background is also a hemisphere which consists of a semitransparent plastic sheet. The stimulus light sources illuminate the bowl from behind the sheet. Light sources are fixed light-emitting diodes (LEDs) or light fibers coming from a common bulb. The number of stimulus locations is more limited compared to other perimeters, but more than 400 locations are possible in modern units (Fig. 1.3B).

Microprojection Perimeter

Basically, this is a projection perimeter with some modifications (inverted projection direction, split ray trace for background and stimulus), but it is miniaturized. The optical system projects stimuli at normal sizes and at an optically infinite distance. Available instruments are limited to an eccentricity of 30° (Fig. 1.3C).

Cathode Ray Tube Perimeter

The cathode ray tube (CRT) is a convenient way to project stimuli of different types and shapes. At present, the examination is limited to an eccentricity of 25° due to the size of the CRT. The maximal luminance is 400 cd/m^2. Based on the scanning principle, the luminance has saw-like temporal characteristics (Fig. 1.3D).

Figure 1.3A. Projection perimeter.

Figure 1.3B. Retroillumination perimeter.

Figure 1.3C. Microprojection perimeter.

Figure 1.3D. CRT perimeter.

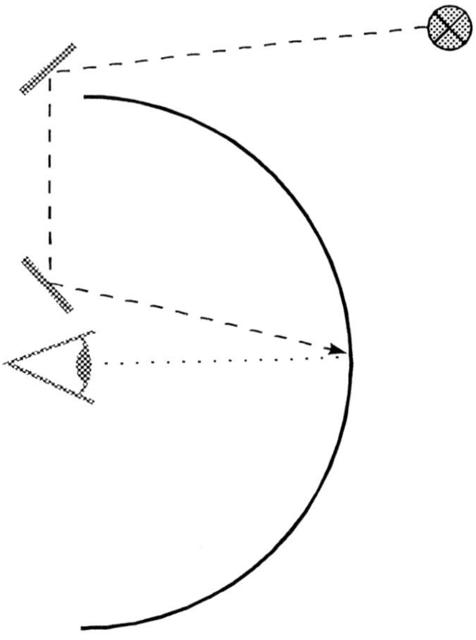

1.3A

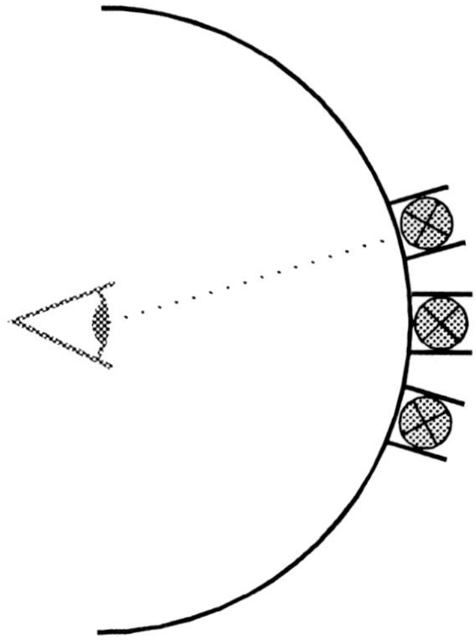

1.3B

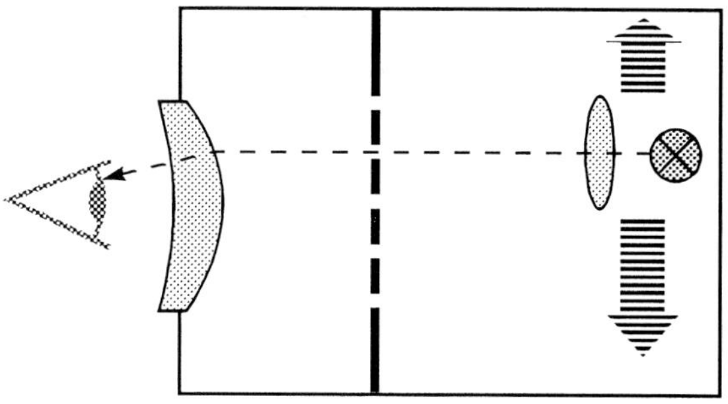

1.3C

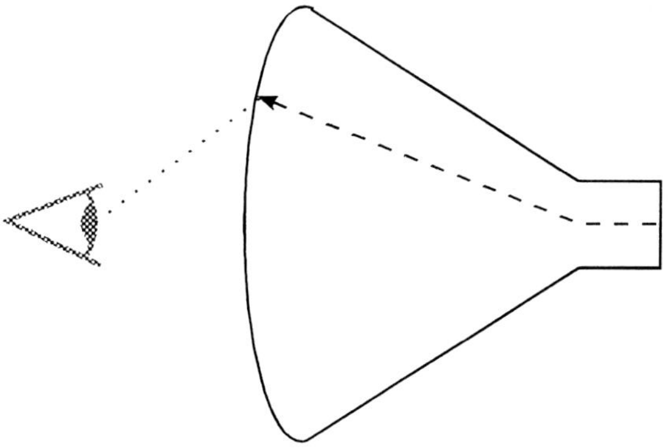

1.3D

1.4 DEFINITION OF STIMULUS POWER AND VISUAL SENSITIVITY

Visual sensitivity in a visual field direction is assessed with stimuli of different sizes and intensities. The stimulus which is just perceived is the *threshold stimulus.* It defines the visual sensitivity. The higher the visual sensitivity, the lower the threshold stimulus.

Stimulus Type

The classical type of stimulus in perimetry is a circular *spot of light* (Fig. 1.4A). Its perceptibility depends on the four physical stimulus factors: brightness, color, size, and duration. In computerized perimetry, variation in stimulus power is created by variation in brightness, while color, size, and duration are kept constant during an examination.

Stimulus Brightness

Brightness is luminance (L) in candelas per square meter (cd/m^2). The older unit, the apostilb (asb), is still frequently used (1 asb = 0.318 cd/m^2). The important dimension for stimulus perception is the *difference between the luminance of the light spot, the stimulus luminance* L_S, *and the luminance of the surround, the background luminance* L_B. Both absolute differential luminance $\Delta L = L_S - L_B$ and relative differential luminance or contrast $\Delta L/L_B$ can be used for measurement.

Scaling of Stimulus Luminance and Sensitivity

In computerized perimetry, *decibel* scales are commonly used. They are characterized by logarithmization and an inversion of the sign: high decibel values represent low luminance contrasts (Fig. 1.4B). Therefore, the visual scale is a scale not only of stimulus intensity with an inverted sign, but also of visual sensitivity with a positive sign. The formula for differential light sensitivity DLS and reverse stimulus intensity I^* is

$$DLS\,[\mathrm{dB}] = I^*[\mathrm{dB}] = 10 \times \left(-\log\left(\Delta L/L_B\right)\right) + \text{constant}$$

The constant differs from perimeter to perimeter and is commonly chosen so that the brightest stimulus of the instrument L_{MAX} corresponds to a visual sensitivity of 0 dB. In this case, the formula can be transformed into

$$DLS\,[\mathrm{dB}] = I^*[\mathrm{dB}] = 10 \times \log\left(L_{MAX}/\Delta L\right).$$

Figure 1.4A. The light spot stimulus has the stimulus luminance L_S, and the surround has the background luminance L_B. The luminance difference $L = L_S - L_B$ is an important parameter with respect to visual perception.

Figure 1.4B. The decibel scale is a scale of both stimulus intensity and visual sensitivity. The logarithmic steps are also commonly used with kinetic techniques, such as those used on the Goldmann perimeter.

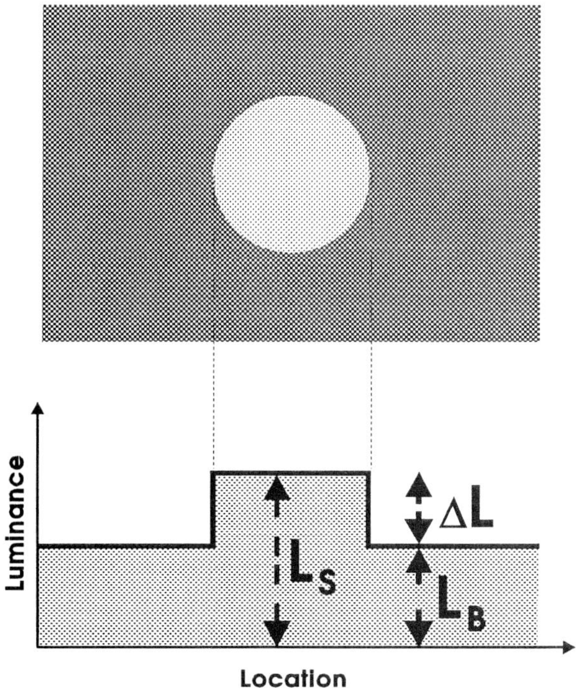

Luminance
ΔL
L_S
L_B
Location

1.4A

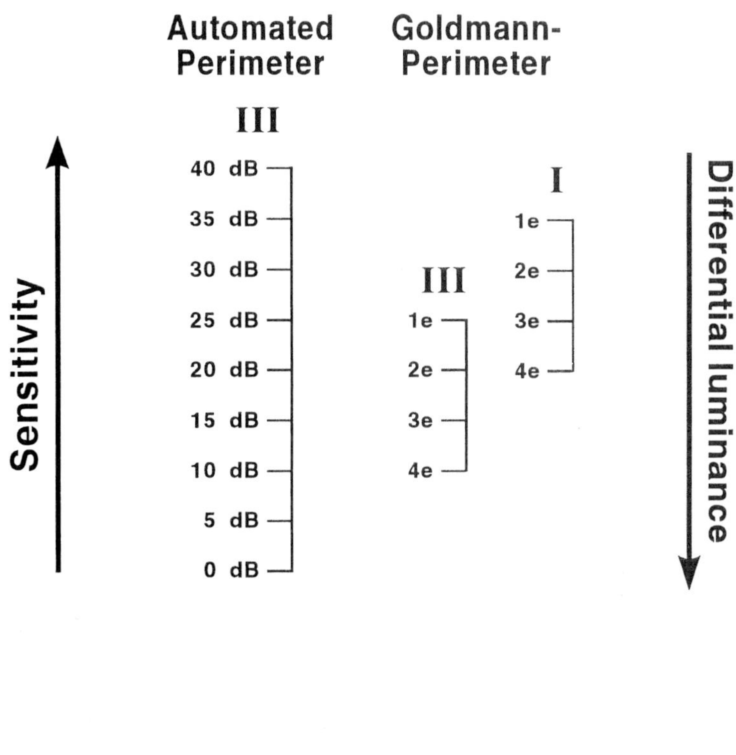

Automated Perimeter
Goldmann-Perimeter
III
40 dB
35 dB
30 dB
25 dB
20 dB
15 dB
10 dB
5 dB
0 dB
III
1e
2e
3e
4e
I
1e
2e
3e
4e
Sensitivity
Differential luminance

1.4B

1.5 PRINCIPLES OF KINETIC AND STATIC MEASUREMENT

Kinetic Perimetry

In kinetic perimetry, the stimulus is moved from nonseeing to seeing areas of the visual field, to the point where the patient first perceives it. This procedure is repeated with a stimulus of the same size and intensity in different regions of the visual field. Thus, numerous threshold positions are identified; these positions are connected and form a line of the equivalent DLS, the isopter. This method is generally used in manual perimetry (Fig. 1.5A).

Static Perimetry

In computerized perimetry, the static method is used almost exclusively. At predefined visual field locations the threshold stimulus is determined. Therefore, a stimulus is shown repeatedly at each location, but with different stimulus intensities (*stimulus sequence;* see measurement procedure, Fig. 1.5B). The size of the stimulus is usually held constant throughout a single test.

Differences Between the Methods

Movement as a stimulus factor: the movement of a stimulus increases its perceptibility. It follows, then, that the sensitivity levels of a kinetic field are higher than those of the corresponding static field. This difference, the *stato-kinetic dissociation,* is increased in some disorders (Riddoch phenomenon) and results in deeper measured defects in the static field.

Position of the measurement locations (Fig. 1.5B): in static perimetry, the measurement locations are predefined. In kinetic perimetry, the directions and speed of stimulus movement can be defined; the locations of the measured thresholds are influenced by the response of the patient and the shape of the visual field. Therefore, the spatial density of measurement locations can vary considerably from test to test and from patient to patient.

Measurement direction (Fig. 1.5C): the sensation of stimuli near the visual threshold is variable and "noisy." If we consider a three-dimensional representation of the visual field, this range of variability extends in the *z*-direction (sensitivity). With static measurements, the range of measurement variation is parallel to this range of variability. The kinetic stimulus, however, crosses this range of variability, either for a long distance in the case of flat defects or for a short distance in the case of deep defects. Therefore, kinetic measurements are less accurate in flat areas and more accurate in steep areas of the visual hill.

Relationship between stimulus presentation and the patient's response (Fig. 1.5D): the patient's response follows perception of the stimulus after a certain reaction time, usually about 0.5 sec, but with large interindividual variation. In kinetic perimetry, the position of the stimulus at the time of response is shifted slightly away from the position at the time of perception. The distance of this shift is the product of reaction time and stimulus velocity. In static perimetry, each stimulus presentation is followed by a waiting interval which is considerably longer than the average reaction time. A response during this interval is correctly related to the previous stimulus and is usually not influenced by the length of the reaction time.

Figure 1.5A. Principles of kinetic (left) and static (right) measurements.

Figure 1.5B–D. Differences between kinetic and static measurements.

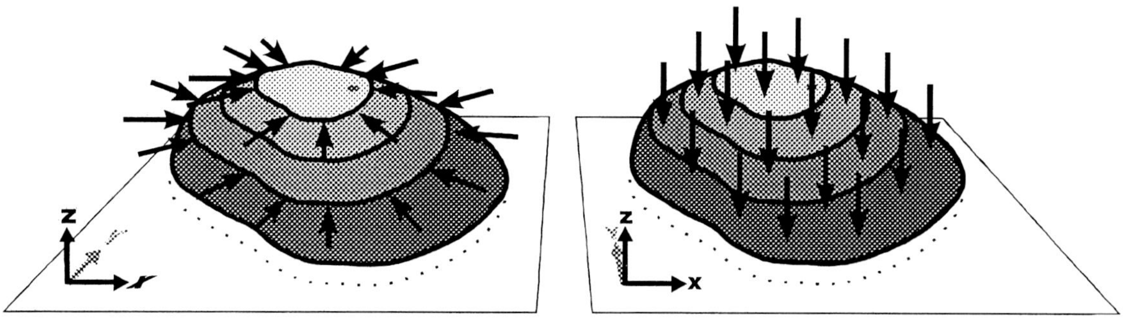

1.5A

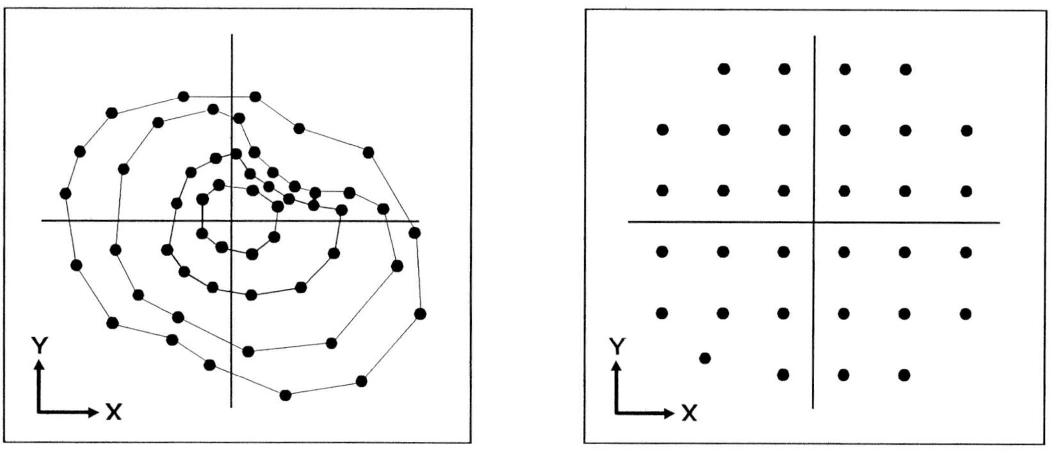

1.5B

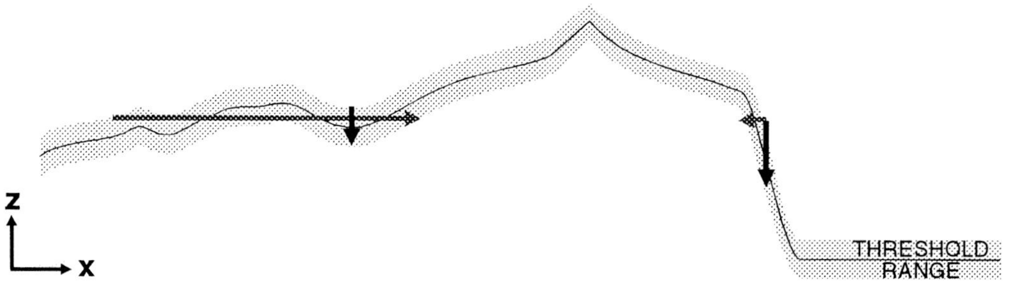

1.5C

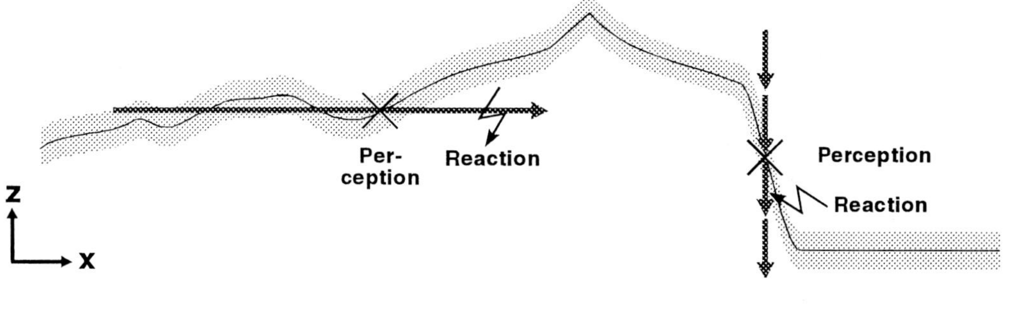

1.5D

1.6 STATIC MEASUREMENTS

Threshold Strategy (Staircase Method)

The most effective method of threshold determination is the staircase method. After presentation of each stimulus, the stimulus intensity is changed toward the direction of the presumed threshold, depending on the patient's response. If the response is positive, the next stimulus is dimmer. If the response is negative, the next stimulus is brighter. The stimulus intensities approach the threshold intensity (threshold convergence) and, after a few stimulus presentations, oscillate around the actual threshold (Fig. 1.6A).

In computerized perimetry, the 4 dB, 2 dB staircase method is most commonly used (Spahr and Fankhauser 1974). First, the stimulus intensity is increased or decreased in steps of 4 dB. After the first change in the patient's response (which presumably corresponds to a crossing of the threshold), the intensity is altered in steps of 2 dB. After the second change in the patient's response (the threshold is crossed again), the stimulus sequence is completed. The threshold intensity is the mean between the last stimulus seen and the last stimulus not seen.

Other methods differ according to the step size used (e.g., 3 dB steps used by the Competer and the Humphrey Fastpac). Variable steps (the *dynamic strategy;* Weber 1989) are also used and can be more efficient if they are tailored to the patient. Other modifications of the staircase method are related to the number of changes in the patient's response that are required to complete the procedure.

Suprathreshold (Supraliminal) Strategy

This procedure, which is also called a *screening strategy* or *scanning strategy,* does not measure sensitivity but instead classifies it into two to four categories. In one modification, only values below a normal range are actually measured or *thresholded.*

The brightness of the first stimulus is 4 to 6 dB brighter than the normal threshold, depending on the program. Thus, the decibel value is reduced by this amount. If this stimulus is perceived, the sensitivity is classified as normal and testing at that location is finished. If the stimulus is not perceived after two presentations, it is recorded as a defect. The simple two-category (one-level) strategy is finished at this point. With the three-category (two-level) strategy, (Fig. 1.6B), a defect will be examined further with the brightest stimulus. If a negative response occurs, this location is recorded as an *absolute defect;* otherwise, it is recorded as a *relative defect.* The four-category strategy continues to test the relative defects and distinguishes *deep relative defects* and *shallow relative defects.* The quantitative suprathreshold strategy measures all defects with a common staircase procedure.

Figure 1.6A. Long staircase method (*threshold strategy*) with five reversals of the patient's response.

Figure 1.6B. Suprathreshold strategy with three categories (two test levels).

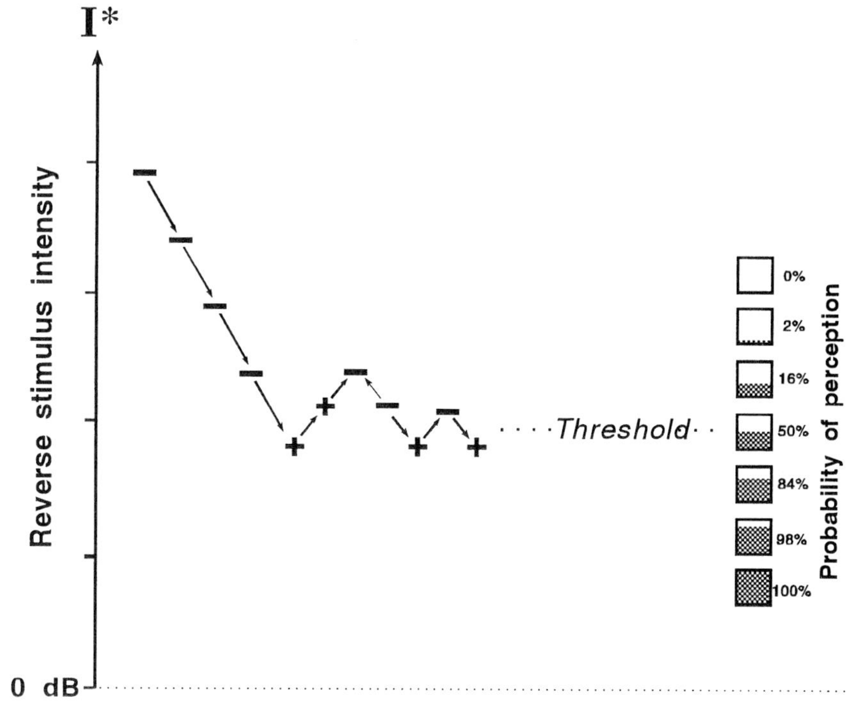
I*
Reverse stimulus intensity
Threshold
0 dB
0%
2%
16%
50%
84%
98%
100%
Probability of perception

1.6A

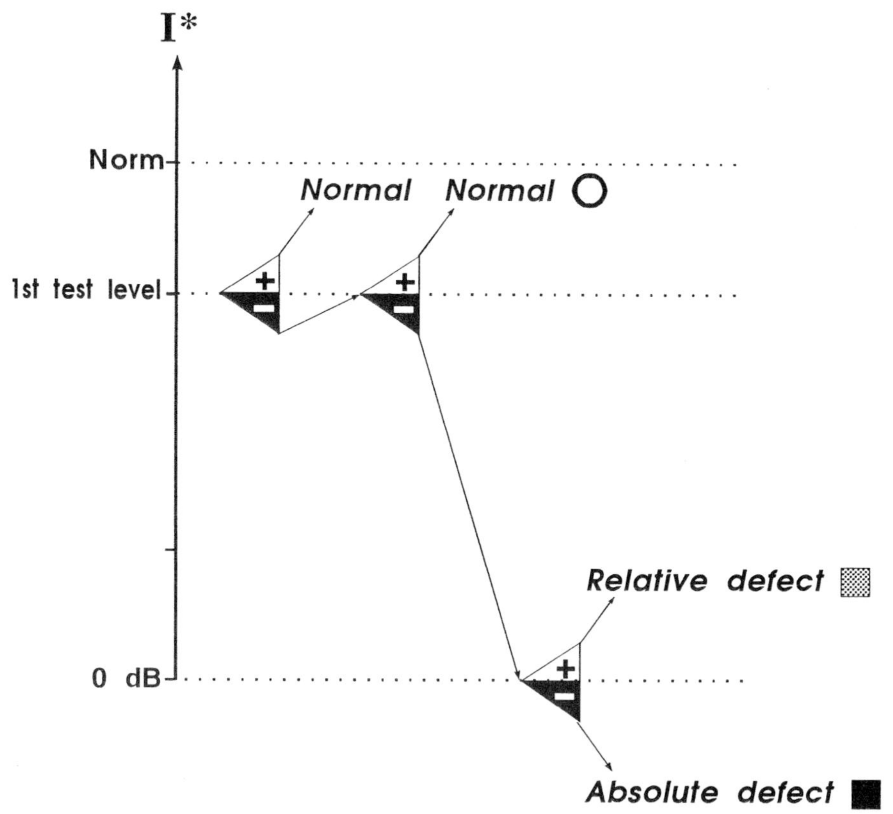
I*
Norm
Normal
Normal
1st test level
Relative defect
0 dB
Absolute defect

1.6B

Variability of the Measured Threshold (Measurement Error)

Like every measurement procedure, the staircase method is associated with measurement error. In psychophysics, this error is partly dependent on the method—especially step size—and partly dependent on the consistency of the patient's response. Inconsistency occurs within a zone around the threshold (*threshold zone*). Within the threshold zone, the frequency of positive responses increases from nearly 0% to nearly 100%. The threshold, by definition, is the stimulus to which the patient responds 50% of the time. This threshold zone is about 8 dB wide in the normal sensitivity zone (from 2% to 98% frequency of seeing). In areas of decreased sensitivity, the threshold zone can be wider than 20 dB. The amount of measurement error with the 4 dB, 2 dB staircase method with normal sensitivity is approximately 2 dB and increases steadily up to 10 dB with decreasing sensitivity (Fig. 1.6C, left). This measurement error is also called *short-term fluctuation.* The measurement of visual thresholds is more properly considered an estimate of visual thresholds.

In the suprathreshold method, the measurement error is substantially larger. Notably, there is a tendency to classify slightly or moderately depressed sensitivities as normal. For example, defects of 4 to 6 dB (where true sensitivity and test intensity are identical) are classified as normal with a probability of 75% due to the "logic of a second chance."

In some perimeters normal values for suprathreshold test software are based on relatively few normal individuals. In addition, the algorithm automatically adjusts the height of the reference hill. Therefore, the results may be misclassified.

Figure 1.6C. Actual and measured sensitivities using the threshold measurement and suprathreshold strategies. The suprathreshold strategy is less accurate and can assign a normal result to suspicious or slightly abnormal points.

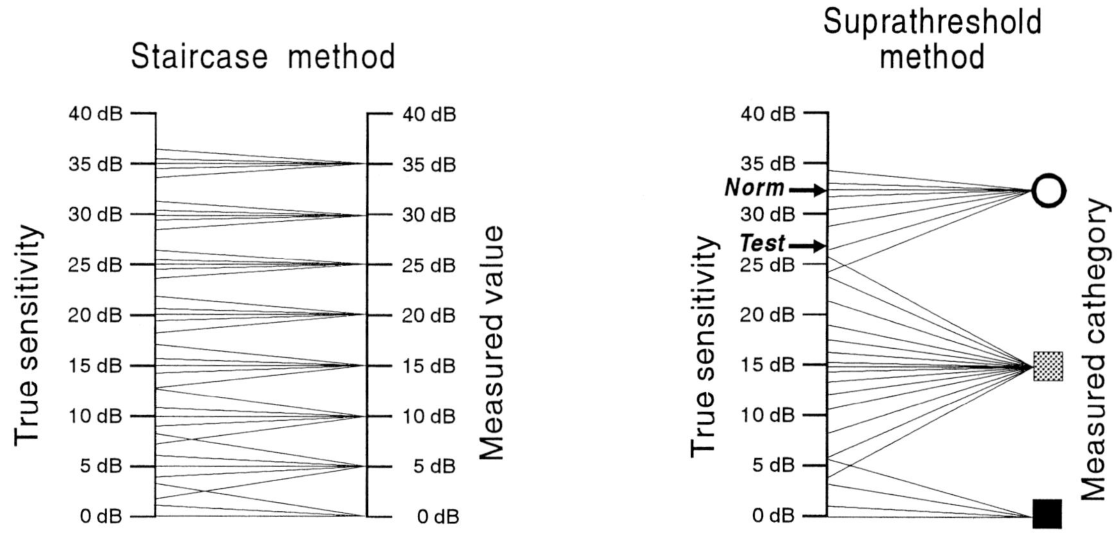
Staircase method
40 dB
35 dB
30 dB
25 dB
20 dB
15 dB
10 dB
5 dB
0 dB
True sensitivity
Measured value
Suprathreshold method
Norm
Test
Measured cathegory

1.6C

1.7 PATTERN OF MEASURED LOCATIONS (TEST POINT PATTERN)

Geometry

The arrangement of measured field locations can be derived from basic geometric patterns as follows (Fig. 1.7A): rectangular, circular, meridional, and irregular. These patterns differ in several respects. The distances between neighboring test points in a region can be equal (equidistant) or unequal. Equidistant locations, if close enough together, are advantageous because the detection of small scotomas is less dependent on their absolute positions. The definition of large defects is also less influenced by their locations (Fig. 1.7B). Only rectangular patterns are entirely equidistant. Circular patterns can be equidistant in certain areas if they are cleverly designed.

The positions of test locations with respect to the axis of the visual field can be centered with respect to fixation (axial, on-axis) or decentered (paraxial, off-axis). For many diseases, measured locations centered on the fixation axis lie just on the border of the scotoma. Points on a scotoma boundary, however, have a high measurement error, and are sensitive to head rotation and unsteady fixation. Paraxial patterns usually include fewer scotoma border points and are generally more efficient (Fig. 1.7C).

An effect which can be found with all patterns is *pseudoshape:* the pattern of test points alters the shape of defects. The perimetric result may show defect patterns which are created solely by the geometric pattern of the measured locations (Fig. 1.7D). Pseudoshapes are most easily recognized in rectangular patterns because there the borders are parallel to the main axes of the visual field.

Figure 1.7A. Types of geometrical patterns in visual field test locations.

Figure 1.7B. Distance of neighboring points: equidistant pattern (left) and pattern with variable distances (right). If the test locations are close enough together, the equidistant pattern can detect small scotomas almost without regard to their position.

Figure 1.7C. Relation to the field axis: axial or on-axis pattern (left) and paraxial or off-axis pattern (right). Usually the paraxial test pattern contains test locations that are less likely to fall on the edges of scotomas.

Figure 1.7D. Pseudoshape: with a circular test pattern, an arcuate scotoma can be artifactually produced.

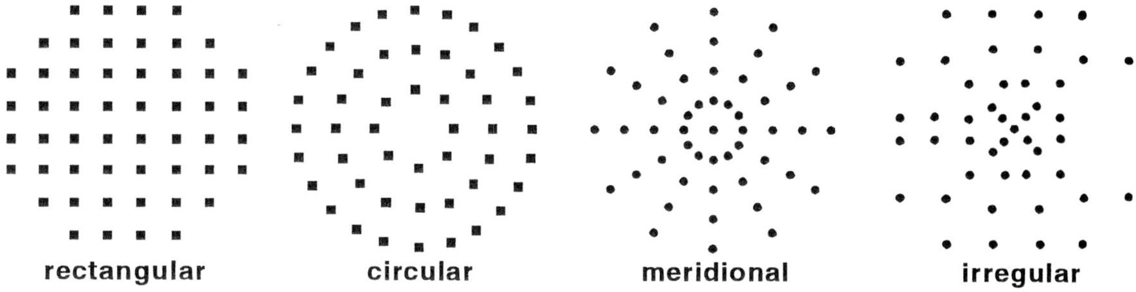

1.7A

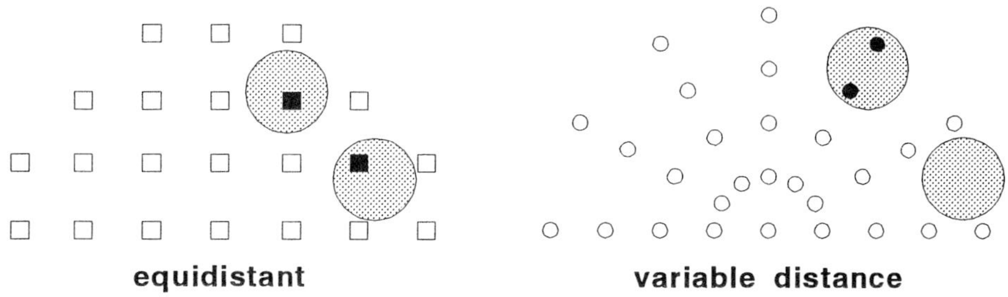

1.7B

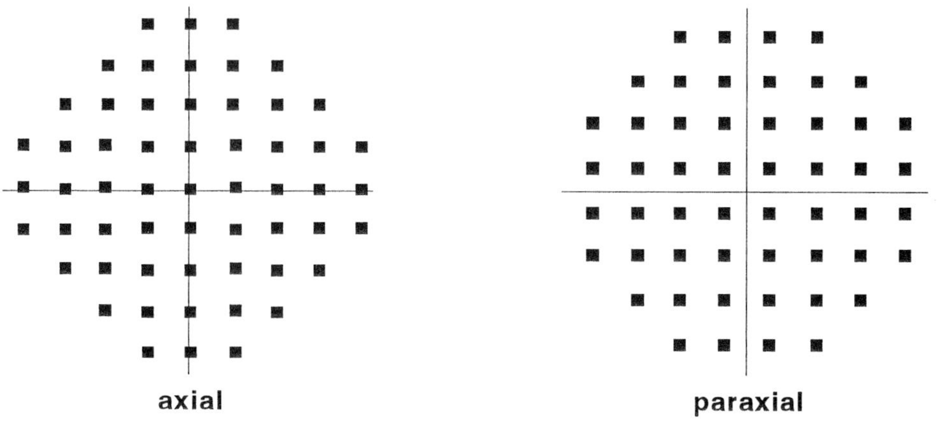

1.7C

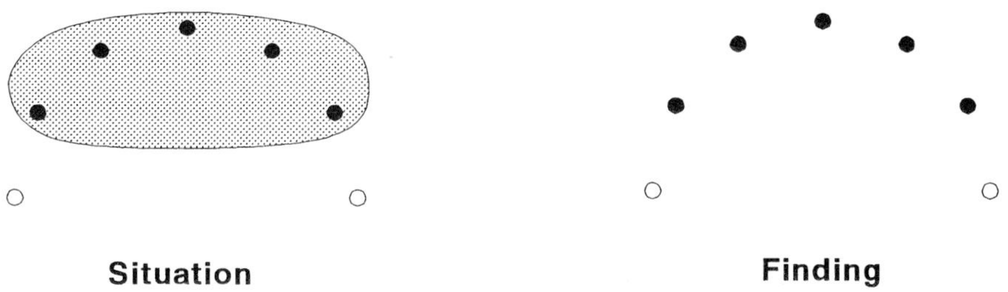

1.7D

Density

The density of the test point pattern can be compressed, either across the entire field or just centrally. Based on the present state of knowledge, equally spaced patterns are suitable for alterations of the central visual pathway and extended retinal disease covering larger areas (e.g., detachments, schisis, chorioretinitis, dystrophies). The classic equidistant pattern is a 6° rectangular pattern introduced by Fankhauser, which is used in programs 31 and 32 of the Octopus and programs 30-1, 30-2, and 24-2 of the Humphrey Field Analyzer. The pattern of programs 31 and 30-1 is axial, whereas that of programs 32, 30-2, and 24-2 is paraxial (Fig. 1.7E). When both types of programs are combined, they form a double-density pattern with a 4.2° spacing. Centrally higher-density patterns are recommended for diseases with small central field defects or important details in the center (e.g., macular disease, vascular diseases of the retina, and others). Concerning alterations of the optic nerve and visual pathway, assessment of the amount of damage is more accurate because the density of nerve fibers increases considerably toward the center of the retina. Therefore, central high-density patterns are recommended for all optic nerve diseases, including glaucoma, and many kinds of alterations of the central nervous system (Fig. 1.7F). Differential diagnosis may also require high central density of the test point pattern.

When comparing the density of different test point patterns, it must be remembered that the number of points per unit area increases with the reciprocal square of the distance between points. For example, when the distance between points is reduced from 6° to 3°, the number of test points in the area quadruples.

Area

Although some programs cover the entire area of the normal visual field, programs with more limited coverage are more commonly used. The central 30° programs are most common. This limitation is appropriate because this area is affected in almost every case of visual field disturbance (there are exceptions, e.g., peripheral retinoschisis). The central 30° area also represents about 60% of all nerve fibers. If there are defects within the center or severely constricted fields with a small central island, programs that test a central area of 10° are preferable.

Combinations

A combination of several patterns can be helpful for increasing either the density (Fig. 1.7G) or the area (Fig. 1.7H). Some perimeters allow the operator to change the density and area even while the program is running.

Figure 1.7E. Pattern of program 32 (Octopus) or program 30-2 (Humphrey Field Analyzer). The test point locations are entirely equidistant.

Figure 1.7F. Pattern GL1 (Rodenstock Peristat 433). The pattern is centrally condensed. Within particular regions, it is rectangular and equidistant.

Figure 1.7G. Combination of two patterns to form a denser pattern.

Figure 1.7H. Combination of two patterns to form a pattern that covers a greater area.

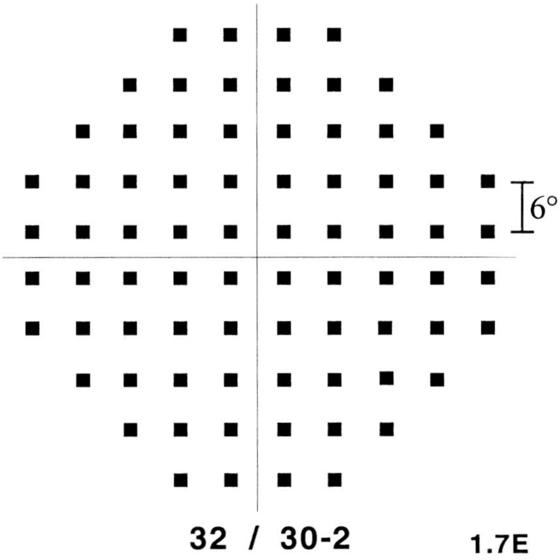

1.7E

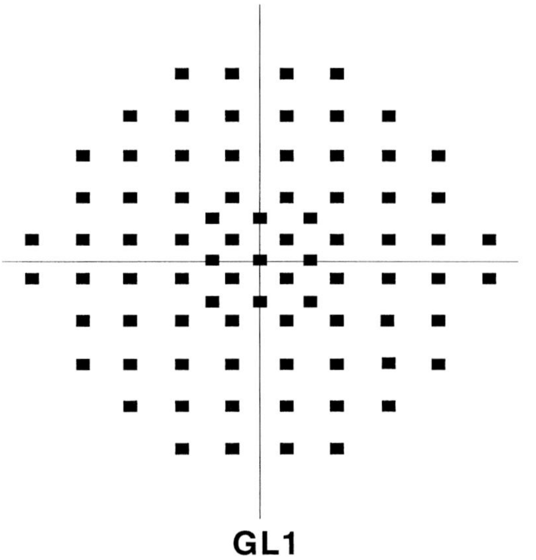

1.7F

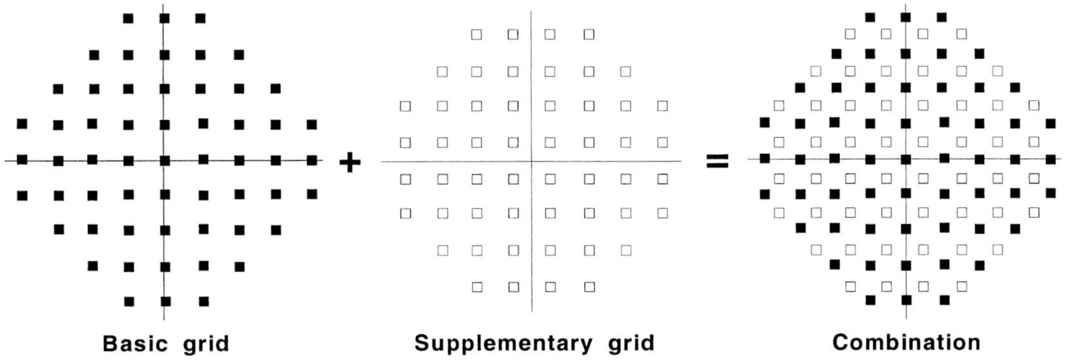

1.7G

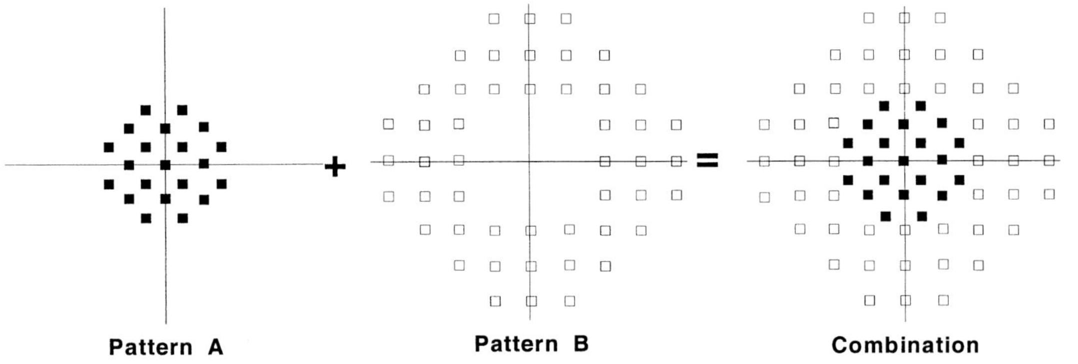

1.7H

1.8 EVALUATION OF PATIENT RELIABILITY

Evaluation of Fixation

Manual optical fixation control is the observation of the patient's eye with a telescope or camera. Automatic electronic-optical fixation control is the observation of the eye with a camera, followed by electronic analysis of the pupil's position (Octopus). When the pupil is moved out of a predefined window, it is detected (Fig. 1.8A). A similar effect occurs with eyelid closure. The last stimulus is repeated to avoid the registration of erroneous results. A newer technique (Humphrey Field Analyzer II) analyzes the light reflex from the cornea relative to the pupil's center. Thus, rotation of the eye can be measured in degrees and distinguished from shifts of the whole head. Automatic sensory fixation control is an indirect method which records the impact of loss of fixation on sensitivity. In the Heijl-Krakau method, bright stimuli are presented at the expected position of the blind spot. If fixation is good, these stimuli are not perceived. If fixation is poor, the blind spot is displaced and the stimuli are seen (Fig. 1.8B). This method is less precise in detecting large defects adjacent to the blind spot. The Tubinger method uses weak, just perceivable stimuli at fixation. Because the center is the most sensitive location in most visual fields, these stimuli are not seen in cases of poor fixation. With sensorial fixation control, the printout will contain the percentage of fixation losses. With electronic-optical control, either the number of repetitions (Octopus) or the angles of eye rotation (Humphrey Field Analyzer II) are printed out.

Catch Trials on False-Positive Behavior

Patients with hypersensitive reaction behavior may press the answer button even when a stimulus is not presented. Nearly all automated perimeters randomly present false-positive catch trials in which the stimulus intensity is in an imperceptible range or is missing altogether. The accompanying noise of the stimulus presentation (motor noise, shutter noise, attention signal), however, is presented. The percentage of false-positive answers ("perception" of a nonpresented or subthreshold stimulus) relative to all catch trials is provided on the printout.

Catch Trials on False-Negative Behavior

Patients with hyposensitive reaction (underreactive) behavior tend not to press the button even though the stimulus is perceived. This behavior can be intended (simulation) or unconscious (psychic, learning, fatigue). Most instruments randomly present stimuli with a luminance which is markedly above the measured threshold at a particular visual field location. The percentage of false-negative answers (no perception of a suprathreshold stimulus) relative to all catch trials is provided in the printout. Unfortunately, the luminance of the test stimuli may lie within the threshold zone, where a negative answer may occur in patients with normal reaction behavior. This occurs very frequently at locations of low sensitivity. Therefore, the significance of false-negative catch trials is limited in damaged fields (Fig. 1.8C).

Figure 1.8A. Electronic-optical fixation control. The sum of luminances in an image window indicates whether the pupil is at its designated position.

Figure 1.8B. Sensory fixation control. The perception of a test stimulus at the position of the blind spot indicates whether the eye is fixating properly.

Figure 1.8C. Stimulus difficulty of catch trials with false-negative reaction behavior.

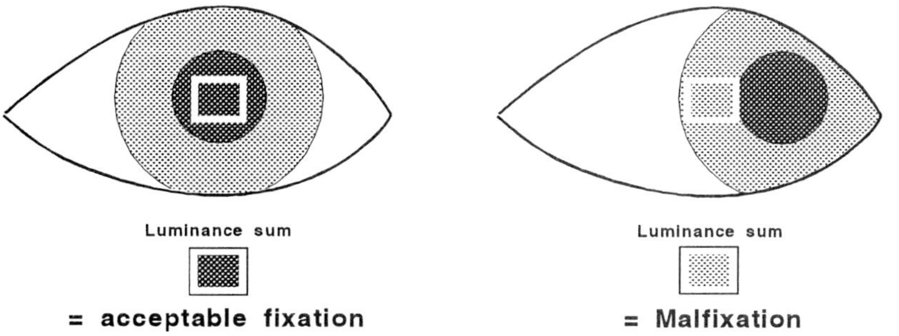
Luminance sum
= acceptable fixation
Luminance sum
= Malfixation

1.8A

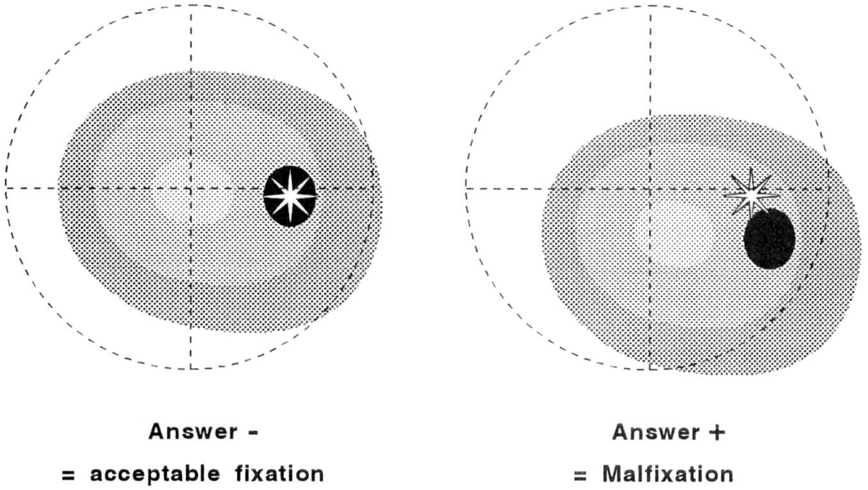
Answer -
= acceptable fixation
Answer +
= Malfixation

1.8B

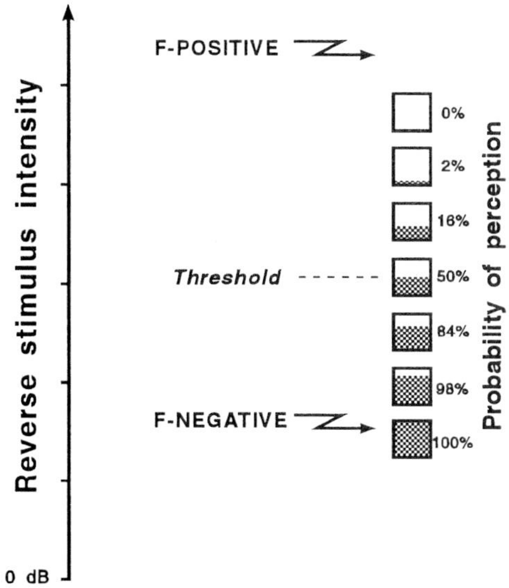
Reverse stimulus intensity
0 dB
F-POSITIVE
Threshold
F-NEGATIVE
0%
2%
16%
50%
84%
98%
100%
Probability of perception

1.8C

2 Representation of the Visual Field

2.1 THE SENSITIVITY VALUE

Normal Sensitivity

The differential light sensitivity (DLS) in the normal visual field depends mainly on two factors: test location and age. It is highest in the center and decreases toward the periphery. The steepest slopes are found nasally and superiorly. With advancing age, the level of sensitivity decreases over the whole visual field. This decline with age is more pronounced in the periphery (Fig. 2.1A).

Absolute Sensitivity

Absolute sensitivity is the actual threshold measurement at a test location. (Fig. 2.1B). It spans decibel values between 0 and about 40 dB (depending on the instrument). Synonyms for absolute sensitivity are *sensitivity* or simply *threshold.* The evaluation of an abnormality based on this value is difficult because age and test location are also factors. Absolute sensitivity at a single test location is generally of little help in clinical evaluation.

Relative Sensitivity

Relative sensitivity is the difference between the measured absolute sensitivity and the age- and location-related normal value of absolute sensitivity (Fig. 2.1C). Therefore, it represents abnormal deviations in sensitivity. In a normal field, relative sensitivity should be 0 dB at every location. In practice, it deviates slightly from 0 dB due to measurement error and interindividual variation. Synonyms for relative sensitivity are *norm-related sensitivity, difference value, total deviation, defect depth,* and *sensitivity loss.*

Abnormally low relative sensitivities are often indicated by negative values, and abnormally high relative sensitivities (often from measurement error or overreactive patients) are indicated by positive values. Some perimeters or programs (e.g., Octopus) use inverted signs: decreased sensitivity has a positive sign, and increased sensitivity has a negative sign. Relative sensitivity is usually the most useful value for clinical use.

Individual Sensitivity

Instead of normal values, some programs use individual reference values which are redefined for each patient and each examination. The basis is the normal value, but the normal hill of vision is shifted until it corresponds to the highest value of the tested field. Thus, the individual sensitivity indicates only the relative depth of sensitivity loss, which may be less than the total defect depth (Fig. 2.1D). Individual sensitivity is usually called *pattern deviation* or sometimes simply *defect;* occasionally it is confused with norm-related defect depth (e.g., Humphrey three-in-one-printout; see Fig. 2.7). Individual sensitivity may be useful for recognizing specific damage patterns, but it masks general depression and effectively reduces the defect depth in fields with combined local and diffuse loss.

Figure 2.1A. Normal sensitivity depends on test location and age (schematic profile).

Figure 2.1B–D. Absolute, relative, and individual sensitivity. Normal values are indicated by the dotted line and measured values by the solid line. The arrows indicate the values described. For individual sensitivity, the normal value is individually adjusted for each field.

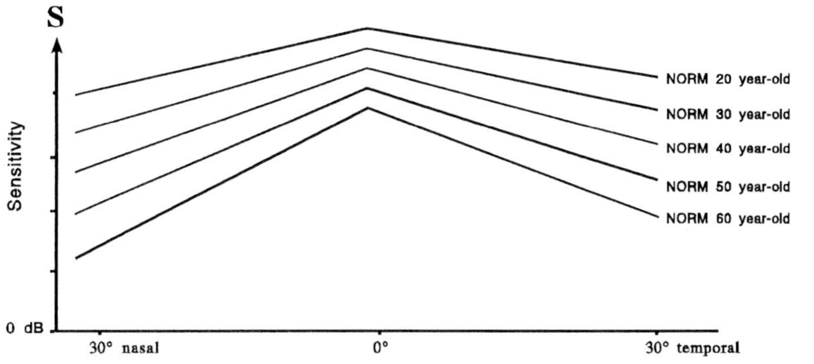

2.1A

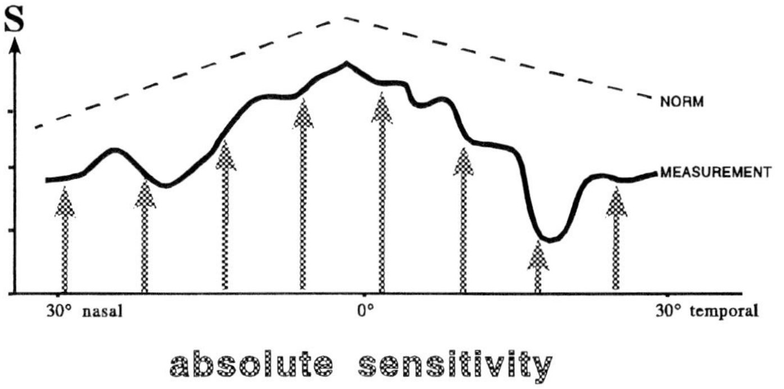

2.1B

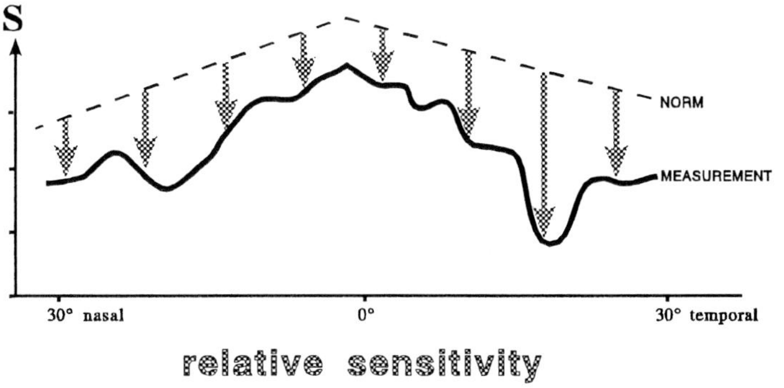

2.1C

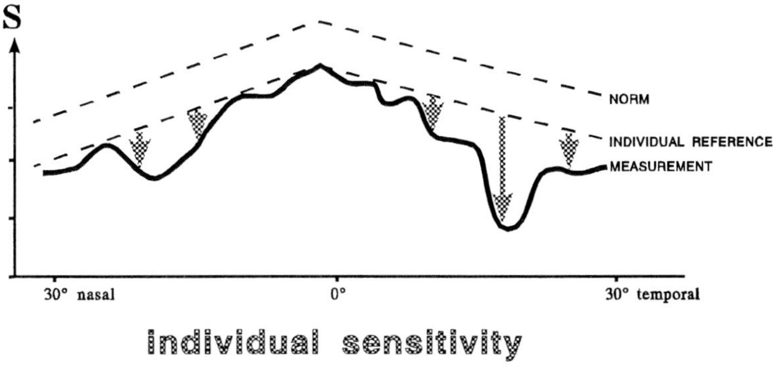

2.1D

2.2 TOPOGRAPHICAL REPRESENTATIONS

Topographical representations usually show the visual field as a two-dimensional map. The coordinates of the map correspond to the coordinates of the visual field. Sensitivity can be shown in different ways.

Numerical Representation (Numerical Map)

A numerical map displays visual sensitivities as numbers. Numerical arrays are created to describe the entire field (Fig. 2.2A). However, assimilation by the examiner of these 50 to 100 numbers is difficult. Numerical maps are easier to read if they are based on relative sensitivities and if all values in a defined normal range (usually from +4 dB to −4 dB) are replaced by a normal symbol (Fig. 2.2B). With this method, the number of numerically displayed thresholds is reduced considerably, usually without the loss of important information.

Grayscale Representation

In a grayscale representation, sensitivity is represented by a graphical scale. Low sensitivities are darker than high sensitivities (Fig. 2.2C). The representation provides a rapidly interpretable graphical impression of the visual field. The detection of defect shapes is improved if the sensitivities are interpolated along the *x*- and *y*-axes (Fig. 2.2D). Interpolation facilitates the interpretation of visual fields. However, the grayscale representation should not be misinterpreted as a high-resolution examination; the possibility that small scotomas are hidden in the gaps between test locations must always be considered.

Figure 2.2A. Numerical representation, absolute sensitivity.

Figure 2.2B. Numerical representation, relative sensitivity. All values between +4 dB and −4 dB are replaced by a normal symbol (o).

Figure 2.2C. Grayscale representation, same field as in Figure 2.2B. The relative sensitivity is replaced by a gray shade with a defined scale. Dark gray represents reduced sensitivity; light gray, normal sensitivity.

Figure 2.2D. Interpolated grayscale representation. In contrast to Figure 2.2C, the gaps between measured points are filled with interpolated sensitivity values before they are converted to grayscales.

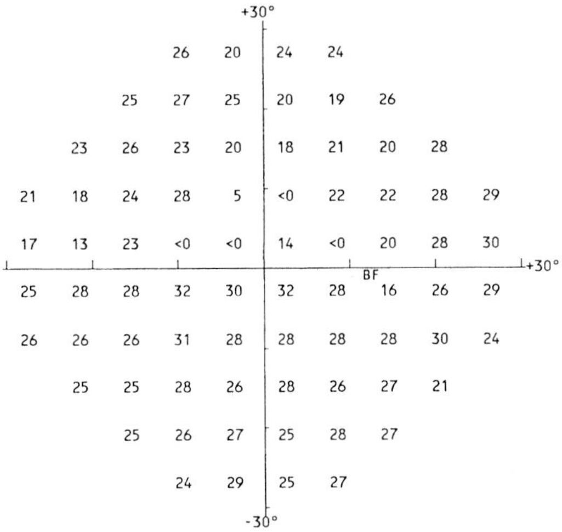

2.2A

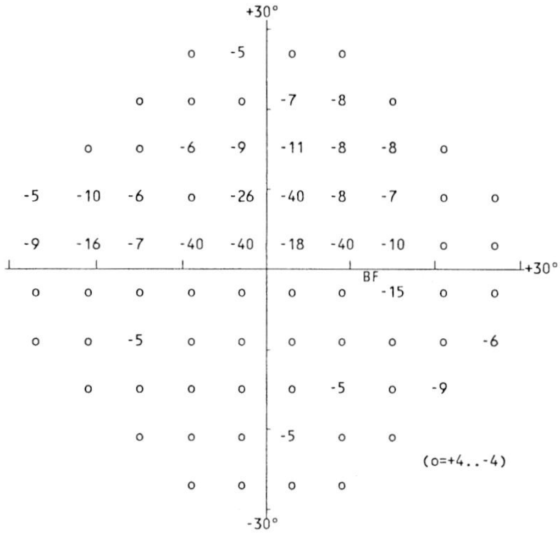

2.2B

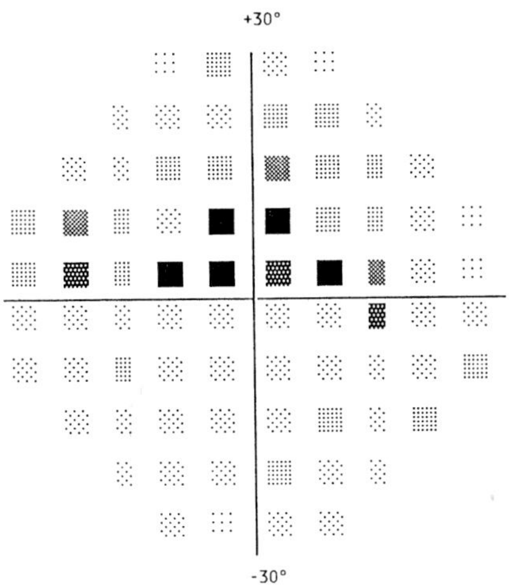

2.2C

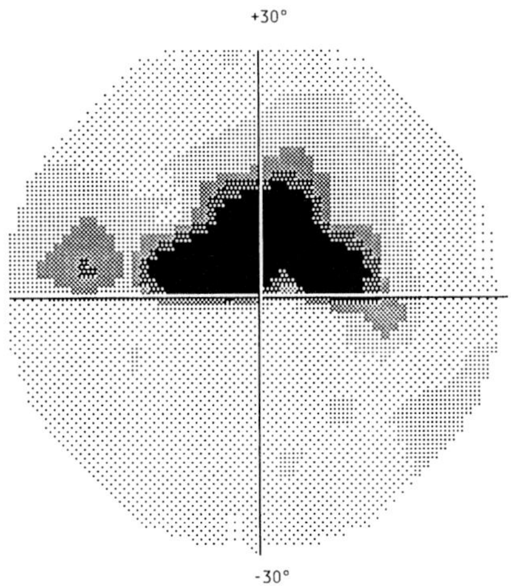

2.2D

Hill of Vision

Displaying sensitivity as height creates the illusion of a three-dimensional hill of vision. On the computer screen and in the printout, this hill is shown in perspective (Fig. 2.2E–F). Every representation demonstrates only one particular vantage point, and higher areas may hide parts of the hill. Several points of view will provide a complete impression of the hill of vision, but this method still has the drawback of perspective foreshortening. Because of this limitation, it is actually a pseudo–three-dimensional representation, and is rarely used in clinical practice.

Profile Cut

In the profile cut, sensitivity is also represented as height. Only one meridian of the hill of vision is shown as a profile at one time. Nothing is hidden, but the profile reflects only a small part of the visual field (Fig. 2.2G–H). The advantage of the profile cut is the simultaneous representation of more than one hill, for example, the normal hill of vision and the measured hill of vision (Fig. 2.2G). Therefore, it is useful for demonstrating the principles of automated perimetry. It is not generally useful in clinical practice.

Figure 2.2E–F. Perspective hill of vision from two different vantage points.

Figure 2.2G. Profile cut through the hill in Figure 2.2E at the 90° meridian. The ordinate represents absolute sensitivity, the solid line is the measured value, and the dashed line is the age-related normal value.

Figure 2.2H. Profile cut as in Figure 2.2G, representing the relative, norm-related sensitivity. The solid line is the measured value, and the dashed line (zero line) is the normal value.

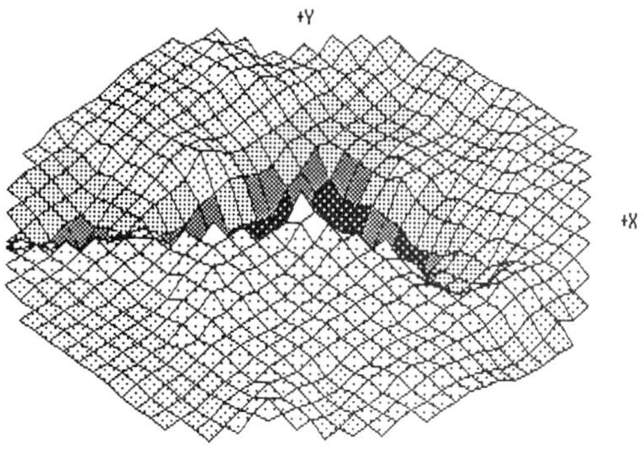

2.2E

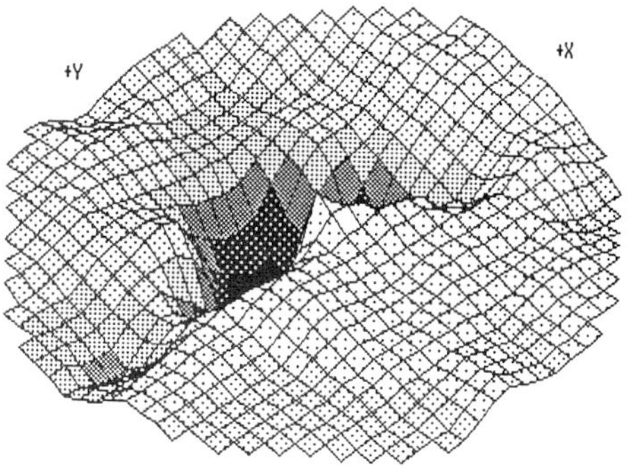

2.2F

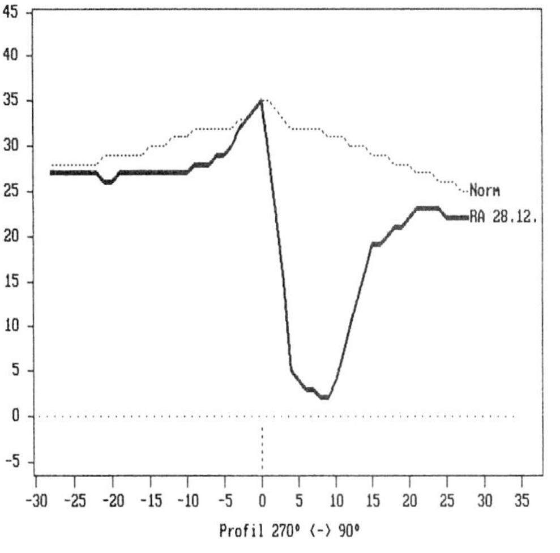

2.2G

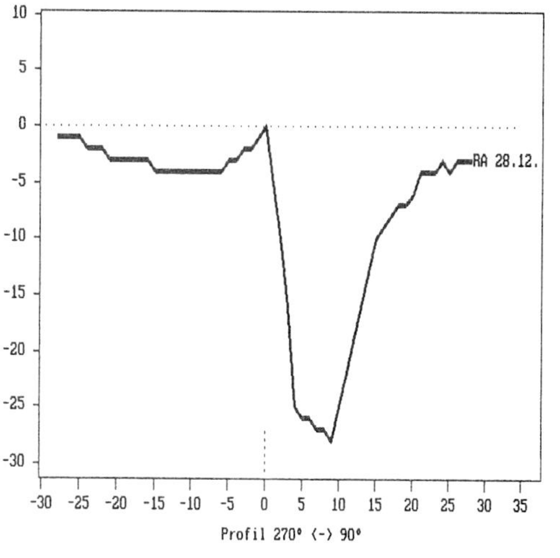

2.2H

2.3 ONE-DIMENSIONAL REPRESENTATIONS

One-Dimensional Transformations (Spatial Deprivation)

Visual field data are three-dimensional. Two dimensions determine the field location, and the third dimension is represented by sensitivity. This format is not suitable for statistical plots. In one-dimensional transformations, visual field data are deprived of their spatial information by deletion of the *x,y* field coordinates. What remains is a collection of one-dimensional data (only sensitivity values) that are displayed with standard statistical plots (Fig. 2.3A). Usually, they are based on norm-related, relative sensitivity values.

Histogram

The histogram (synonyms: *bar diagram, frequency plot*) represents the frequency of sensitivity values as bars. For this purpose, sensitivity is divided into classes. The abscissa represents frequency and the ordinate sensitivity. This orientation deviates from statistical convention but provides sensitivity using the vertical direction (height), as in the profile cut or the hill of vision (Fig. 2.3A).

Cumulative Curve

The cumulative curve (synonyms: *cumulative defect curve* or *Bebié curve*) displays the cumulative frequency of sensitivity values. The abscissa and ordinate are oriented according to the histogram: lower sensitivities will lower the curve (Fig. 2.3A). Cumulative curves allow plotting of a normal range for comparison.

Examples of Different Degrees of Damage

Figures 2.3B–D show visual fields with different amounts of damage. The displayed values are relative sensitivities. The normal visual field (Fig. 2.3B) has a histogram with a bell-shaped curve. The normal cumulative curve is an S-shaped curve. With increasing damage, the histogram and cumulative curves will shift downward (Figs. 2.3C and 2.3D).

Figure 2.3A. Topographical representation (numerical), spatial deviation, histogram, and cumulative curves. For better understanding, the bars and curve are drawn using the numerals on which they are based.

Figure 2.3B–D. Different representations (topographical maps, histogram, and cumulative curve) for visual fields without damage (B), with moderate damage (C), and with severe damage (D).

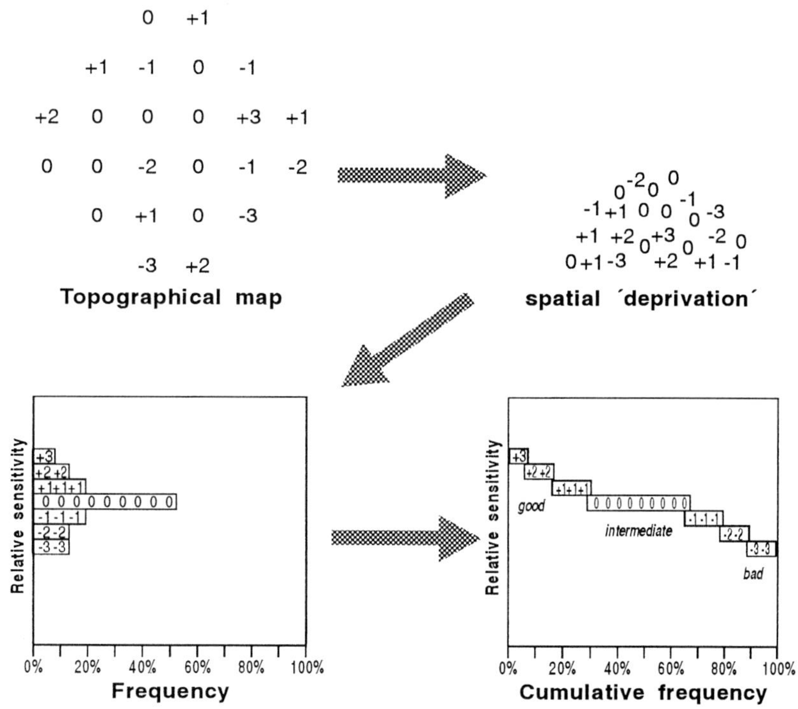

2.3A

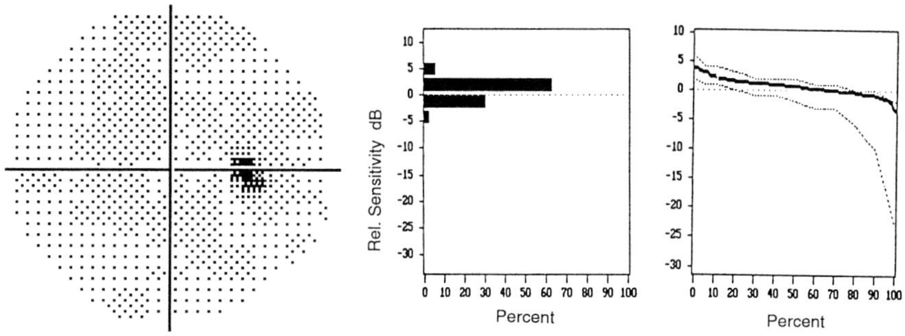

2.3B

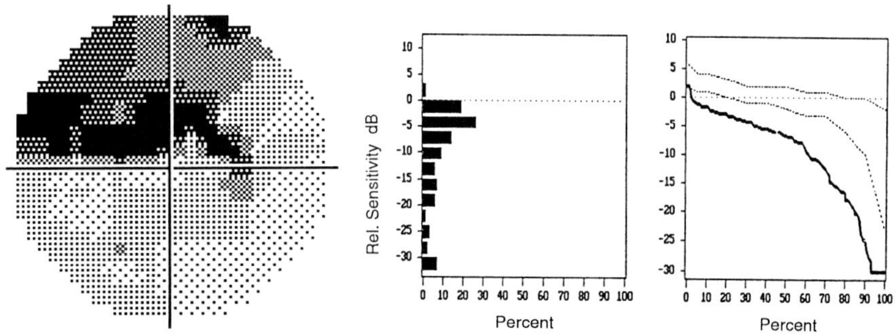

2.3C

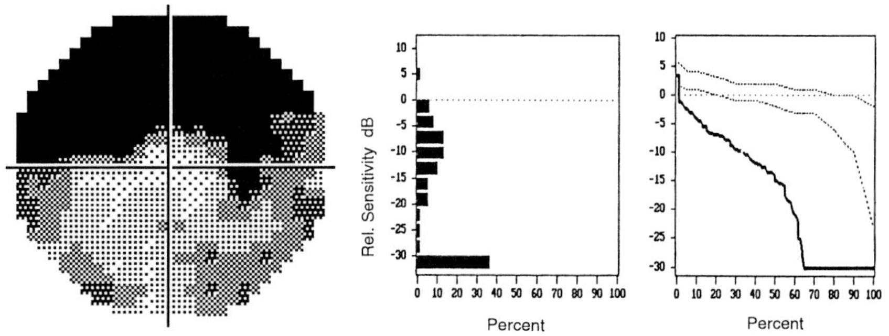

2.3D

Box Plot

A space-saving alternative to the cumulative curve is the box plot (Fig. 2.3E). Five points on the cumulative curve are chosen and displayed in a box with vertical arms. The box extends from the 20th to the 80th percentile (Humphrey Statpac) or from the 16th to the 84th percentile (Peridata). The bar in the middle of the box represents the 50th percentile (median). The arms reach out to the best (0 percentile) and worst (100th percentile) values. Compared to the cumulative curve the data are considerably reduced, but the box plot allows the convenient display of a series of fields (see Chapter 5).

Graphical Bar

The graphical bar shows sensitivity not as a number or height, but as a grayscale (Fig. 2.3F). These grayscale squares are stacked after being sorted into groups (*stacked histogram*). The width of each gray scale represents its frequency in the visual field. The graphical bar also has a shape that makes it suitable for follow-up. In comparison to the box plot, it displays all values, but the values are shown less exactly by the division into groups of 5 dB.

Examples of Different Degrees of Damage

Figures 2.3G–I show visual fields with different amounts of damage using reduced, one-dimensional representations. The normal visual field (Fig. 2.3B) has a short box plot which lies along the zero line. The graphical bar represents grouped sensitivities of +5 dB through +1 dB and 0 dB through −4 dB. With increasing damage, the box plot is shifted downward. With the graphical bar, lower sensitivity classes are given additional space (Fig. 2.3H). With severe damage, a considerable part of the visual field is an absolute defect (0 dB). The lower margin of the box is at the bottom, and the lower arm is invisible (Fig. 2.3I). The graphical bar shows large portions of black grayscale.

Figure 2.3E. Relation between the cumulative defect curve and the box plot.

Figure 2.3F. Topographical representation (grayscale), spatial deviation, and graphical bar.

Figure 2.3G–I. Several representations (topographical map, cumulative curve, box plot, and graphical bar) for visual fields without damage (G), with moderate damage (H), and with severe damage (I).

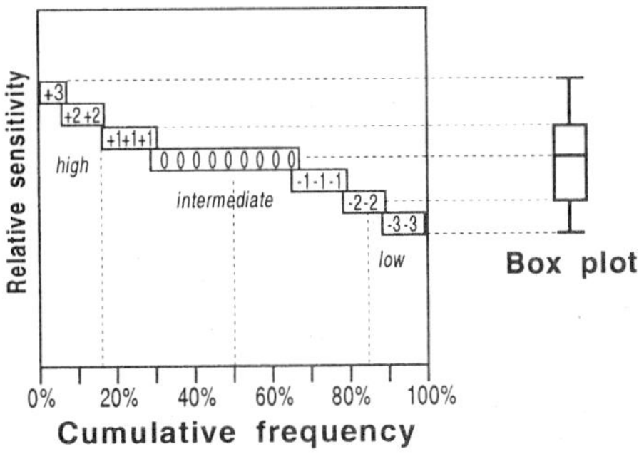

2.3E

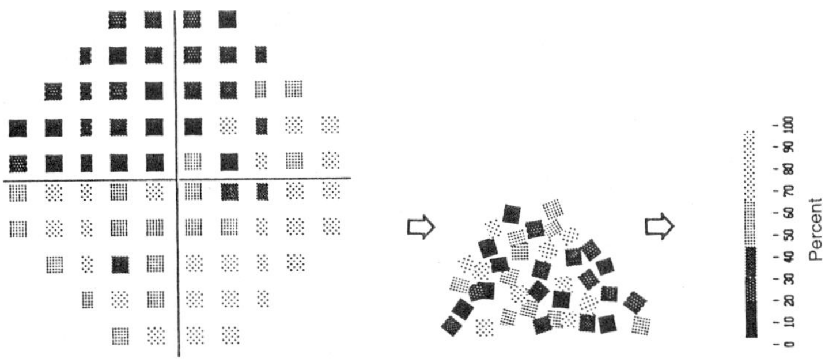

2.3F

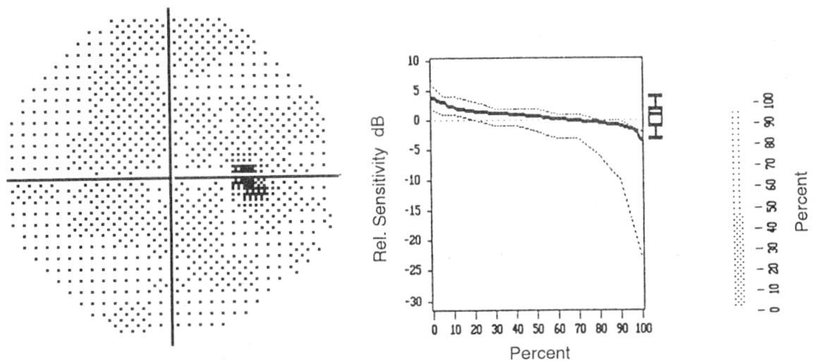

2.3G

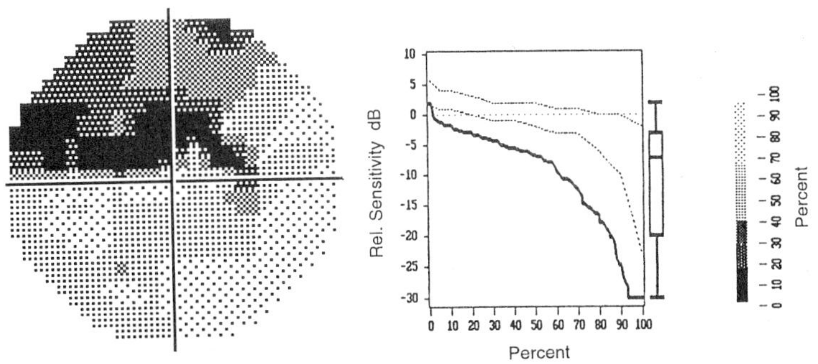

2.3H

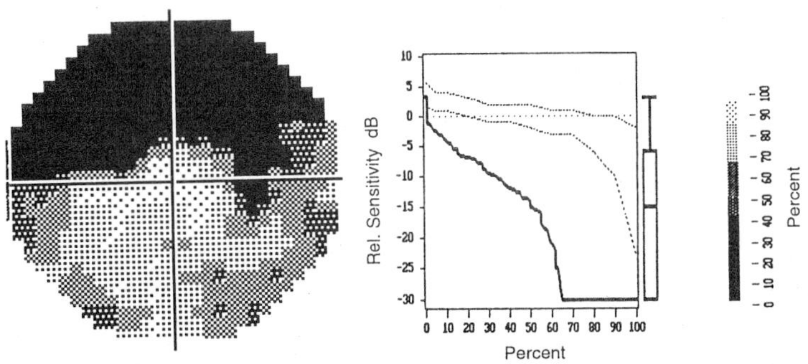

2.3I

2.4 STATISTICAL INDICES

Visual field indices are mathematical and statistical indices which are calculated with the sensitivity values of the visual field.

Global Indices

The calculation of global visual field indices is based on sensitivity values from the entire (global) visual field. Historically, the oldest index is the mean of all local (absolute) sensitivity values, *mean sensitivity* (*MS*). Later, indices were introduced based on relative, norm-related sensitivities, which are more useful for clinicians. Like any other distribution of values, they can be described by the statistical values: *mean value (MV), standard deviation (SD),* and *variance (VA),* where variance is the square of the standard deviation (Fig. 2.4A). Because of their successive introduction to perimetry, the terminology is not systematic. Their names and relations are:

MV:	MD	mean defect or mean deviation
SD:	PSD	pattern standard deviation
VA:	LV	loss variance

Corrected Global Indices

The measures of the scatter of visual field thresholds (PSD and LV) indicate not only the scatter of true values, but also the scatter created by measurement error (Fig. 2.4B). Subtracting this error (estimated from the short-term fluctuation) from the total value provides an estimate of the true scatter. Such indices are called *corrected* indices and are indicated by an additional *C* in the acronym.

SD:	CPSD	corrected PSD
VA:	CLV	corrected LV

Examples of Different Degrees of Damage

Figures 2.4C–E show visual fields with different amounts of damage. With increasing loss, the mean (MD) falls below 0. The standard deviation (PSD) initially increases with increasing damage but declines again when it reaches the measurement limits of the instrument.

Figure 2.4A. The global mean and global standard deviation are derived from one-dimensional values.

Figure 2.4B. Increase in the scatter of visual field thresholds by the measurement error. PSD (measured) is always larger than CPSD (true).

Figure 2.4C–E. Topographical map, cumulative curve, and indices of visual fields with no damage (C), moderate damage (D), and severe damage (E).

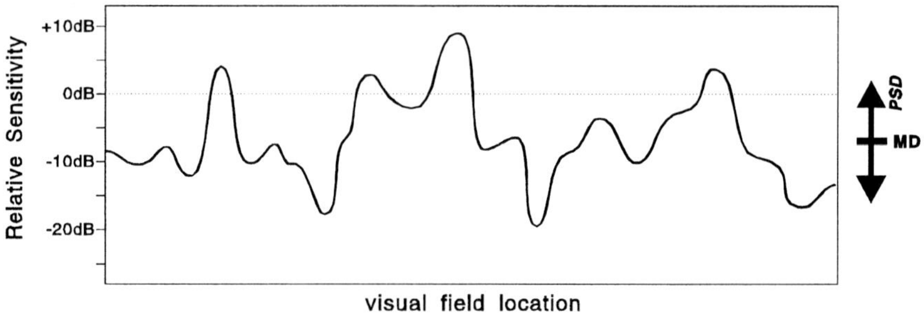

2.4A

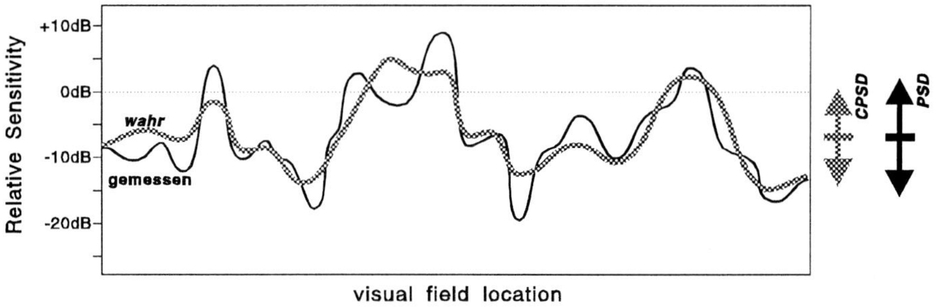

2.4B

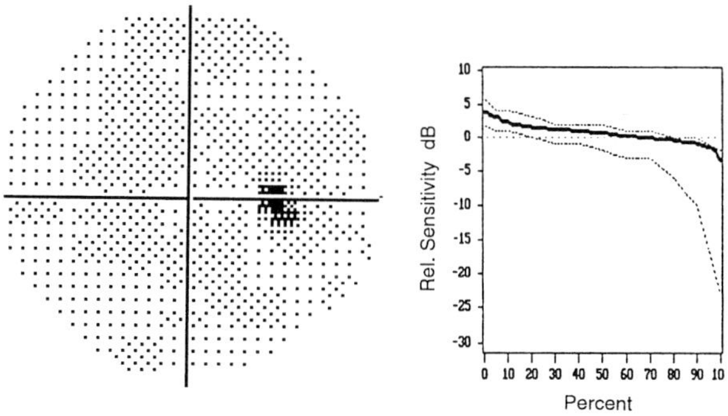

MD	+0.6
PSD	1.3
CPSD	0.2
LV	1.7
CLV	0.0

2.4C

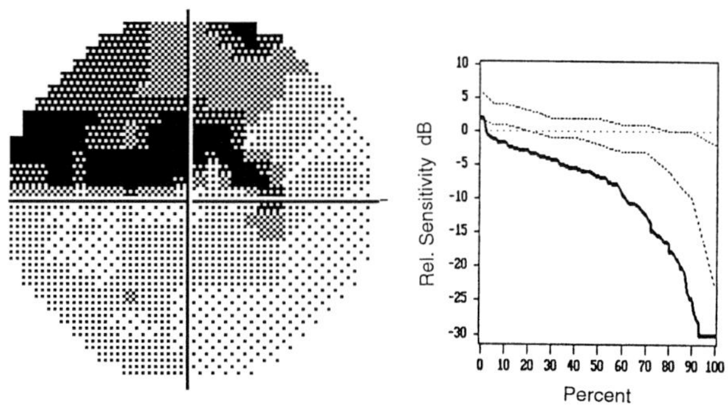

MD	-10.2
PSD	8.7
CPSD	8.5
LV	75.5
CLV	71.9

2.4D

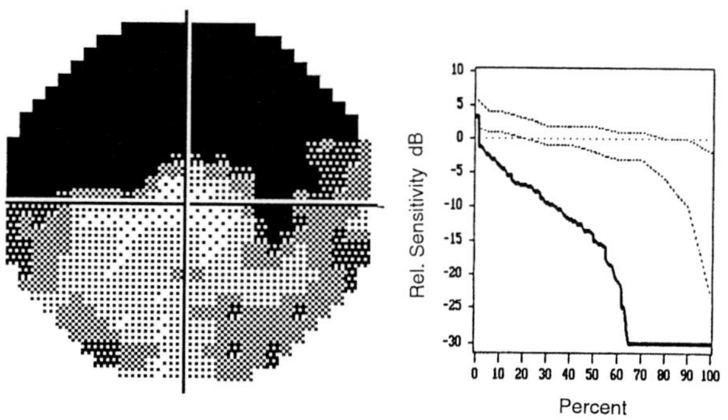

MD	-17.7
PSD	14.9
CPSD	14.8
LV	221.7
CLV	218.5

2.4E

Fluctuation

Fluctuation is the variation over time (temporal variation) in sensitivity measurements. It can be calculated as the standard deviation of repeated measurements at identical visual test locations.

Short-Term Fluctuation (Measurement Error)

Short-term fluctuation (SF) is the temporal variation of measured values during an examination. Two sensitivity measurements at some or all test locations are made. When the local fluctuation values at these doubly determined locations are averaged (Fig. 2.4F), the global SF is calculated. This global SF is the average variation in the visual field and is displayed on the printout. For statistical purposes, this average is determined as a geometric mean (root of the mean squares, RMS).

SF is an estimate of the measurement error. But measurement error in perimetry is not due solely to physical variations in the apparatus. Instead, it is mostly an effect of the measurement method (e.g., the staircase method) and the patient's uncertainty about the threshold. Using constant staircase methods, SF correlates with the uncertainty about the threshold (Fig. 2.4G). It is increased in unreliable patients and in those with damaged fields.

Long-Term Fluctuation

Long-term fluctuation (LF) is the variation in measurements made at successive examinations (Fig. 2.4H) on separate visits. Not all analysis programs calculate this index. It is very important in evaluating the significance of visual field changes (see also Chapter 5).

Figure 2.4F. Calculation of global fluctuation SF for examination program 30-2 (Humphrey Field Analyzer). Based on 10 double measurements (left), 10 local fluctuation values (right) are computed. The geometric mean of these values is the global SF fluctuation.

Figure 2.4G. Calculation of global fluctuation SF for examination program G1 (Octopus). In this program, phase 2 consists of second measurements at all locations (left). This allows the calculation of 59 local fluctuation values (right) and a more robust estimate of the global SF fluctuation.

Figure 2.4H. Long-term fluctuation (LF) from a series of four visual fields calculated by the Peridata program.

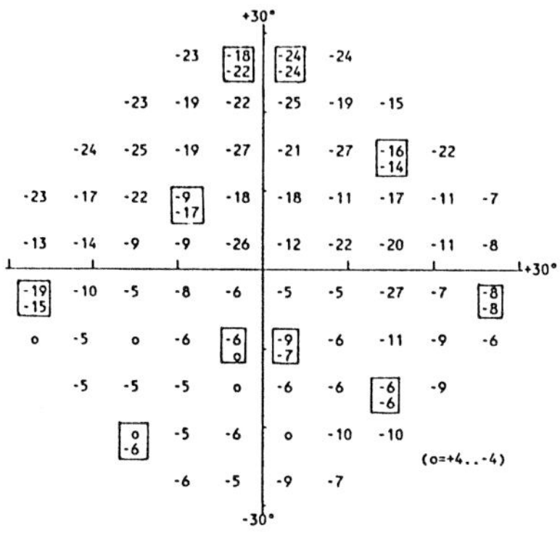

measured values

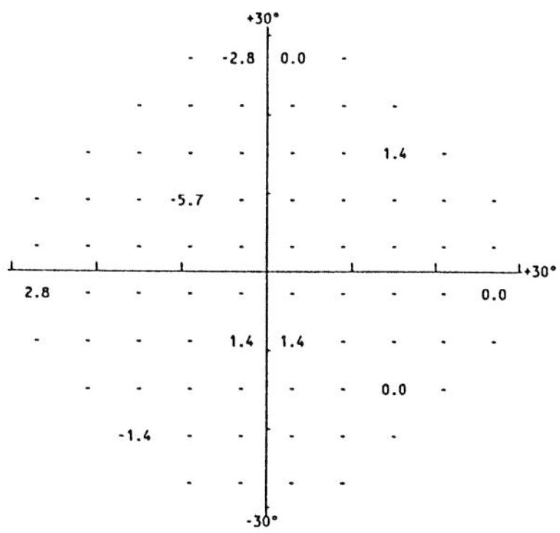

local fluctuation

SF=2.5 dB

2.4F

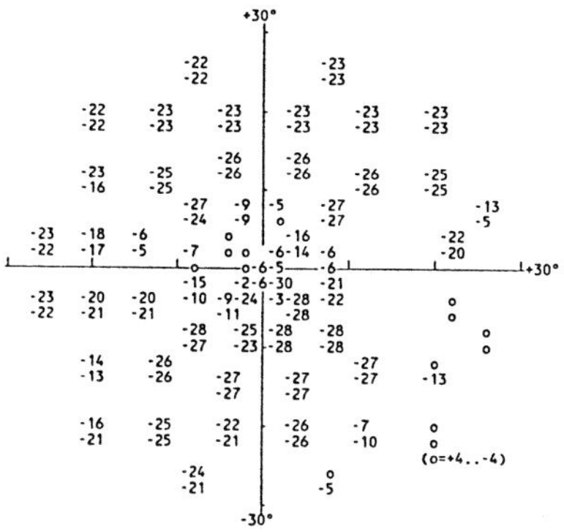

measured values

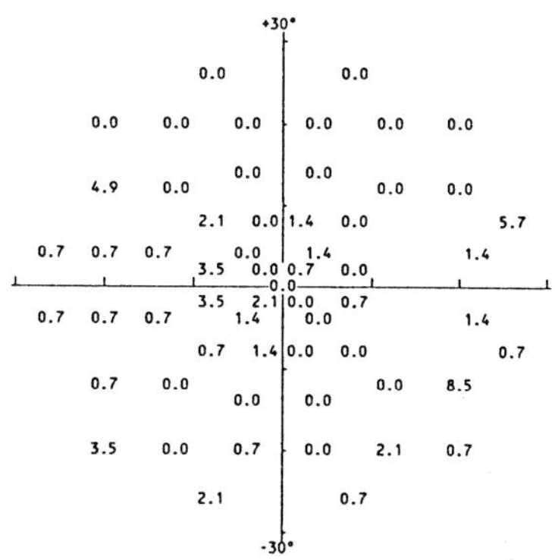

local fluctuation

SF=2.4dB

2.4G

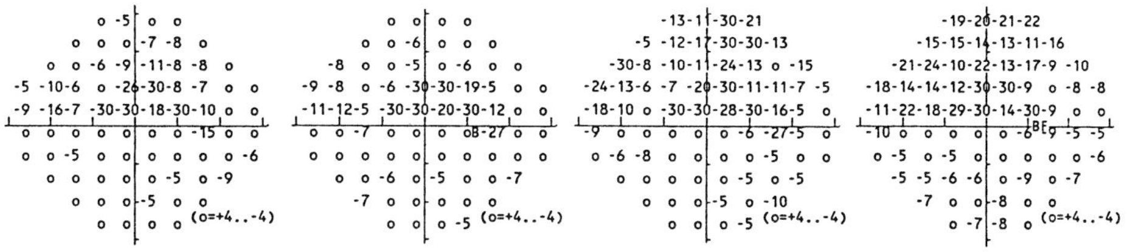

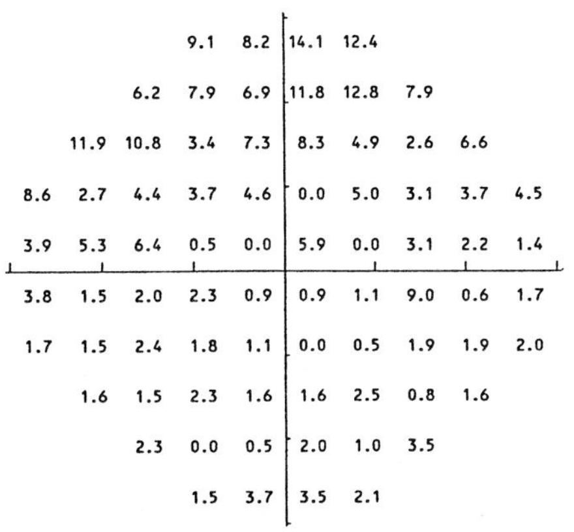

LF= 5.1 dB

local long-term fluctuation

2.4H

2.5 PROBABILITY PLOTS

Normal Range

Sensitivity values of normal eyes vary not only by location and age, but also among individuals. The normal values, which are used to calculate norm-related relative sensitivities (defect or deviation), are mean values for a given location and age group. Around this mean, the individual values scatter: the normal range is narrower in the center than in the periphery, and narrower in younger persons than in older ones (Fig. 2.5A). For example, the 5th to 95th percentile normal range of the Humphrey Field Analyzer in the center of a 20-year-old person's visual field is about +4 dB through −4 dB, and in the periphery of an 80-year-old person it is about +6 dB through −10 dB. Under the measurement conditions of the Octopus perimeter (lower background/variance), these differences are somewhat less pronounced.

Analysis of Normality

The normal limits are especially important when considering whether relatively small departures from normal sensitivity loss are actually normal or abnormal. A sophisticated analysis not only uses a single definition but also estimates the probability that a given sensitivity loss departs from a normal range (Fig. 2.5B). Such values of the probability of normality are usually displayed on a grayscale map. In this case, the grayscale map is called a *probability plot* (Fig. 2.5C). The percentage value provides either the percentage of normal individuals who have values above the measured value at that location or the percentage of normal individuals who have lower values. It should be stressed that such a map visualizes abnormalities very well, but it does not always reflect the amount of damage accurately. A uniform deviation due to cataract, for example, is not displayed as a uniform gray area but is darker in the center because of narrower normal limits there (Fig. 2.5D). Complete evaluation of a visual field also requires the use of a grayscale map and a numerical map based on relative sensitivity (deviation).

Probability maps can also be used for follow-up (see Chapter 5).

Figure 2.5A. Scheme of normal ranges (normal percentiles) in a visual field profile. The normal ranges are wider toward the periphery and are asymmetric.

Figure 2.5B. Translation of sensitivity values into probability of normality. The defect depths on the left are equal, but the probabilities are different. The same is true of the defects on the right.

Figure 2.5C. Normal probability plot: display of the probability of normality as a grayscale.

Figure 2.5D. Relative sensitivity (left) and a normal probability plot (right) in a case of cataract.

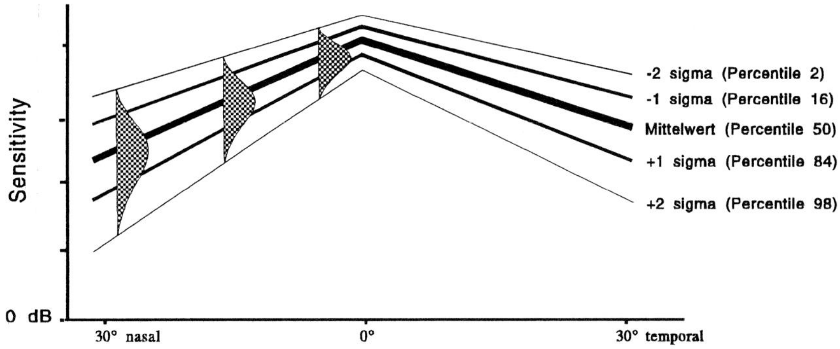

2.5A

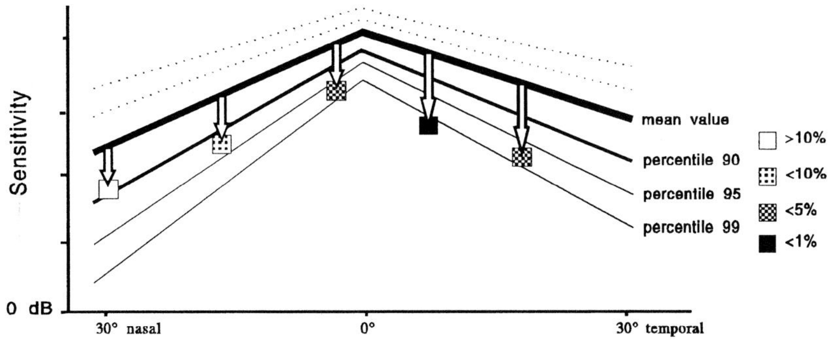

2.5B

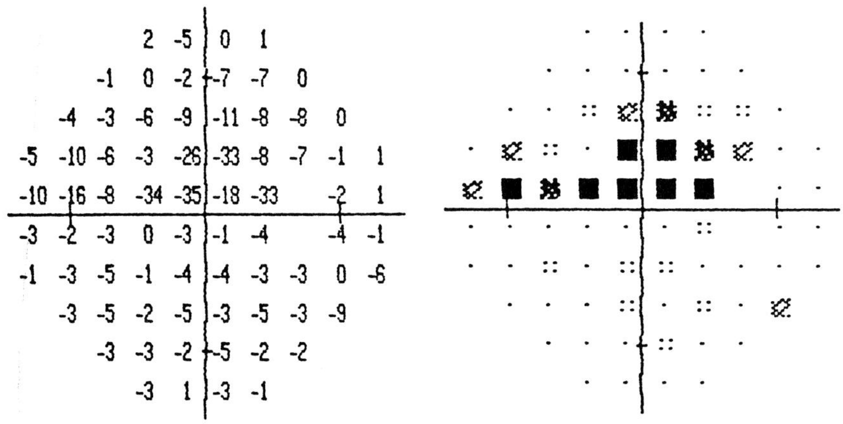

2.5C

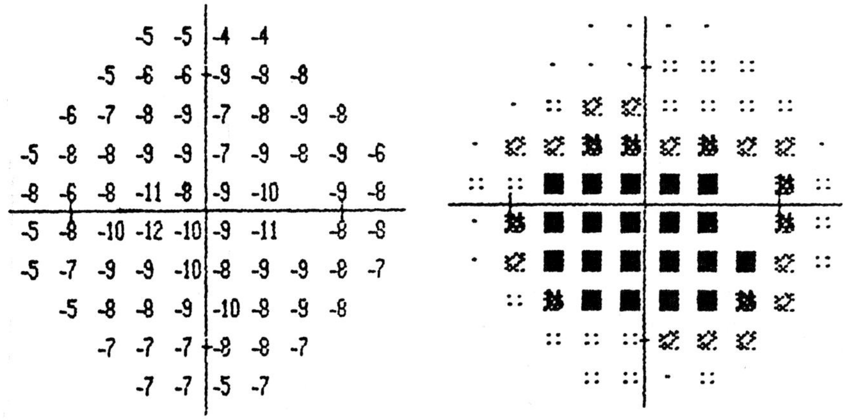

2.5D

2.6 REPRESENTATION OF SUPRATHRESHOLD MEASUREMENTS

Two-Category Method

The two-category method (synonyms: *one-level-test, standard strategy* [Humphrey Field Analyzer]) tests each visual field location with one stimulus intensity. This intensity is brighter (lower decibel value) than the expected normal value. Possible results fall into two categories: normal or abnormal *(defect).* The normal symbol depends on the perimeter and may be a point, a small circle, or a cross. The defect symbol is usually a black square (Fig. 2.6A).

Three-Category Method

The three-category method (synonyms: *scanning strategy, two-level test, three-zone test)* tests a location with the normal expected intensity and the instrument's maximum intensity. Thus, the two defect categories, *relative defect* and *absolute defect,* can be distinguished and are depicted by different symbols (Fig. 2.6B).

Four-Category Method

The four-category method (synonym: *three-level test)* uses three stimulus intensities. Consequently, the results can fall into either the normal range or into one of three defect categories. For example, in the Rodenstock Peritest and Perimat perimeters, the first defect level contains defects between –6 dB and –12 dB, level 2 covers –12 dB to –18 dB, and level 3 contains defects below –18 dB. These defects are represented by square symbols with different intensities of gray.

Quantitative Suprathreshold Method

With the quantitative suprathreshold method (synonyms: *quantify defects, fast strategy, smart mapping*), all defects detected by the presentation of the initial stimulus intensity are then measured with a staircase method. Possible results include "normal" or a numerical value which corresponds to the depth of the defect in decibels (Fig. 2.6C). The reference depth level is either the age-related normal value (e.g., Octopus) or an individually adapted normal value (e.g., the Humphrey perimeter, Peritest, Perimat, and Tubinger Automatic Perimeter).

Significance of Suprathreshold Results

All numerical and symbolic results are the outcome of a measurement or test and are affected by measurement error, which can be enormous (see Chapter 1). The normal level, for example, includes test locations which have a sensitivity loss of up to 6 dB and sometimes up to 10 dB. The displayed results invariably look better than the actual visual field. Regions with severe damage and absolute defects are represented accurately.

Figure 2.6A. Two-level method, principle (left) and example of a result (right).

Figure 2.6B. Three-level method, principle (left) and example of a result (right).

Figure 2.6C. Quantitative suprathreshold method, principle (left) and example of a result (right).

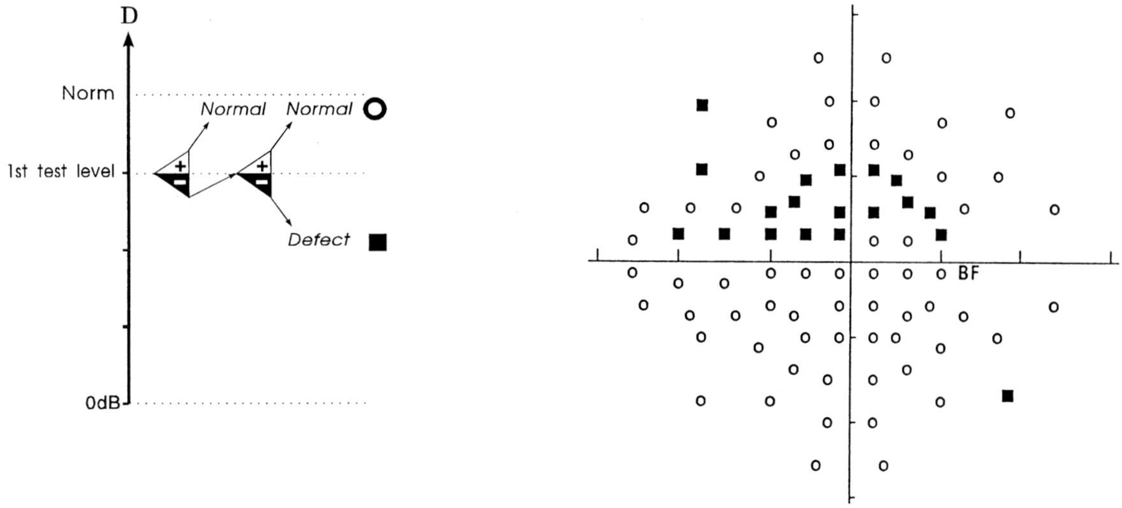
D
Norm
Normal
Normal
1st test level
Defect
0dB
BF

2.6A

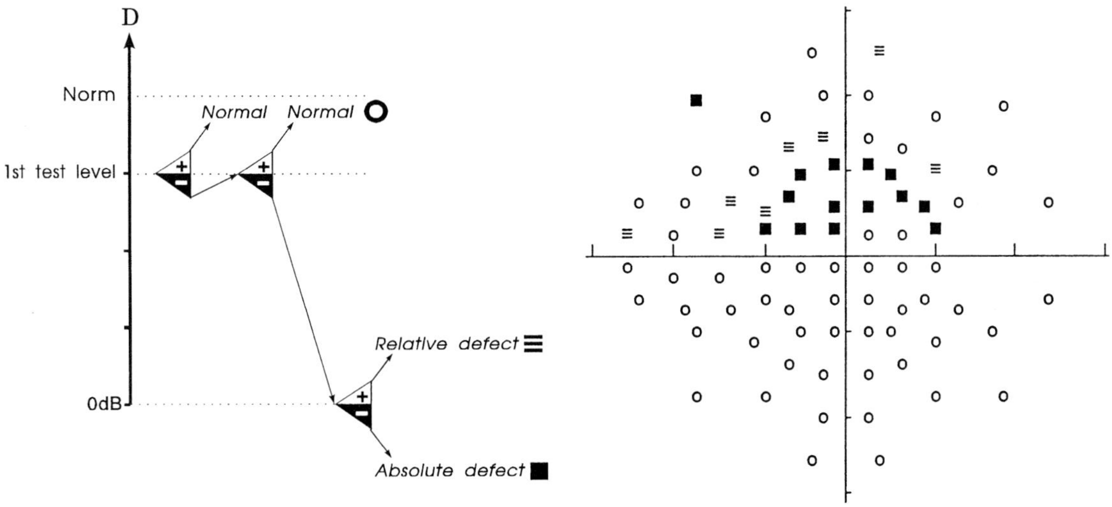
D
Norm
Normal
Normal
1st test level
Relative defect
0dB
Absolute defect

2.6B

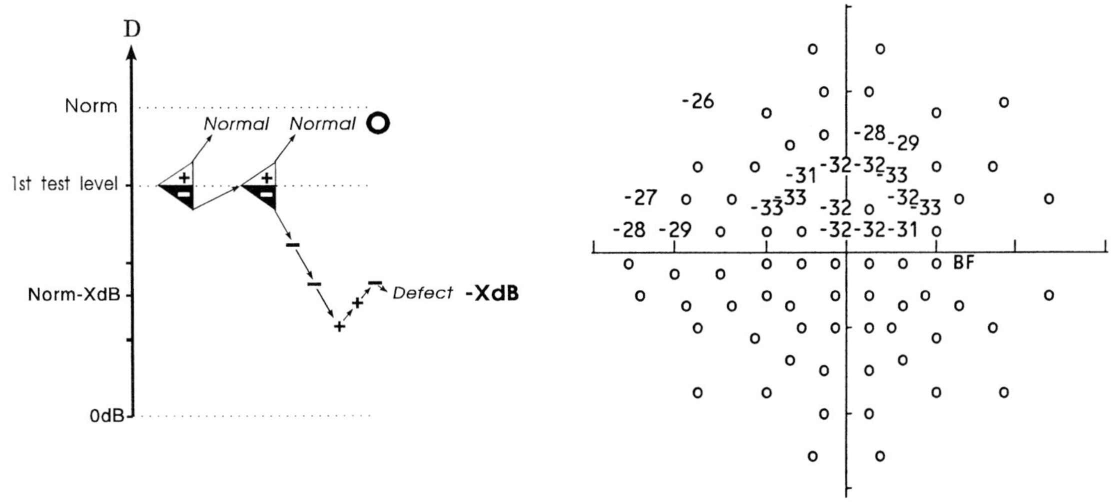
D
Norm
Normal
Normal
1st test level
Norm-XdB
Defect -XdB
0dB
-26
-28
-29
-31
-32
-32
-33
-27
-33
-33
-32
-32
-33
-28
-29
-32
-32
-31
BF

2.6C

2.7 EXAMPLE: HUMPHREY FIELD ANALYZER THREE-IN-ONE PRINTOUT

The standard software of the Humphrey Field Analyzer offers three visual field representations, which are combined in the three-in-one printout (Fig. 2.7): an interpolated grayscale of thresholds (absolute sensitivity) (A), threshold numbers (absolute sensitivity) (B), and defect depths (numbers) relative to an individual reference (individual sensitivity) (C). The topography of damage is represented by the grayscale. The actual results (thresholds) are raw data. The figures on the left side (defect depth) are based on individual sensitivity, meaning that they are derived not from age-related normal values but from individually adjusted normal values (see Section 2.1). The level of this individual norm is indicated by the peak of this hill in the center, the *central expected normal value (CEN)*. This individual CEN may differ by up to 10 dB from the age-related CEN, which is about 36 dB for ages 10 through 30 years, 35 dB for 30 through 50 years, 34 dB for 50 through 70 years, and 33 dB for 70 through 80 years. The identification of field damage is difficult with this printout. Follow-up is also difficult because the CEN may change from examination to examination.

Figure 2.7. Humphrey Field Analyzer: three-in-one printout of an examination (program 30-2).

THREE-IN-ONE	Name: SFW-DEMO, 10	Eye: RIGHT
Central 30 - 2	Birthdate: 10 Jun 1935	ID:

Stimulus: III, WHITE	Background: 31.5 asb	Test Date: 8 May 1990	Age: 55
Blind Spot Check Size: III	Fixation Target: CENTRAL	Test Time: 07:24:06	
Strategy: FULL	RX Used: +3.00 DS DC x °	Pupil Diameter: 2.0 mm	VA: 20/20

THRESHOLD GRAYTONE

Fixation Losses:	1/30
False Pos Errors:	0/20
False Neg Errors:	1/17
Test Duration:	18:10
Fluctuation:	1.01 dB
Fovea:	35 dB

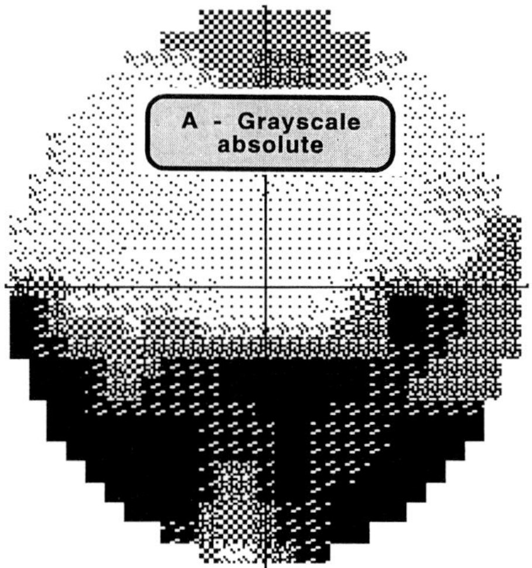

30°

DEFECT DEPTH (dB)

C - Numerals Individual

			11	8	▪	13			
		◇					▪		
	▪	◇					▪	◇	
◇	▪	◇	▪	◇	▪	◇	▪	7	▪
◇	▪	◇	▪	◇	▪	◇	▪	◇	18
23	9	9	7	▪	▪	5	26	20	18
23	25	12	26	28	28	27	18	13	17
	24	25	26	20	27	19	26	26	
		24	25	7	25	26	26		
			8	◇	13	25			

▪ = within 4 dB of Expected

Central Reference Level: 31 dB

THRESHOLD DATA (dB)

B - Numerals absolute

Quad Total 433 (upper left); Quad Total 400 (upper right); Quad Total 164 (lower left); Quad Total 118 (lower right)

			10	13	17	7			
		23					22		
	21	24					25	25	
19	24	24	25	29	26	28	24	18	22
23	23	27	28	31	30	30	23	23	9
<0	16	18	21	30	31	22	<0	6	8
<0	<0	15	3	<0	<0	<0	8	13	9
	<0	<0	<0	7	<0	8	<0	<0	
		<0	<0	19	1	<0	<0		
			15	21	12	<0			

Humphrey Instruments, Inc.
A Carl Zeiss Company

SFW version 1.0

Graytone Symbols HFA S/N: 630-3972

>40	>35	>30	>25	>20	>15	>10	>5	>0	≤0

SFW-DEMO, 10	RIGHT

2.8 EXAMPLE: HUMPHREY FIELD ANALYZER STATPAC PRINTOUT

The software of the Humphrey Field Analyzer can be extended with Statpac 1. This software provides the instrument with age-related normal values. The Statpac printout "Single Field Analysis" (Fig. 2.8) shows threshold (absolute sensitivity) (A), a grayscale of thresholds (B), total deviation (relative sensitivity) (C), pattern deviation (individual sensitivity) (D), a total probability plot (E), a pattern probability plot (F), and indices (G).

The measured sensitivities (thresholds) are raw results. The topography of the damage is represented by absolute grayscales, which also contain age effects and eccentricity effects. The amount of local damage can be seen in the relative numerals (total deviation). The individual numerals (pattern deviation) are related to an individually shifted normal hill of vision. They enhance the identification of focal defects but ignore the component of diffuse loss (see Section 2.1). The probability plot displays the degree of abnormality of these numbers. The global damage is shown by the standard indices.

Figure 2.8. Humphrey Field Analyzer, Statpac 1, printout "Single Field A

SINGLE FIELD ANALYSIS	Name: SFW-DEMO, 10	Eye: RIGHT
Central 30 - 2	Birthdate: 10 Jun 1935	ID:

Stimulus: III, WHITE	Background: 31.5 asb	Test Date: 30 Aug 1990	Age: 55
Blind Spot Check Size: III	Fixation Target: CENTRAL	Test Time: 08:17:46	
Strategy: FULL	RX Used: +3.00 DS DC x °	Pupil Diameter: 2.0 mm	VA: 20/20

Fixation Losses: 3/30
False Pos Errors: 0/30
False Neg Errors: 1/16
Test Duration: 18:17
Fovea: 34 dB

A - Numerals absolute

```
               4  15 | 15   5
           12  ?     |          ?
       14  17        |             23
15  16  26  29  27   | 26  24  26  22  20
15  25  25  30  31   | 28  28  23  21  17
----------------------------------------- 30°
<0   9  11  <0  27   | 31  27  <0   5  10
<0  <0  <0  <0  <0   |  2   5  16  21  10
    <0   6  <0  <0   | 12  14   5  12
         14  <0  22  | 21  18   8
             10  18  | 18   7
```

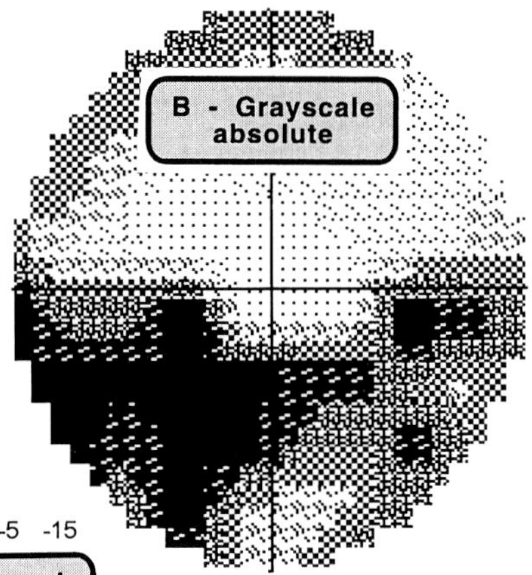

C - Numerals relative

```
          -19  -9 | -7  -18
     -12                    -3
-10 -11  -3  -1  -3 | -4  -5  -3  -6  -7
-11  -3  -5  -1  -1 | -4  -2      -8 -11
----------------------------------------
-28 -20 -20 -32  -5 | -1  -4     -24 -19
-28 -30 -32 -33 -33 |-29 -26 -14  -8 -18
    -29 -23 -32 -32 |-18 -16 -25 -17
        -13 -30  -7 | -8 -11 -20
            -16  -9 | -9 -20
```

Total Deviation

D - Numerals individual

```
          -17  -6 | -5  -15
     -10                    -1
 -8  -9  -1   1  -1 | -2  -3   0  -4  -5
 -9  -1  -3   1   1 | -1   0      -6  -9
----------------------------------------
-26 -17 -17 -30  -3 |  1  -2     -22 -17
-26 -28 -30 -31 -31 |-27 -23 -11  -6 -16
    -27 -20 -29 -30 |-16 -14 -22 -14
        -11 -28  -4 | -6  -9 -18
            -14  -6 | -7 -18
```

Pattern Deviation

Glaucoma Hemifield Test:

WNL	BL	ONL

Outside Normal Limits

MD: -14.00 dB P < 0.5%
PSD: 12.87 dB P < 0.5%
SF: 3.61 dB P < 2%
CPSD: 12.20 dB P < 0.5%

G - Standard Indices relative

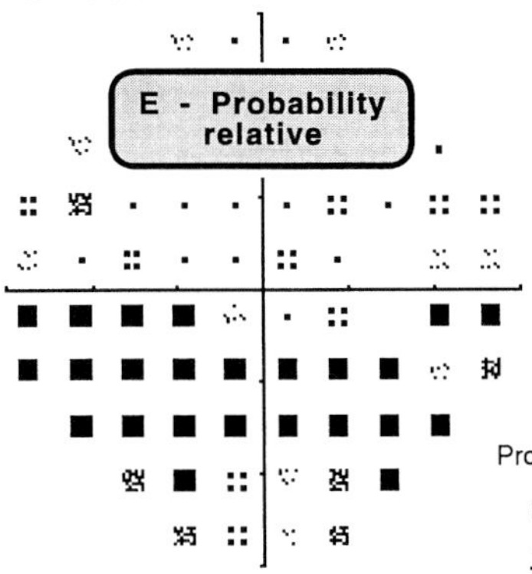

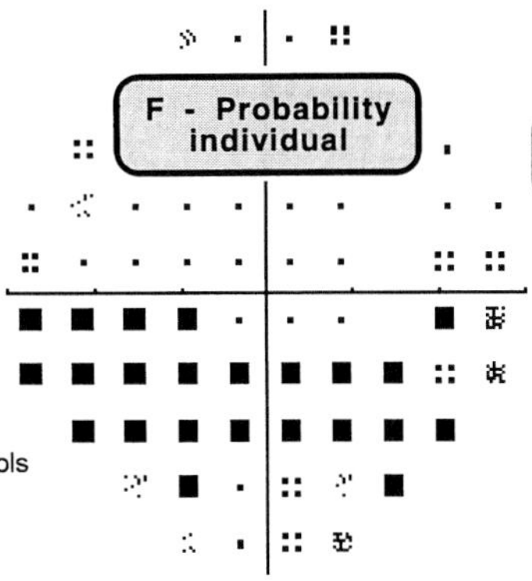

Probability Symbols
:: P < 5%
⁖ P < 2%
▩ P < 1%
■ P < 0.5%

Graytone Symbols

>40	>35	>30	>25	>20	>15	>10	>5	>0	≤0

HFA S/N: 630-2709

Humphrey Instruments, Inc.
A Carl Zeiss Company
SFW version 1.0

SFW-DEMO, 10	RIGHT

2.8

2.9 EXAMPLE: OCTOPUS 101 SEVEN-IN-ONE PRINTOUT

The Octopus 101 (Interzeag Company) is controlled by a personal computer program. The same program is used for storage and printout. The seven-in-one printout combines similar representations as the Humphrey Statpac printout, with an additional cumulative curve (Fig. 2.9). These include a detailed grayscale of thresholds (absolute sensitivity) (A), threshold values (B), comparison with normal (relative sensitivity) (C), corrected comparisons (individual sensitivity) (D), probability plot (E), corrected probability plot (F), cumulative defect curve (G), and indices (H). The threshold values are the raw results. The topography of the damage is represented by a grayscale of thresholds, which also contains age effects and eccentricity effects. The amount of local damage can be seen in the relative numbers (comparison). The probability plot displays the degree of abnormality of these numbers. The individual numerals (corrected comparison) are related to an individually shifted normal hill of vision. They enhance the identification of focal defects but mask the component of diffuse loss (see Section 2.1). The same is true of the corrected probability plot. The global damage is readily appreciated on the cumulative curve and summarized by the standard indices.

Figure 2.9. Octopus 101: combination printout of an examination with program 32.

INTERZEAG	OCTOPUS 101	V 2.21a
Seven-in-One		

Name:	**STEIN**	Eye / Pupil[mm]:	**Left (OS) / 7.1**
First name:	MARY	Date / Time:	09/17/1997 01:24 PM
ID #:	224-37-16	Test duration:	12: 8
Birthdate:	09/18/1942	Program / Code:	32 / 0
Age:	55	# Stages / Phases:	4 / 1
Sex:	female	Strategy / Method:	Normal / Normal
Refr. S / C / A:	+5.00 / -2.00 / 176	Test target / duration:	III / 100 ms
Acuity:		Background:	4 asb
IOP:		# Questions / Repetitions:	373 / 1
Diagnostics:	GLAUCOMA	# Catch trials:	pos 0 / 19, neg 1 / 19

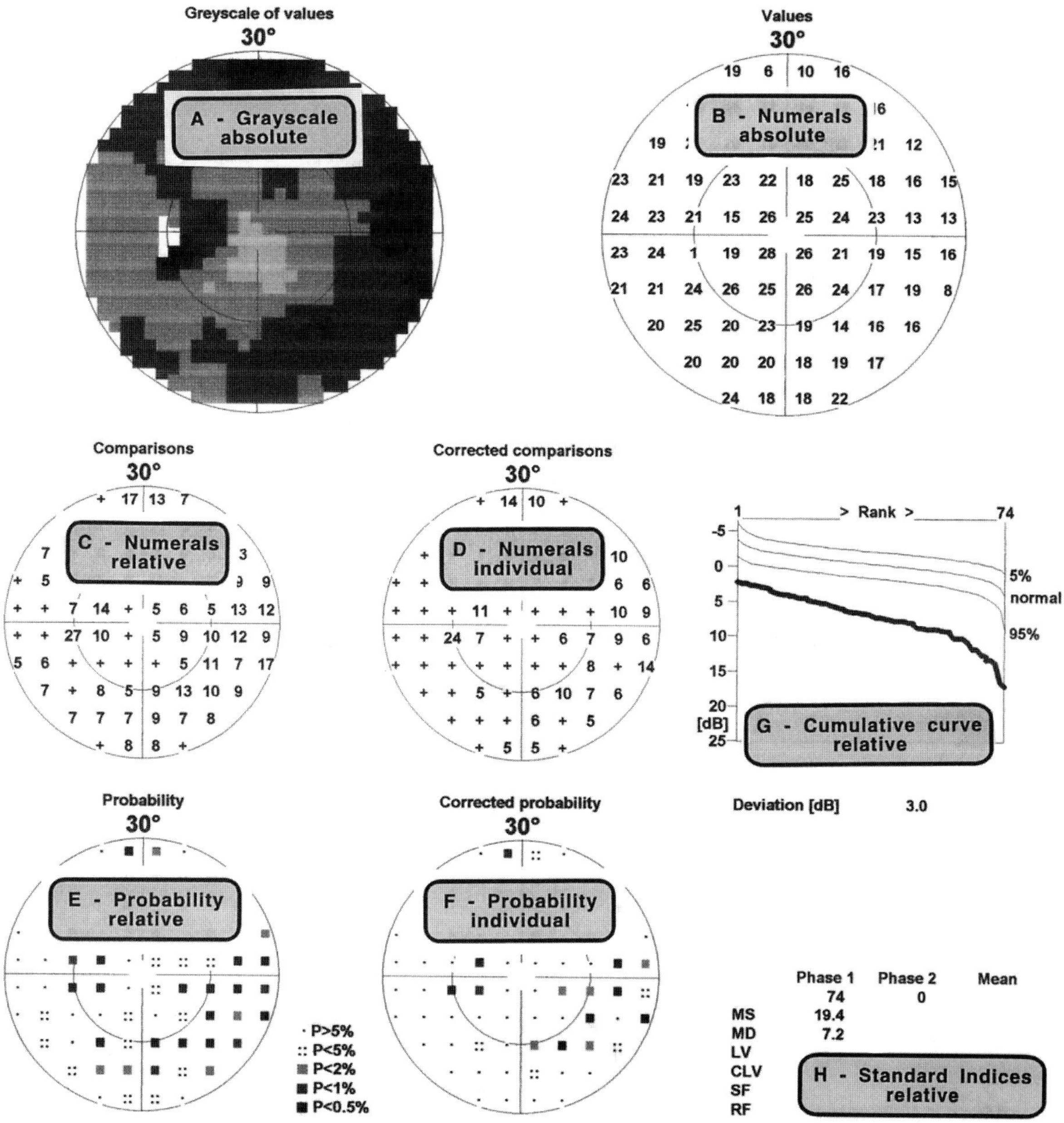

2.10 EXAMPLE: OCTOPUS 1-2-3 COMBINATION PRINTOUT

The Octopus 1-2-3 (Interzeag Company) uses incorporated analysis software. The combination printout can be arranged by the user. Figure 2.10 shows a combination of absolute grayscale (A), absolute sensitivities (B), cumulative defect curve (C), relative defects (D), and standard indices (E). The grayscales help the examiner recognize the topography of the damage, biased by the effects of age and eccentricity. The absolute sensitivities are the raw data, and the relative defects show the amount of local damage. The global damage is readily appreciated on the cumulative curve and summarized by the standard indices.

Figure 2.10. Octopus 1-2-3: combination printout of an examination with program G1 (courtesy of J. Flammer, M.D., University of Basel).

INTERZEAG OCTOPUS 1-2-3 V 3.15g
Combination central

Name:	**Case 15**	Eye / Pupil[mm]:	**Left (OS) / 5.2**
First name:	Chorioret.Les.	Date / Time:	29.08.1995 09:52
ID #:		Test duration:	9:14
Birthdate:	01.06.1931	Program / Code:	G1X / 3
Age:	64	# Stages / Phases:	4 / 1
Sex:	male	Strategy / Method:	Normal / Normal
Refr. S / C / A:	/ /	Test target / duration:	III / 100 ms
Acuity:	20/30	Background:	31.4 asb
IOP:		# Questions / Repetitions:	287 / 0
Diagnostics:	Chorioretinal lesions	# Catch trials:	pos 0 / 18, neg 1 / 18

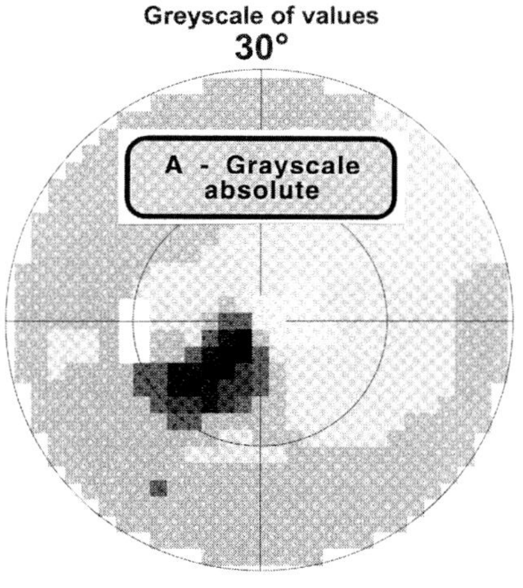

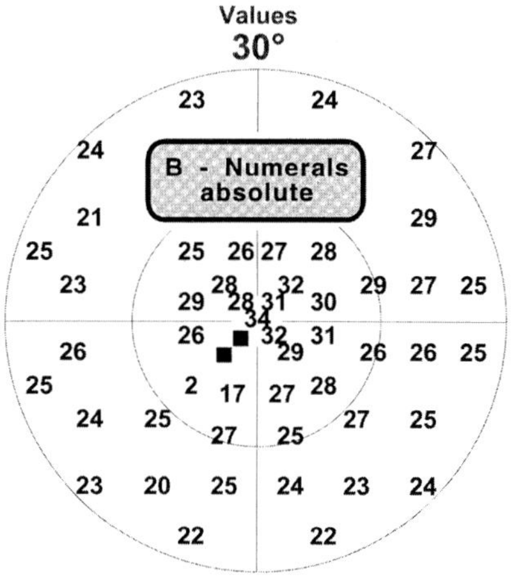

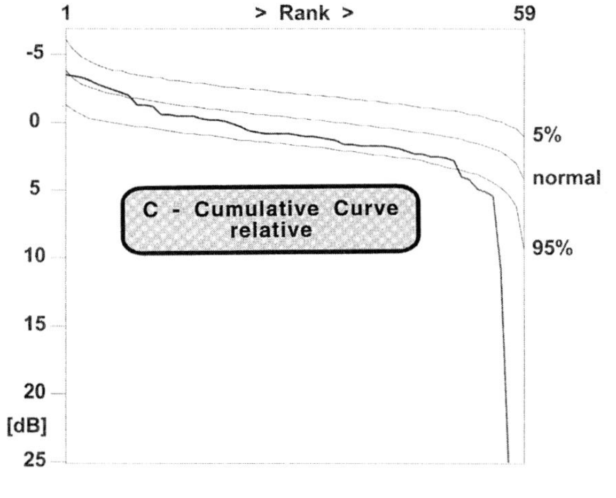

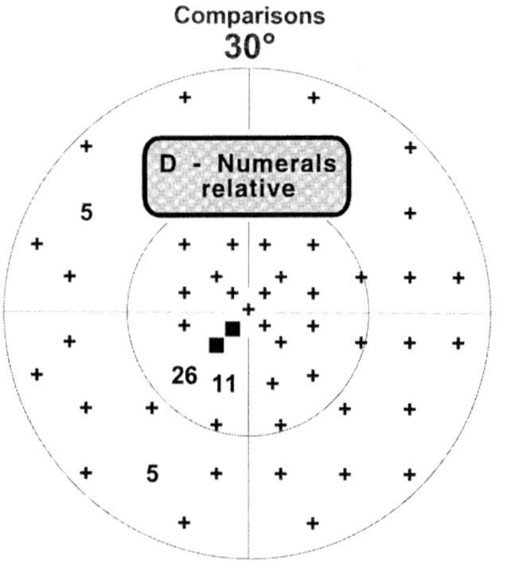

E - Standard Indices relative

			Normal	Phase 1	Phase 2	Mean
Number of test locations				59	0	0
Mean sensitivity	MS	[dB]		24.6		
Mean defect	MD	[dB]	-2..2	2.2		
Loss variance	LV	[dB²]	0..6	42.5		
Corrected loss variance	CLV	[dB²]	0..4			
Short term fluctuation	SF	[dB]	0..2			
Reliability factor	RF	[%]				2.8

2.10

2.11 EXAMPLE: PERIDATA STANDARD PRINTOUT

The Peridata program is a multi-instrument standard program which stores data from different perimeters and analyzes them. At the time of this printing, data from all Octopus perimeters, all Humphrey perimeters, the Opthimus Ring Perimeter, the Rodenstock Perimat 206, and the Rodenstock Peristat 433 can be read. The display is independent of the perimeter used. The standard printout (Fig. 2.11) combines several representations which are all based on relative, norm-related sensitivity: sensitivities (A), interpolated defect grayscale (B), cumulative defect curve (C), Intellitext (D), and standard global indices (E). The grayscale helps the examiner to recognize the topography of the field damage, having eliminated the effects of age and eccentricity with the use of relative sensitivities. The amount of local damage can be seen from the grayscale and the numerals. The global damage is indicated by the cumulative defect curve and the standard indices. The newly introduced Intellitext is a descriptive analysis of the entire field based on mathematical calculations and rules (artificial intelligence) and offers an alternative approach to visual a field evaluation (second opinion).

Figure 2.11. Peridata standard printout of an examination (program 30-2) performed with the Humphrey Field Analyzer. For details, see text.

PERIDATA Professional 7.0

1 TEST * SINGLE RESULT (06-21-98 D:\PROJEKTE\ATLAS\ATLAS.PHF)

2.11A M., A. *12-16-39 ID: +9168 (RE: Low-tension glaucoma)

RE 12-28-84 20.11 HFA1 30-2 ZENTRALFELD SCHWELLENTEST Stim III (200ms) Full threshold

Pupil 5.0 mm VA 0.50 Fixation Target Central RX Used 3.00 DS 0.00 DC 0° axis

Test Duration 17:31 min Questions 605 MalFixation [III] 5% (3/55) FalsePos 0% (0/21) FalseNeg 6% (1/18)

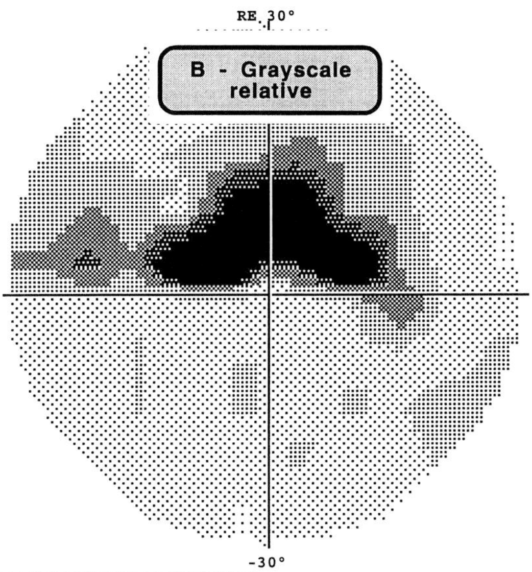

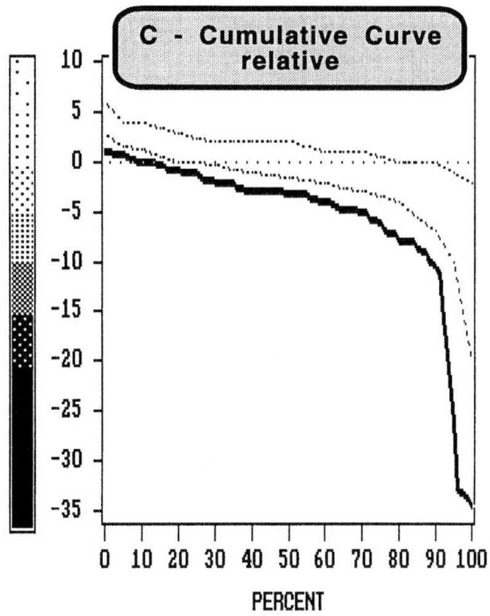

D - Intellitext

The visual field is not normal. 100% of the measured values are below normal limits. The average damage (MD) is -5.7 dB. The neuro-functional score (FS) is changed by -34%.

The damage is not evenly distributed. The damage topography correlates with the pattern: NerveFibreBundles. The damage is found mainly in the following region(s): short upper arcuate, long upper arcuate. The greatest damage is in the following region: short upper arcuate.

Mathematical analysis does not assess every kind of abnormality.

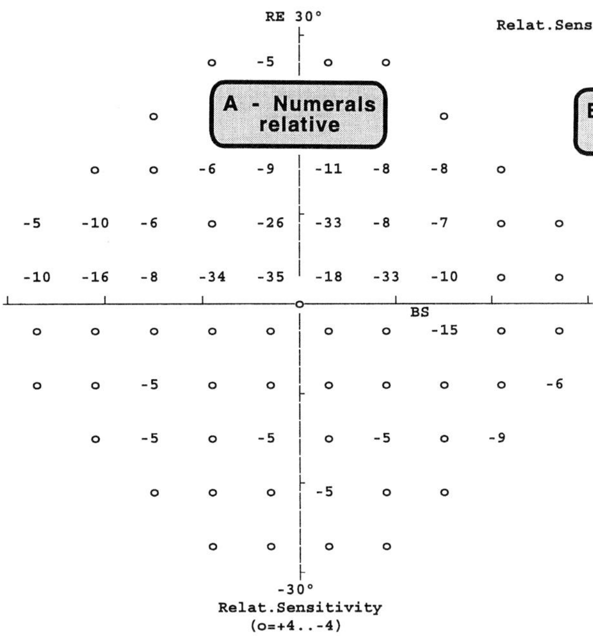

E - Standard Indices relative

MD	-5.7
LV	64.0
CLV	54.6
PSD	8.0
CPSD	7.4
SF	3.4
N	75.0
MS	23.5
FS	66.0

2.12 EXAMPLE: DICON 6-PLUS-2 PRINTOUT

The Dicon perimeter 5000 offers a printout which contains nearly every item of the Humphrey Field Analyzer Statpac Single Field Analysis (Fig. 2.12). Only some of the standard indices are missing. There are threshold data (absolute sensitivity) (A), a grayscale of thresholds (B), difference from age-related normals (ARN–Delta = relative sensitivity) as numerals (C) and a probability plot (D), difference from a shifted hill of vision (HOV–Delta = individual sensitivity) as numerals (E) and a probability plot (F), regional indices for quadrants, a hemifield and the global field based on relative sensitivity (G), and individual sensitivity (H).

The actual measured sensitivities (thresholds) are raw results. The topography of the damage is represented by absolute grayscales, which also contain age effects and eccentricity effects. The amount of local damage can be seen in the relative numerals (ARN–Delta). The individual numerals (HOV–Delta) are related to an individually shifted normal hill of vision. They enhance the identification of focal defects but ignore the component of diffuse loss (see Section 2.1). The probability plots display the degree of abnormality. The global and regional damage is shown by the regional indices.

Figure 2.12. Dicon 6-plus-2 printout, program FieldView Omega.

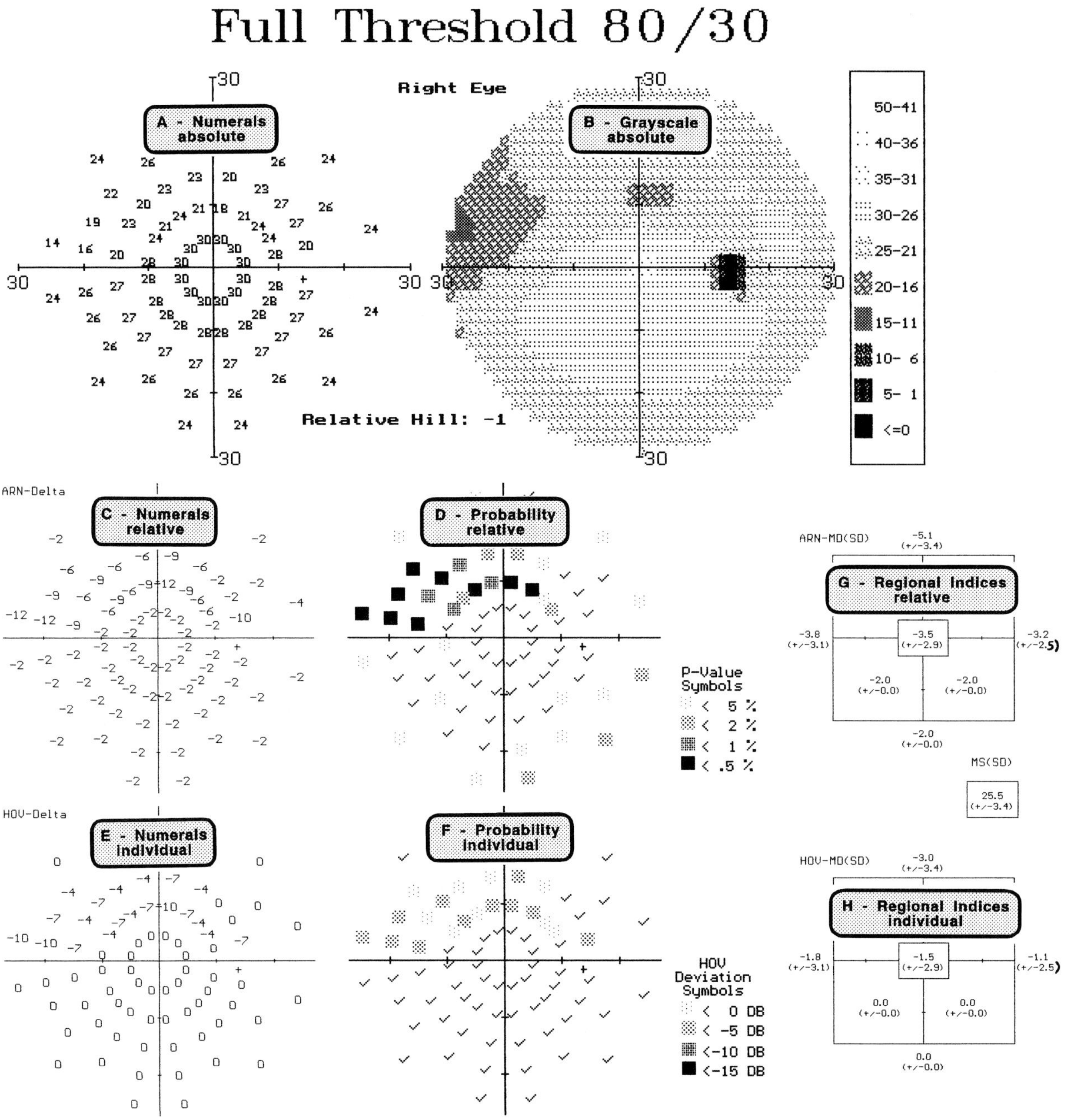

Exam Conditions	
Stimulus	: Single
Strategy	: Threshold
Macula	: Off
Background Luminance	: 31.5 ASB
Stimulus Duration	: 0.25
Stimulus Min Interval:	0.50

Exam Results	Right Eye
Points Tested	80
False Positives	0
False Negatives	0
Presentations	190
Fixation Losses	0/12
Exam Time	7:00

Exam Date: 10/30/1996
Birthdate: 03/03/1977
Age : 19
Patient : FieldLink Test
ID# : Unknown

Perimeter: TKS4K Version 2.50
Serial Number 200

Program: FieldView Omega 1.22 FL 1.2
Serial Number 12685

Licensed to: For Demo Purposes Only

2.12

3 Perimetric Findings

3.1 TOPOGRAPHY OF THE OPTICAL PROJECTION AND THE VISUAL PATHWAY

The Principle of Optical Projection

Our ability to orient ourselves by our visual system derives from the fact that every light-emitting point in our visual world falls on a single corresponding point on the retina, and stimulates a defined area in the visual cortex. This correspondence is based partly on optical principles which ensure an inverted image of the visual world on the retina and partly on the neuronal connections between retinal photoreceptors and the visual cortex. Along the course of three optical surfaces and four neurons, the cross-sectional topography of visual information—related to the original location in space—changes. Figure 3.1 shows the projection tracks, including cross-sectional cuts, in a perspective view from above and behind.

Physico-optical Part

All light rays converge at the optical plane (nodal point) of the eye, which is positioned at the posterior of the crystalline lens. Behind the nodal point the image is inverted. Images are focused on the retina in emmetropia.

Nervous Part

The retina transforms light impulses into electrical impulses. The optic projections are nerve fibers that connect the retinal photoreceptors to the cells of the visual (occipital) cortex. They originate from the various retinal regions and take either a straight path (nasal fibers) or an arcuate-shaped path (temporal fibers) to the optic nerve head. Therefore, at the optic nerve head, fibers from neighboring retinal areas lie together. In the subsequent course of the optic nerve the original orientation at the retina, the retinotopy, is restored. At the optic chiasm, the nerve fibers of the nasal retina cross to the opposite side. There they join the temporal retinal nerve fibers of the contralateral eye so that fibers of corresponding retinal regions lie beside each other. Each optic tract consists of the projection of one-half of the visual field. Inside the tract, fibers are rotated inward. In addition, central and peripheral fibers change their location. The retinal nerve fibers end at the lateral geniculate nucleus and synapse with the last neuron of the optic projection. Its axons spread out widely and form the optic radiations. The anterior arch extends more inferiorly than shown in Figure 3.1. Finally, the visual electrical impulses reach the primary visual cortex at the calcarine sulcus in the occipital lobe of the brain.

Sufficient damage to the optical projections leads to visual field loss. The pattern of visual field loss results from the topography of the projections at the damaged site.

Figure 3.1. Overview of the optical projection and the visual pathway viewed from the rear above. The hemispheres of the occipital brain are set aside to visualize the optical cortex at the calcarine sulcus.

Note: For all figures in Chapter 3, the letters I and O have been skipped in numbering to avoid confusion with digits.

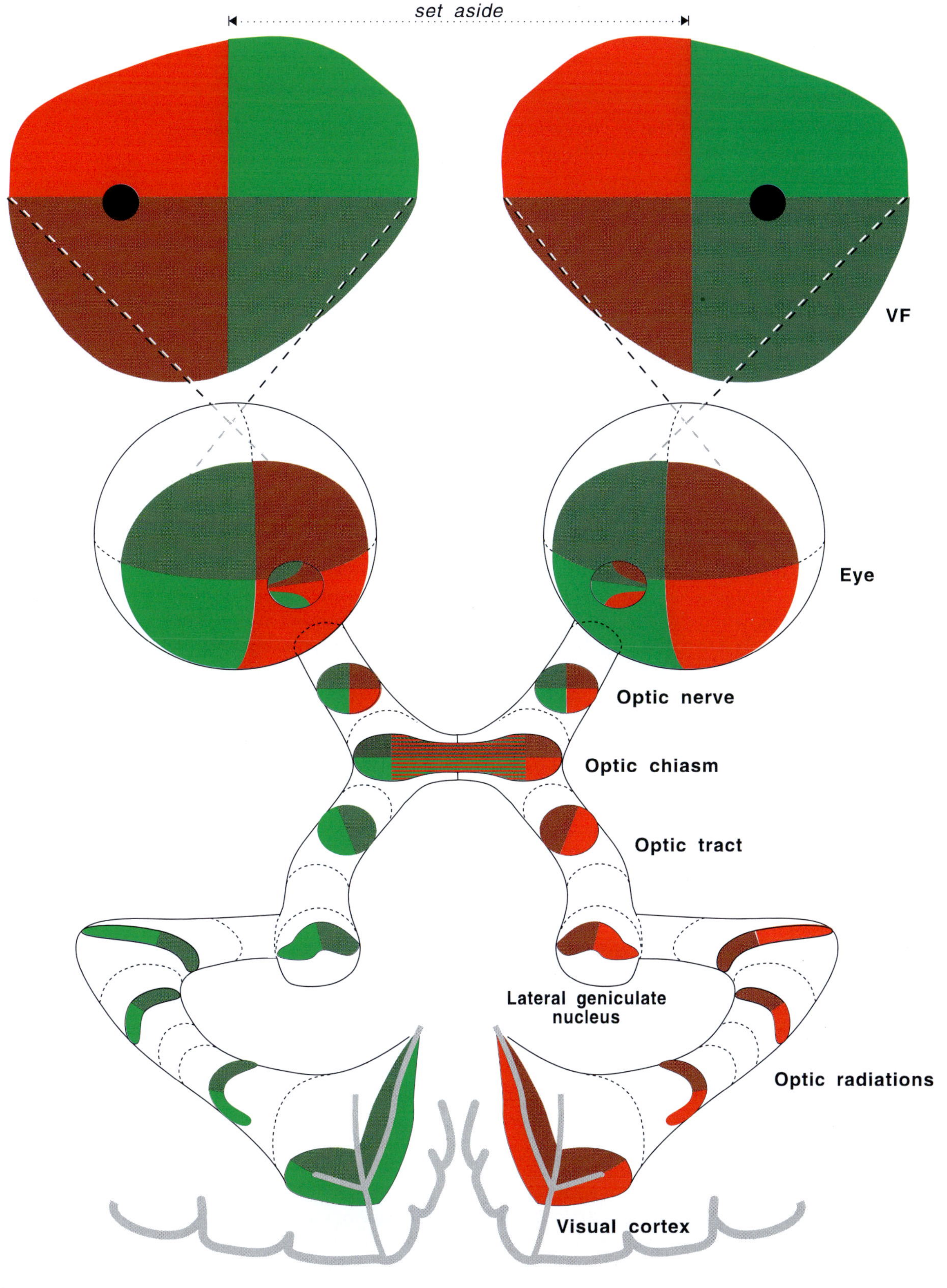
set aside
VF
Eye
Optic nerve
Optic chiasm
Optic tract
Lateral geniculate nucleus
Optic radiations
Visual cortex

3.1A

3.2 EFFECTS OF DISTORTION OR OBSCURATION OF LIGHT ENTERING THE EYE

Principle

Light rays which enter the eye linearly converge at the nodal point of the eye. Any distortion or obscuration will cause a corresponding visual field defect like a shadow that is projected onto the field (Fig. 3.2A).

Nose

A large nose may cause visual field constriction in the lower nasal quadrant. The margin of this absolute defect is usually seen between 35° and the limit of the normal field at 50°. The shadow of the nose usually does not cause visual field defects in standard examination programs which measure up to 30° of eccentricity. This nose artifact can be avoided with a slight rotation of the head during testing.

Eyebrows and Skin of the Eyelid

In patients with brow ptosis or deep-set eyes, the upper orbital margin causes an absolute visual field constriction from above, which may come as close as 20° from fixation. It is important to distinguish these conditions from other diseases that cause superior field defects, such as glaucoma. When an eyebrow defect is suspected, perimetry should be repeated with the patient's head reclined. If the forehead rest cannot be adjusted, a cushion between the forehead and the headrest may suffice. In such cases, the trial lens also requires appropriate repositioning.

Redundancy and relaxation of the eyelid skin (dermatochalasis) affects visual field results only if the skin fold falls over the lashes. Because such skin folds fall more over the temporal side of the lid, the visual field constriction is usually from above on the temporal side (Fig. 3.2B). Lid-skin field defects can be avoided by fixing the skin above the lid margin with tape.

Spectacle Lens Margin

Decentered spectacle lenses produce absolute visual field defects. The defect may occur almost anywhere, depending on the direction of decentration, but it nearly always has a half-moon shape (Fig. 3.2C). If the lens is too far from the eye, a full ring scotoma may also be seen. To avoid lens rim artifacts, large lenses with thin frames should be used and positioned near the eye; the position of the head should be checked frequently during the examination. If a suspected lens rim artifact persists during a second examination, another perimetric exam should be performed with no lens at all. In this case, the effect of defocusing (see below) must be considered. For this reason, it is preferable to omit weak spectacle corrections (1.5 diopters of spherical correction and 1.5 diopters of cylindrical correction) as long as large stimuli (Goldmann size 3 or more) are used.

Figure 3.2A. Topographical principle of optical interference. The visual field defect is equivalent to the cross-sectional optical abnormality.

Figure 3.2B. Dermatochalasis with visual field constriction from above, especially from the temporal side.

Figure 3.2C. Lens rim artifact with the typical geometrical shape of the absolute defect. Islands of vision within the absolute scotoma can sometimes occur during test intervals when the head is correctly positioned (program: Humphrey Field Analyzer [HFA] 30-2, representation: Peridata norm-related grayscale).

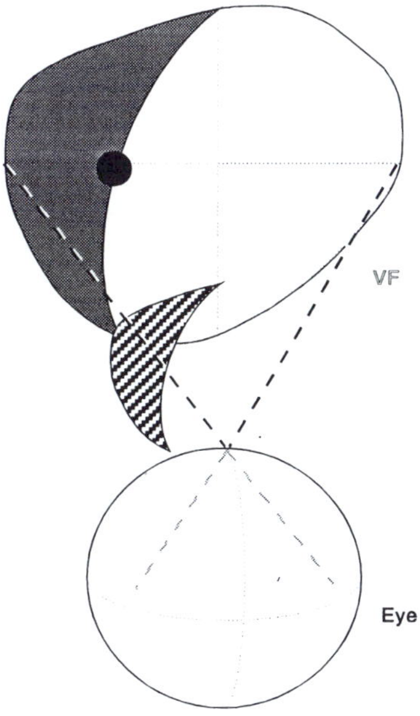

3.2A

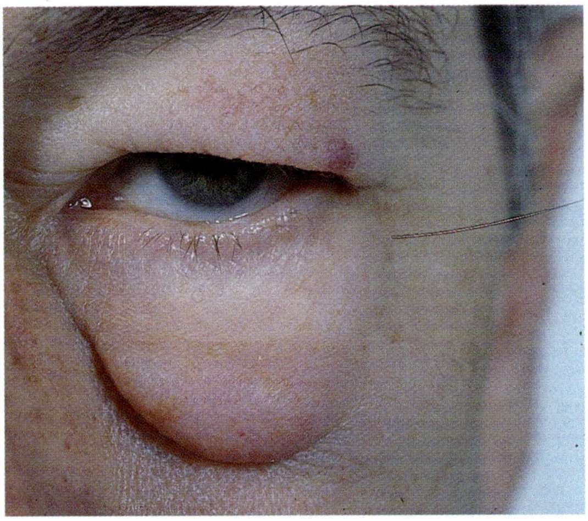

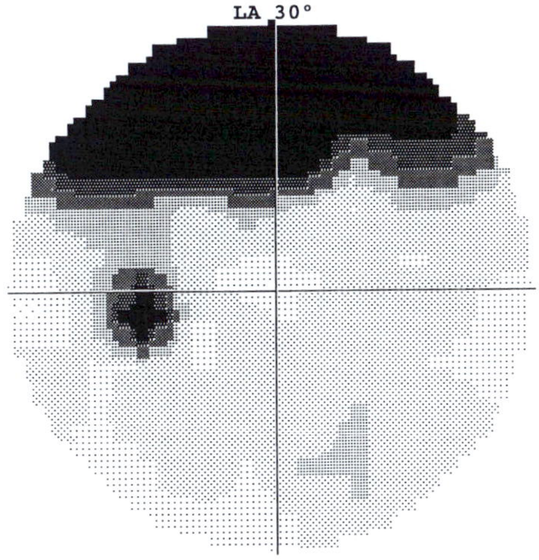

3.2B

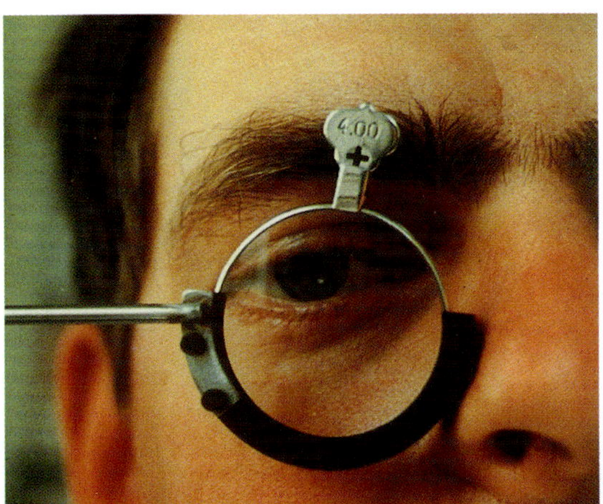

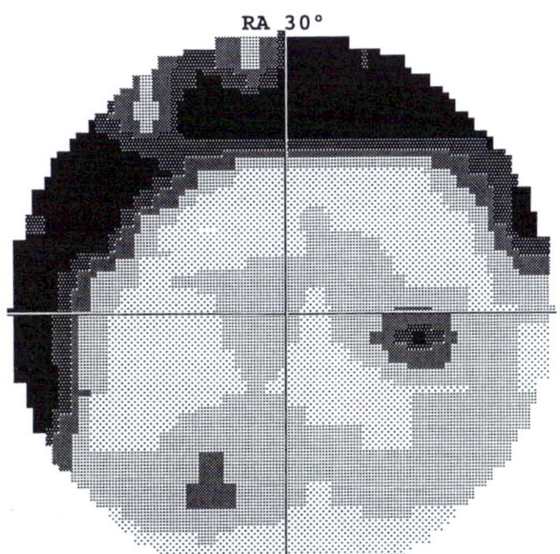

3.2C

Optical Effects of Spectacle Correction

Not only the lens rim but also the lens itself can influence the visual field because of optical effects. A single weak trial lens allows the patient to view the visual field accurately up to 40° to 45°. With powerful plus lenses (e.g., in aphakia) the image is magnified, while the extent of the tested visual field becomes smaller. An absolute ring scotoma is thereby created (Fig. 3.2D,E). A lens of up to +15 diopters which is properly positioned near the eye and well centered permits visual field testing of up to 30°.

The visual angle, however, is effectively reduced by high-powered plus lenses. Light stimuli which enter the eye at a subjective angle of 30° may be located at 20° in the perimeter bowl. The blind spot, all other visual field zones, and the visual field borders are shifted toward the center, increasing the steepness of the hill of vision (Fig. 3.2D). Therefore, relative depressions in the periphery are rather common in spectacle-corrected aphakia.

In contrast, strong minus lenses reduce image size, and the visual field is correspondingly enlarged. Ring scotomas do not occur, but the objective visual angle is increased. The blind spot and all scotomas are shifted peripherally.

Note: Refractive effects can be markedly reduced by using properly fitting contact lenses during perimetry.

Effects of Incorrect Spectacle Lenses

Incorrect spectacle lenses produce a blurred image of the stimulus. The ability to perceive the stimulus is diminished, and the measured sensitivity is reduced. The effect is very similar at all visual field locations and causes a homogeneous depression (Fig. 3.2F). With the commonly used stimulus size 0.43° (Goldmann III), the depression is approximately 1 dB per diopter of uncorrected refractive error. With smaller stimulus sizes the reduction in sensitivity is larger, and vice versa. If low-powered correcting lenses are omitted to avoid lens rim artifacts, the effect of the uncorrected refractive error should be taken into account.

Figure 3.2D. The effect of hyperopic spectacle correction: absolute limits of the visual field (hatched) and reduction of the objective visual angle.

Figure 3.2E. The effect of spectacle correction in an aphakic patient with an 18 diopter lens. The blind spot is slightly shifted toward fixation. In the periphery, an absolute positive lens defect is found (program: HFA 30-2, Peridata norm-related grayscale).

Figure 3.2F. The effect of miscorrection of +7 diopters in a normal emmetropic eye. The field is homogeneously depressed by 8 dB (program: HFA 30-2, Peridata norm-related grayscale; the predominant grayscale in this figure is at the −5 dB to −10 dB level).

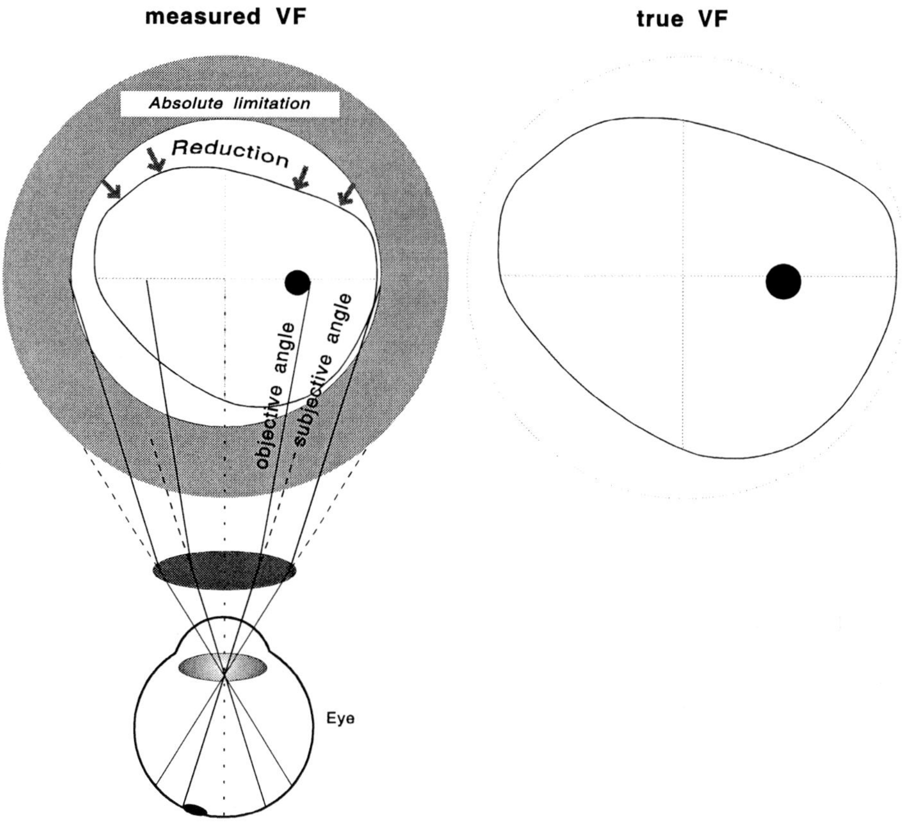
measured VF
true VF
Absolute limitation
Reduction
objective angle
subjective angle
Eye

3.2D

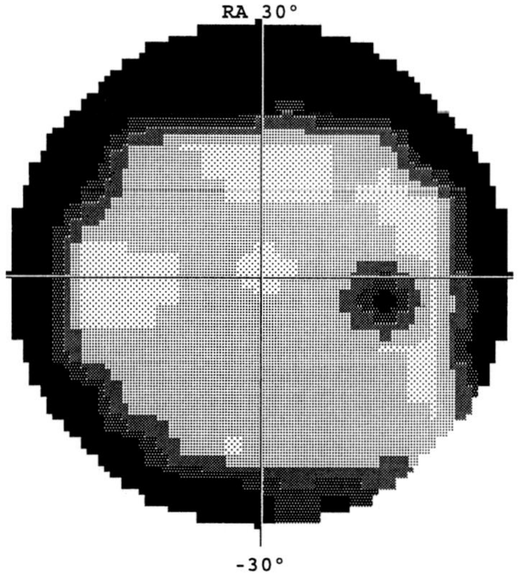
RA 30°
-30°

3.2E

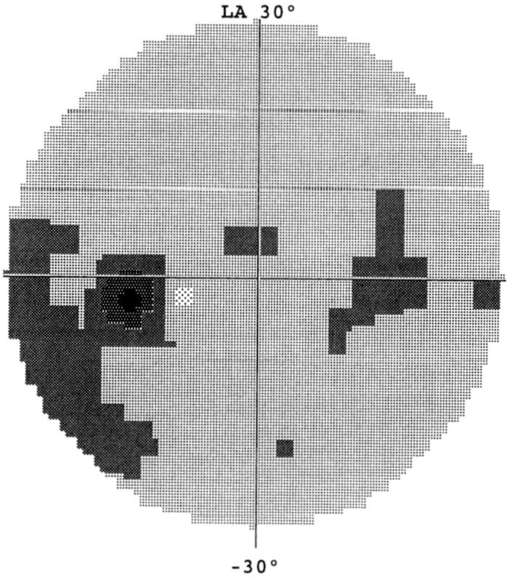
LA 30°
-30°

3.2F

3.3 OPTICAL DISTORTION OR OBSCURATION BY THE EYELIDS AND ANTERIOR SEGMENT STRUCTURES

Principle

In the crystalline lens of the eye, light rays from all visual field objects cross over. The central rays pass through the nodal point, which is positioned near the posterior pole of the lens, and the other rays pass through neighboring points in this plane. Therefore, any optical interference in this plane disturbs rays from all directions and causes a homogeneous, diffuse loss of sensitivity throughout the whole visual field. The image of the interfering object cannot be recognized in the visual field (Fig. 3.3A). Any form of optical interference close to the lens has a similar effect. By contrast, a shape can be recognized with increasing distance from the nodal point, which resembles, with considerable blur, the cross section of the interfering object.

Eyelids

The eyelids are only about 8 mm anterior to the nodal point. Therefore, the visual field defect is a rough approximation of the shape of the eyelid (Fig. 3.3B).

Cornea

The perimetric stimulus is blurred and dimmed by central corneal opacities throughout the whole visual field. Diffuse visual field defects can be seen. Irregular astigmatism and other irregularities of the corneal surface diminish the clarity of the stimulus and can cause visual field loss. These effects are more pronounced with small stimulus sizes.

Pupil

A small pupil reduces the luminance of the retinal image of the stimulus. However, the contrast of the stimulus against the background is not affected if the media are clear. The differential light sensitivity does not change as the absolute luminance levels change under ordinary testing conditions. This is stated as Weber's law: differential light sensitivity (the ratio of stimulus luminance to background luminance) is constant over a wide range of luminances. If the ocular media are not clear, pupil sizes less than approximately 3 mm will significantly reduce the differential light sensitivity. This deepens scotomas and enlarges the area of absolute defects (Fig. 3.3C). If the pupil diameter is less than 3 mm, pupils should be dilated whenever possible before a perimetric exam. However, mydriatics will not dilate small, rigid pupils with extensive posterior synechia formation. Pupil size should always be recorded at the time of perimetric examination.

Figure 3.3A. Effects of optical interference at the nodal point of the eye. The visual field defect is diffuse, and the cross-sectional topography of the damage cannot be recognized.

Figure 3.3B. Effect of blepharoptosis on the visual field: diffuse sensitivity loss which is deeper in the superior visual field (program: HFA 30-2, representation: Peridata grayscale and numerals, based on norm-related sensitivity).

Figure 3.3C. Change of pupil size in a 54-year-old glaucoma patient with cataract. Visual activity is 20/25. Left, the visual field examined with a pupil size of 2 mm. Right: 3 days later, without miotics and a pupil size of 3 mm (program: HFA custom program, Peridata norm-related grayscale).

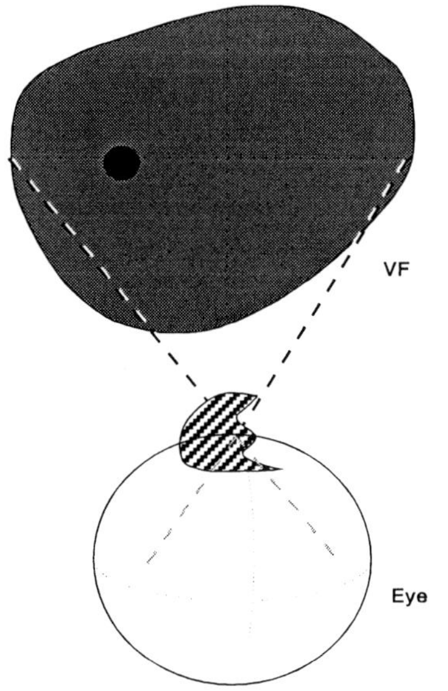
VF
Eye

3.3A

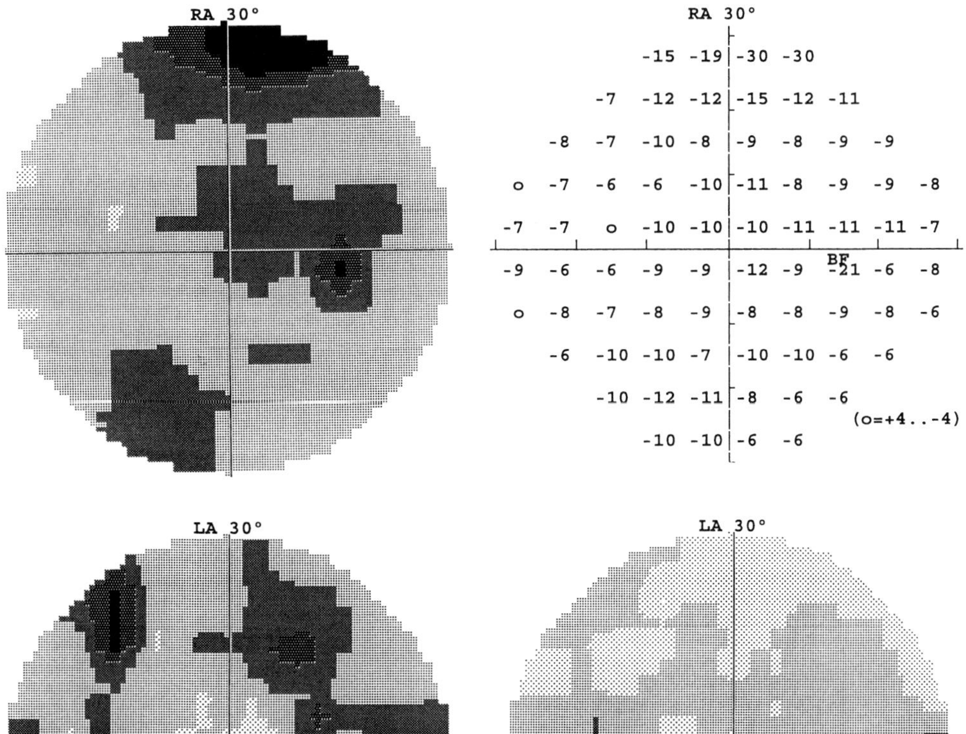
RA 30°
RA 30°
-15 -19 -30 -30
-7 -12 -12 -15 -12 -11
-8 -7 -10 -8 -9 -8 -9 -9
o -7 -6 -6 -10 -11 -8 -9 -9 -8
-7 -7 o -10 -10 -10 -11 -11 -11 -7
BF
-9 -6 -6 -9 -9 -12 -9 -21 -6 -8
o -8 -7 -8 -9 -8 -8 -9 -8 -6
-6 -10 -10 -7 -10 -10 -6 -6
-10 -12 -11 -8 -6 -6
(o=+4..-4)
-10 -10 -6 -6

3.3B

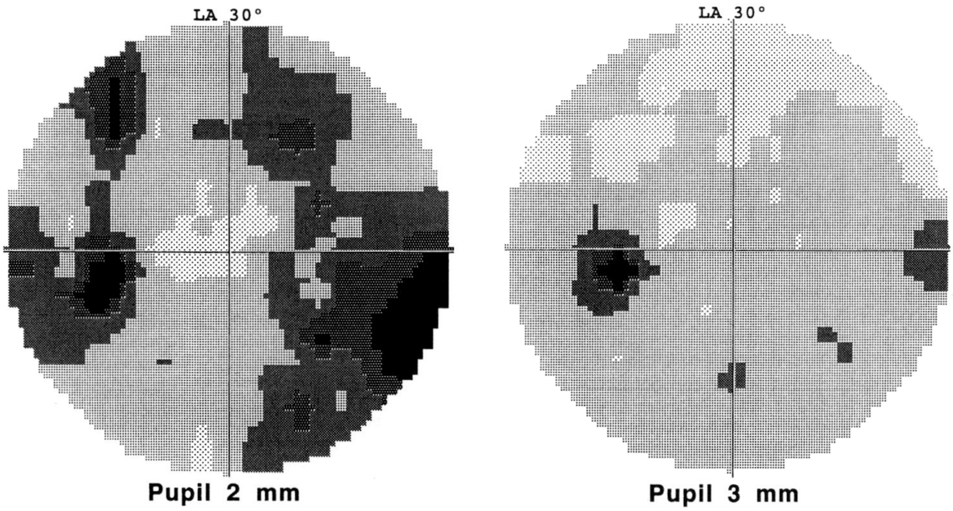
LA 30°
LA 30°
Pupil 2 mm
Pupil 3 mm

3.3C

Lens

Lens opacification (cataract) causes diffuse loss of sensitivity across the entire visual field (Fig. 3.3D). Areas of high sensitivity like the central field are more susceptible to optical degradation. Therefore, the defect depth is greater in the center (Fig. 3.3D right).

The effect of cataract is added to perimetric defects from other causes (Fig. 3.3E). The ability to distinguish between visual field abnormalities from both diseases is often claimed, but this is difficult or impossible in diseases like glaucoma, which also may have a generalized (diffuse) component of field loss. The cataract component may often be overestimated. According to recent studies, the average defect depth caused by a cataract prior to surgery (visual acuity 20/40 to 20/200) is only about 4 dB.

Figure 3.3D. Effect of cataract in a 67-year-old man with a visual acuity of 10/200 on the visual field. Diffuse loss of sensitivity is more pronounced in the center. Absolute sensitivities show a flattened profile (right eye, program: HFA 30-2, Peridata norm-related grayscale and profile; the dotted line indicates the normal profile for a patient of this age).

Figure 3.3E. Visual fields of a 60-year-old man with open-angle glaucoma before and after cataract surgery with lens implantation. The patient's visual acuity increased from 20/200 to 20/30. The visual field improved, especially in areas where deeper defects occurred (program: HFA 30-2, representation: Peridata norm-related grayscale and absolute profile).

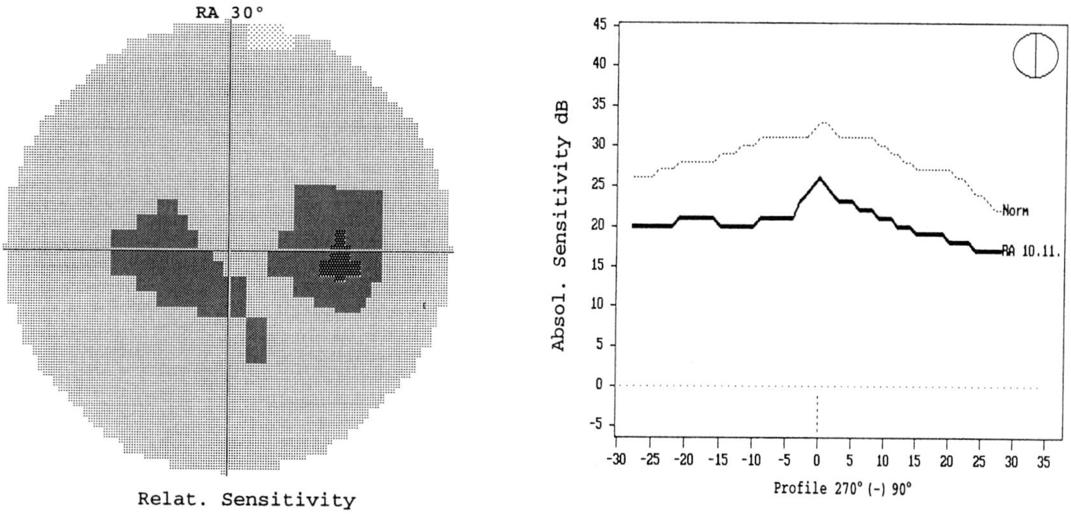
RA 30°
Relat. Sensitivity
Absol. Sensitivity dB
Norm
RA 10.11.
Profile 270° (-) 90°

3.3D

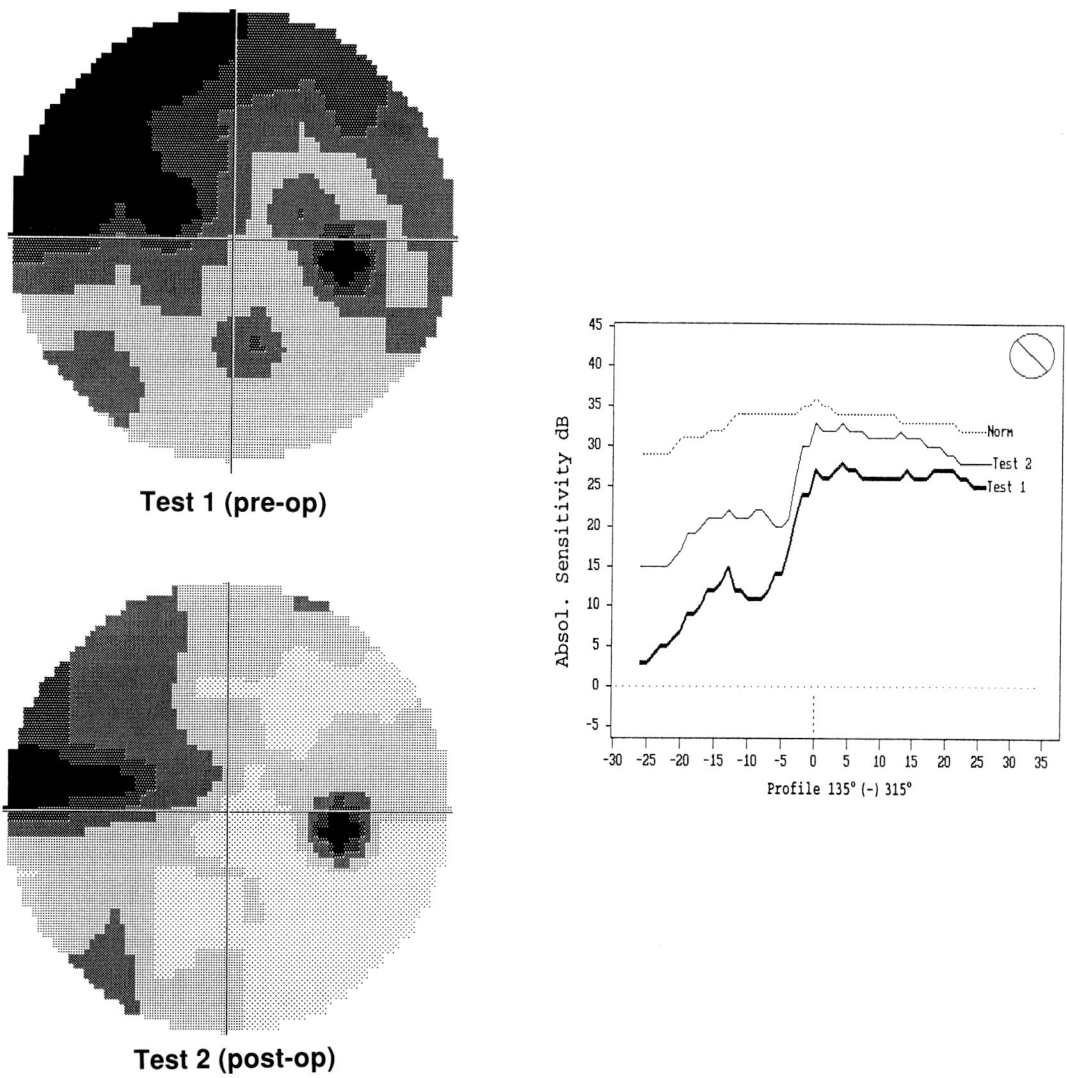
Test 1 (pre-op)
Test 2 (post-op)
Absol. Sensitivity dB
Norm
Test 2
Test 1
Profile 135° (-) 315°

3.3E

3.4 OPTICAL DISTURBANCES IN THE VITREOUS

Principle

Light rays from an object diverge behind the nodal point of the eye, where the image is inverted. Any optical disturbance in this area creates a visual field defect of the same but inverted shape (Fig. 3.4A).

Vitreous

Vitreous opacities can cause relative visual field defects (Fig.3.4B). The closer the vitreous opacities are to the retina, the more clearly their topography is reflected in the visual field. Preretinal visual field disturbances are usually perceived by the patient as "floaters" and are caused by minimal vitreous condensations. They are very common but usually cannot be detected by conventional perimetry.

Tumors in the vitreous cavity create shadows which appear inverted in the visual field. Discrimination between shadows cast on the retina and actual tissue damage is not possible because both can cause absolute defects.

Figure 3.4A. Effects of optical disturbances behind the crystalline lens. The visual field defect is an inverted image of the cross-sectional shape of the disturbance.

Figure 3.4B. Vitreous hemorrhage caused by a peripheral retinal break. The bleeding reaches into the optical axis from above and lowers the visual acuity to 20/30. The shape of the relative field defect is the mirror image of the hemorrhage (right eye, program: HFA 30-2, representation: Peridata norm-related grayscale).

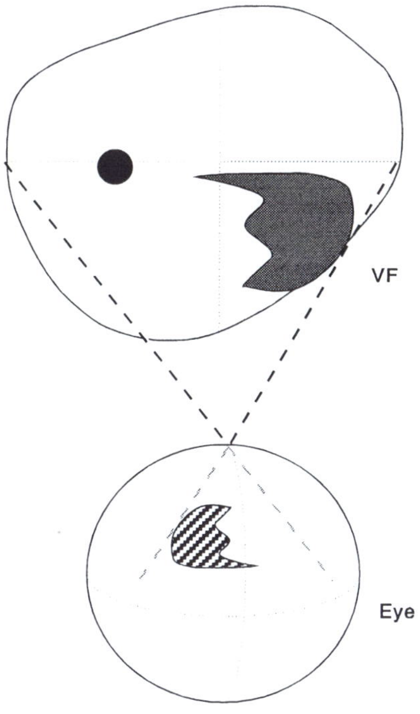

3.4A

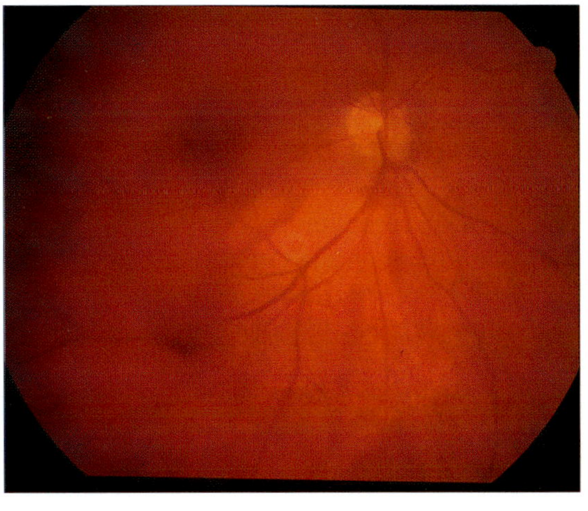

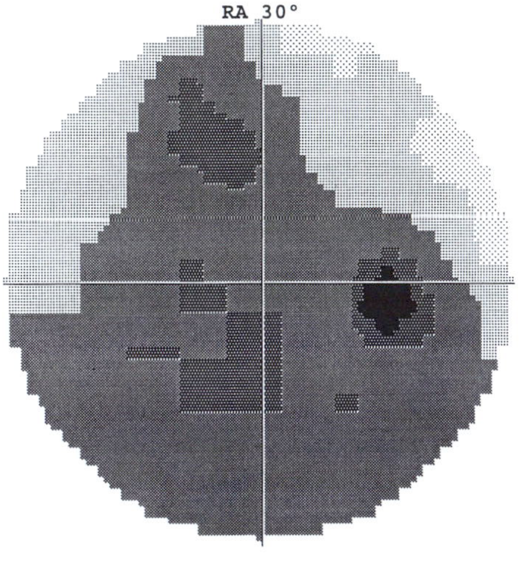

3.4B

3.5 DISEASES OF CHOROID AND OUTER RETINA

Principle

The emmetropic eye produces a focused, inverted image on the retina. At each retinal location, light is transformed into neural impulses by the photoreceptors (rods and cones). The photoreceptor cell transmits these impulses to the subsequent nerve cell (second-order neuron), which stimulates the ganglion cells (third-order neuron). The axons of the ganglion cells leave the retina and run through the optic nerve head. Diseases of the choroid and the outer retina generally interfere with photoreceptor and second-order neuron function. Thus, perception is disturbed at the retinal locations involved. The resulting visual field defect is inverted and shaped similarly to the area of retinal damage (Fig. 3.5A).

In comparing the retinal image and the visual field, it is crucial to consider that the visual field usually is represented from the patient's point of view but the fundus is represented from the examiner's point of view. When this additional mirroring is considered, the visual field defect and the funduscopic image of the altered area are understood to be mirror images of each other about the horizontal axis.

The broad spectrum of patterns of retinal and choroidal diseases is expressed in the variety of related visual field defects. Diagnoses are facilitated more by the funduscopic appearance than by the shape of the visual field defect. Subtle funduscopic changes, however, may be revealed more clearly by their corresponding visual field defect; the degree of functional damage may facilitate evaluation of the abnormality.

Tumors

The most common malignant tumor of the eye is the choroidal melanoma. The visual field defect corresponds to the extent of the tumor. The depth of the defect depends on the extent of damage to the choroid, choriocapillaris, and outer retina. Commonly, the defects are absolute in the center and relative at the edges, with a transition zone to normal sensitivity. Additional field defects occur in the form of shadow effects, serous retinal detachments and concurrent retinal or subretinal hemorrhage. After successful local radiation therapy the scotoma often becomes more absolute, indicating destruction of the underlying choriocapillaris. In addition, the scotoma may enlarge due to radiation damage to adjacent areas. Perimetry will help determine whether the goal of local radiation therapy, the preservation of the central vision, has been achieved (Fig. 3.5B).

Figure 3.5A. Visual field damage in diseases of the choroid and the outer retina. The visual field defect is an inverted image of the damaged region.

Figure 3.5B. Choroidal melanoma with subretinal hemorrhage and adjacent retinal detachment. The visual field shows a corresponding scotoma. One month after radiation therapy with a ruthenium/rhodium applicator the defect had enlarged, but fixation was preserved. Visual acuity decreased from 20/30 to 20/50 (right eye, program: HFA 30-2, representation: Peridata norm-related grayscale).

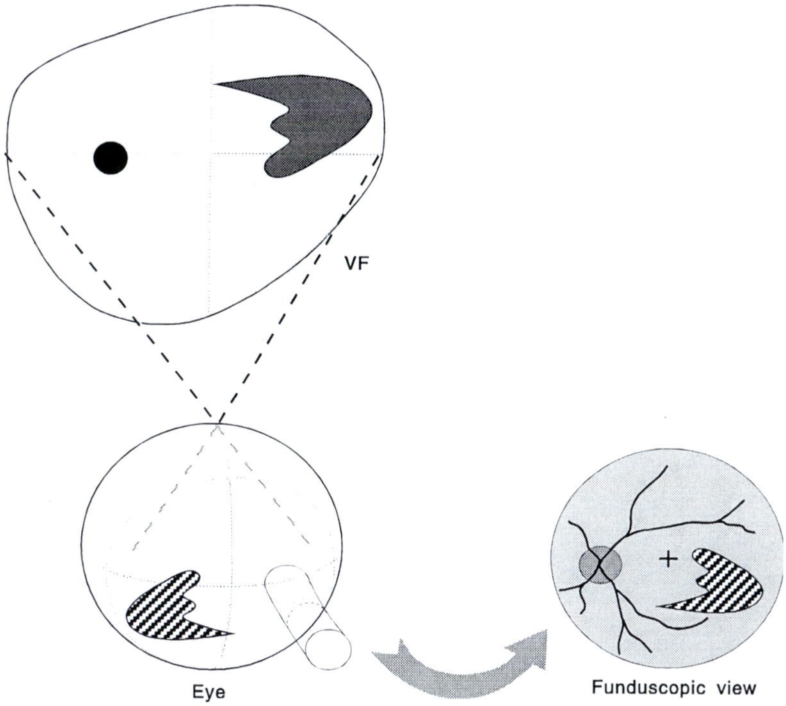
VF
Eye
Funduscopic view

3.5A

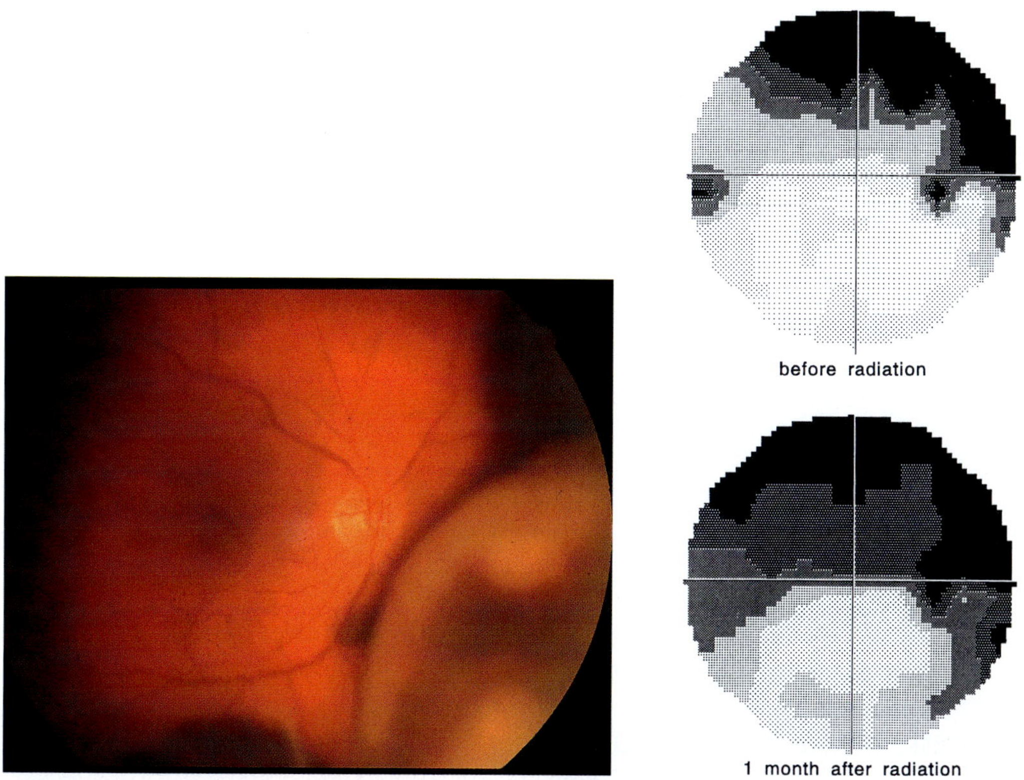
before radiation
1 month after radiation

3.5B

Retinal Detachment

In retinal detachment, the outer segments of the receptors are separated from the pigment epithelium. While neural transmission is not directly damaged, malfunction of the detached tissue or optical effects of the displacement (such as from defocusing or shadowing), relative defects, or absolute defects are found in the visual field (Fig. 3.5C). There is no need for perimetry as a diagnostic instrument in highly elevated rhegmatogenous detachments. In subtle shallow detachments, however, it can be helpful (Fig. 3.5D). In severe cases (proliferative vitreoretinopathy), the visual field can often provide information about anatomical and functional status (Fig. 3.5E). The preferred method of perimetry depends on the indication. Automated perimetry is more suitable for the central visual field and exact follow-up. Kinetic perimetry is often preferable for screening the full visual field.

Figure 3.5C. Highly elevated rhegmatogenous retinal detachment in the left eye. Fundus and 30° field (program HFA 30-2, representation: Peridata norm-related grayscale).

Figure 3.5D. Shallow inferior redetachment 6 months after placement of an encircling band. The patient noticed a decrease in vision from 20/25 to 20/30 and a shadow in the superior field (program: HFA 30-2, representation: Peridata norm-related grayscale).

Figure 3.5E. Myopia after retinal detachment with a hole near the macula, after vitrectomy with silicone oil, followed by proliferative vitreoretinopathy and revitrectomy. Large functional defects were present after membrane peeling with intraoperative bleeding (program: HFA 30-2, representation: Peridata norm-related grayscale).

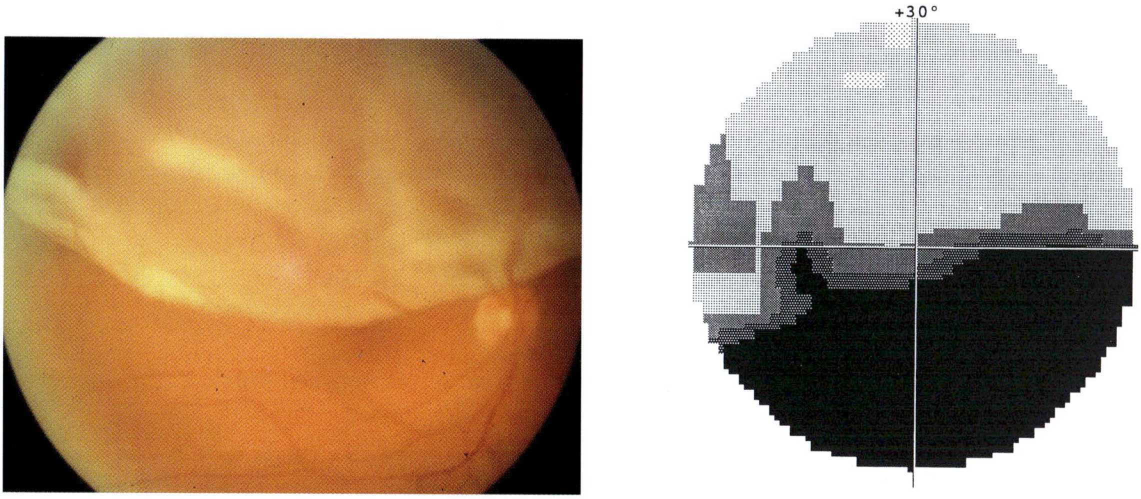

3.5C

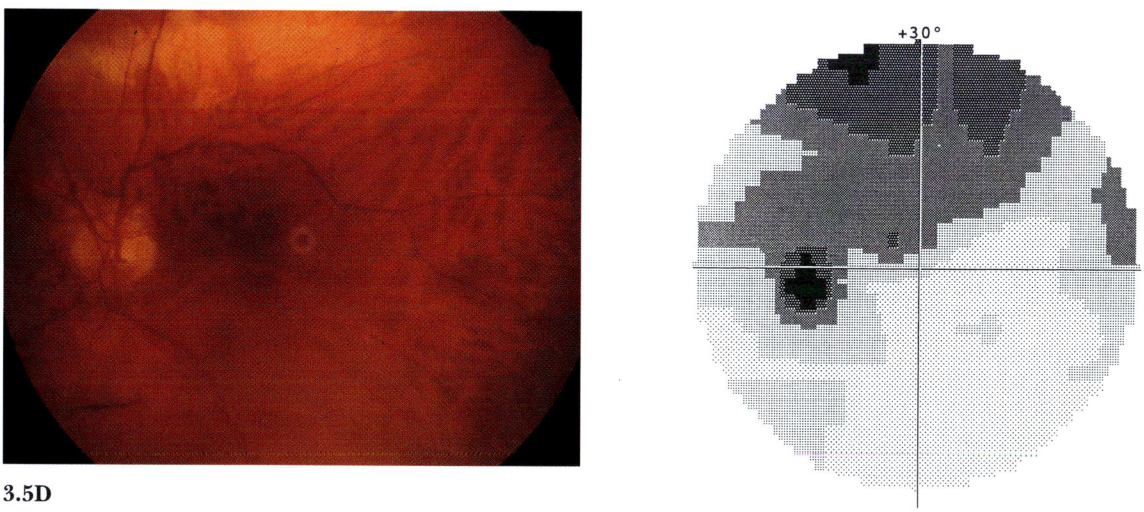

3.5D

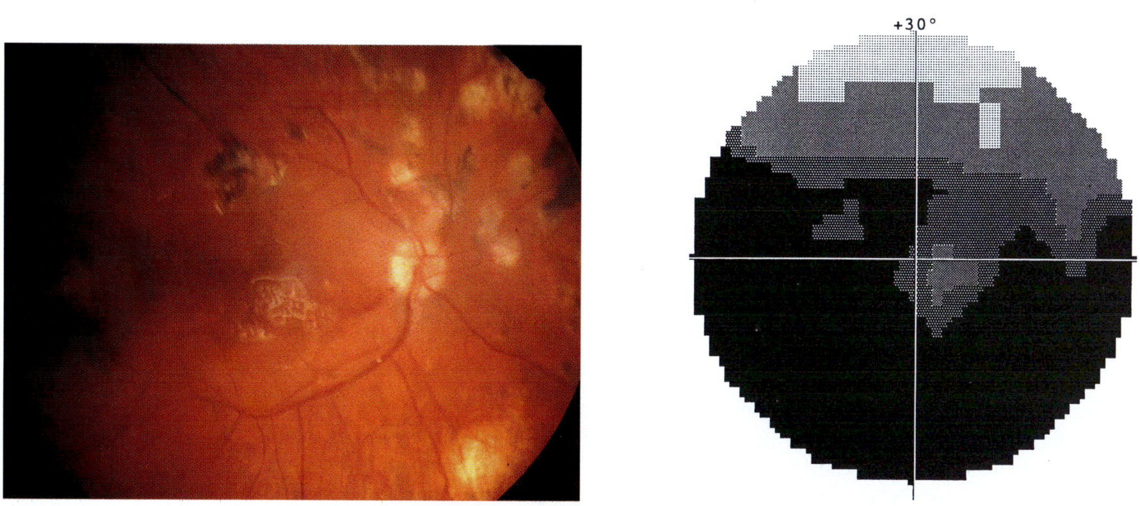

3.5E

Retinoschisis

In senile retinoschisis the retina is split between the receptors and the bipolar cells, interrupting neural transmission between the first and second visual neurons. In juvenile retinoschisis, the disconnection is situated between the second and third neurons. Due to the complete interruption, the visual field defect is always absolute (Fig. 3.5F).

Retinitis Pigmentosa

Like other tapetoretinal diseases, retinitis pigmentosa causes widespread functional loss (Fig. 3.5G). The amount of pigment change varies among individuals and is not well correlated with the amount of tissue damage. This is well demonstrated by the *sine pigmento* type of retinitis pigmentosa (Fig. 3.5H).

Figure 3.5F. Retinoschisis in the temporal lower quadrant. The 60° field shows a sharp border between normal sensitivity and absolute defects, indicated by a sensitivity of <0 dB (right eye, program: HFA 30-S combined with 30/60-2, representation: Peridata numerals and grayscale of absolute values).

Figure 3.5G. Retinitis pigmentosa in the left eye of a 43-year-old man, with visual acuity of 0.7 and a flat (ERG) (program: HFA 10-2, representation: Peridata norm-related grayscale).

Figure 3.5H. Retinitis pigmentosa sine pigmento in the left eye of a 19-year-old man with visual acuity of 20/30 and a flat ERG. The 30° field shows a small central island which is more or less equivalent to the central, more normally pigmented retinal area. The other eye was very similar (program: HFA 30-2, representation: Peridata norm-related grayscale).

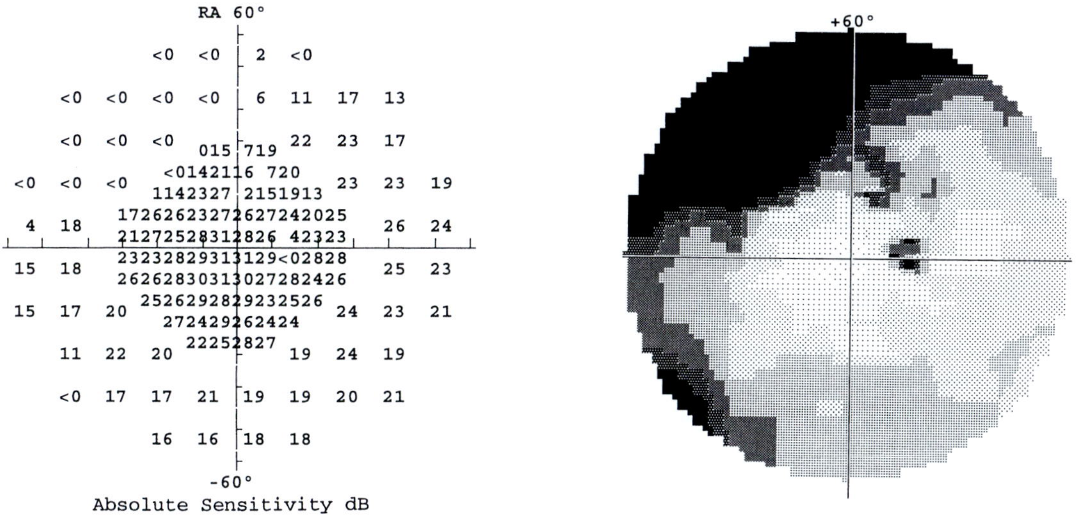

3.5F

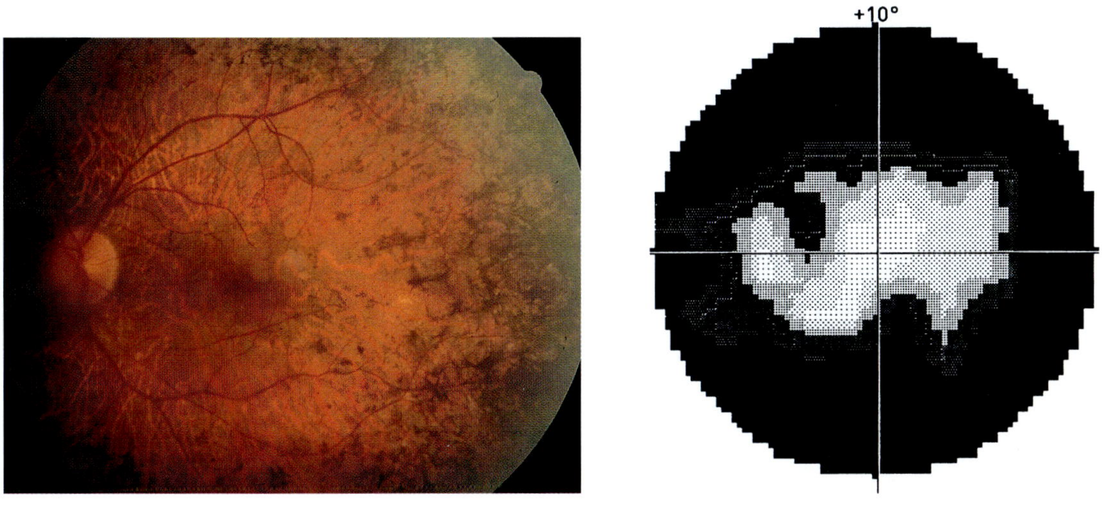

3.5G

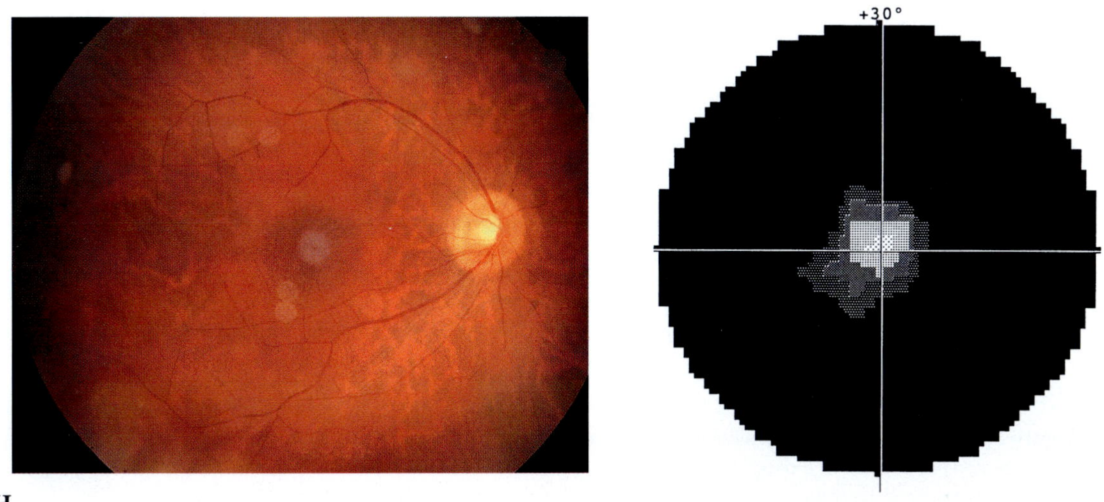

3.5H

Myopic Alterations of the Retina and Choroid

Temporal conus and circular conus are peripapillary tissue defects. In a choroidal conus, the retinal pigment epithelium is hypotrophic and causes a relative scotoma around the blind spot (Fig. 3.5J). In a scleral (white) conus, the choroid is missing completely and causes an absolute scotoma. Because the atrophy is adjacent to the optic disc, it appears on perimetry as an enlargement of the blind spot (Fig. 3.5K).

In myopic staphyloma, defocusing leads to relative scotomas called *refraction scotomas.* With the use of large targets (Goldmann sizes III through V) and with a change in corrective glasses (more minus) the refractive effect can be neutralized, but the thinning of the choroid in the staphyloma remains, and with it a shallow relative scotoma. Their classic refraction scotoma, more accurately called *scotoma of staphyloma,* is situated in the upper temporal area adjacent to the blind spot. In general, it crosses the vertical axis, a criterion used to distinguish it from central nervous system disorders (Fig.3.5L).

In eyes with very large staphylomas, spotty full-thickness choroidal defects can be found. They cause absolute visual field defects. Ruptures in Bruch's membrane are visible as areas of leakage on fluorescein angiography. They can lead to subretinal neovascularization and severe functional impairment (Fig. 3.5M).

Figure 3.5J. Circular conus and surrounding circular choroidal thinning in myopia (left eye, program: HFA 30-S custom program, representation: Peridata norm-related grayscale).

Figure 3.5K. Large white (scleral) circular cone in myopia (left eye, program: HFA 30-S custom program, representation: Peridata norm-related grayscale).

Figure 3.5L. A staphyloma scotoma in mild myopia (–5 diopters) and a narrow temporal conus, with pronounced myopic choroidal thinning in the lower nasal quadrant (left eye, program: HFA 30-S custom program, representation: Peridata norm-related grayscale).

Figure 3.5M. Leakage and edema due to degenerative myopic alterations in a 52-year-old patient (refraction –12 diopters, visual acuity 20/70). Fluorescence angiography and 30° visual field (left eye, program: HFA 30-1 combined with 30-2, representation: Peridata norm-related grayscale).

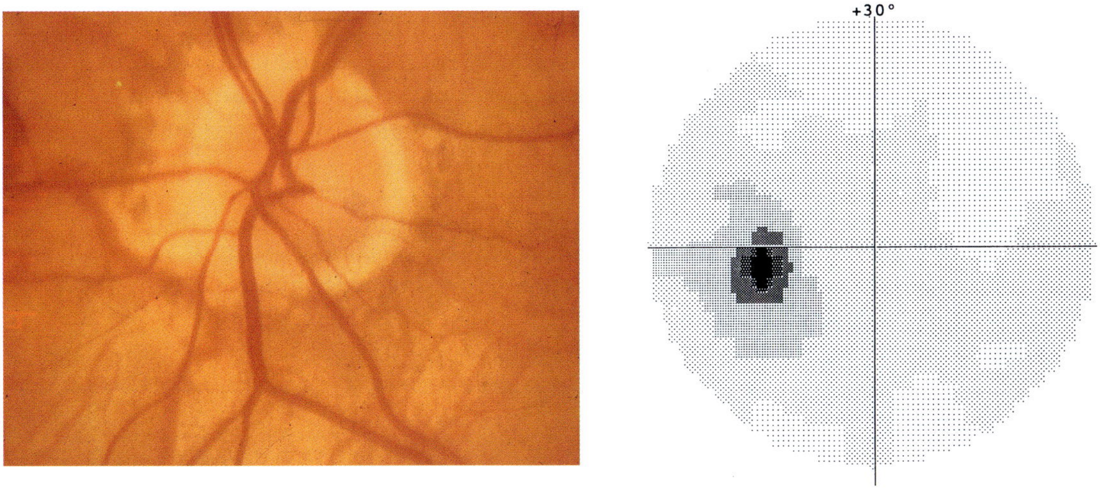

3.5J

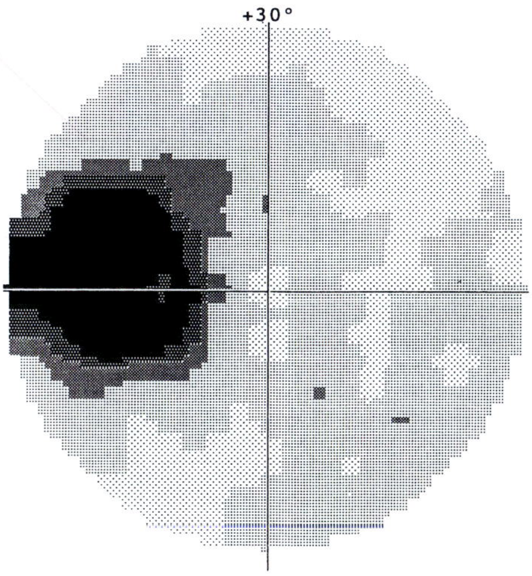

3.5K

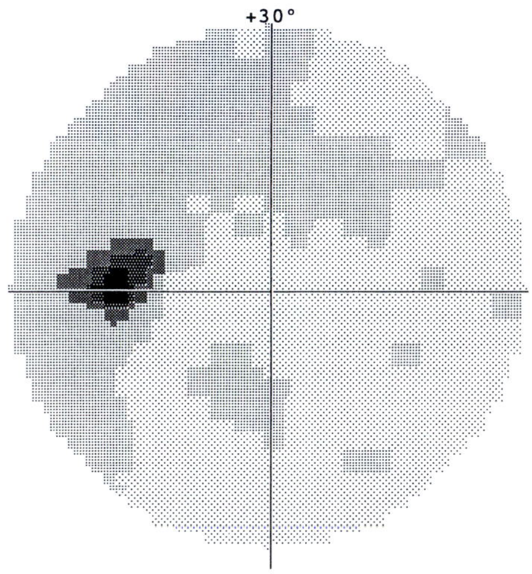

3.5L

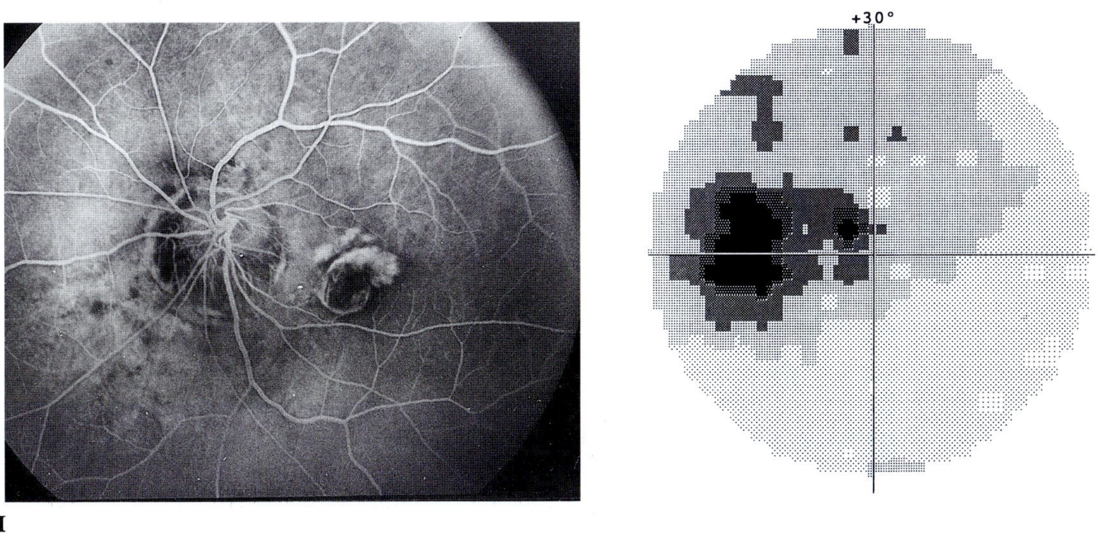

3.5M

Hereditary Dystrophies of the Macula

All hereditary dystrophies of the macula are characterized by central scotomas. The depth of the scotoma correlates with the degree of visual acuity. The relation between the ophthalmoscopic findings and functional loss, however, is not always clear.

Stargardt's disease creates deep or absolute defects and a considerable loss of visual acuity (Fig. 3.5N). In cases of vitelliform macular degeneration (Best's disease), defects tend to be shallow and the loss of visual acuity is less severe (Fig. 3.5P). The appearance of cone dystrophies is not striking on ophthalmoscopy. In addition to reduced visual acuity, a relative central scotoma is clearly demonstrable (Fig. 3.5Q).

Figure 3.5N. Stargardt's disease in the left eye of a 29-year-old man. Horizontal-oval, hypopigmented flake-like areas with darker centers and a central scotoma (displaced to the upper right) are seen. Visual acuity is 20/100. The findings in the other eye were similar (program: HFA 30-S custom program, representation: Peridata norm-related grayscale).

Figure 3.5P. Vitelliform macular degeneration (Best's disease) in the left eye of a 31-year-old woman (the findings in the other eye were identical). Yellow spots with a horizontal-oval area containing submacular fluid and a relative central scotoma are seen. Visual acuity was 20/30 (program: HFA 30-2, representation: Peridata norm-related grayscale).

Figure 3.5Q. Cone dystrophy in the right eye of an 18-year-old woman. The fundus shows mild pigmentary irregularities. In the visual field is a central scotoma of about 5 dB. Visual acuity was 20/60. The findings in the other eye were similar (program: HFA 30-2, representation: Peridata norm-related grayscale).

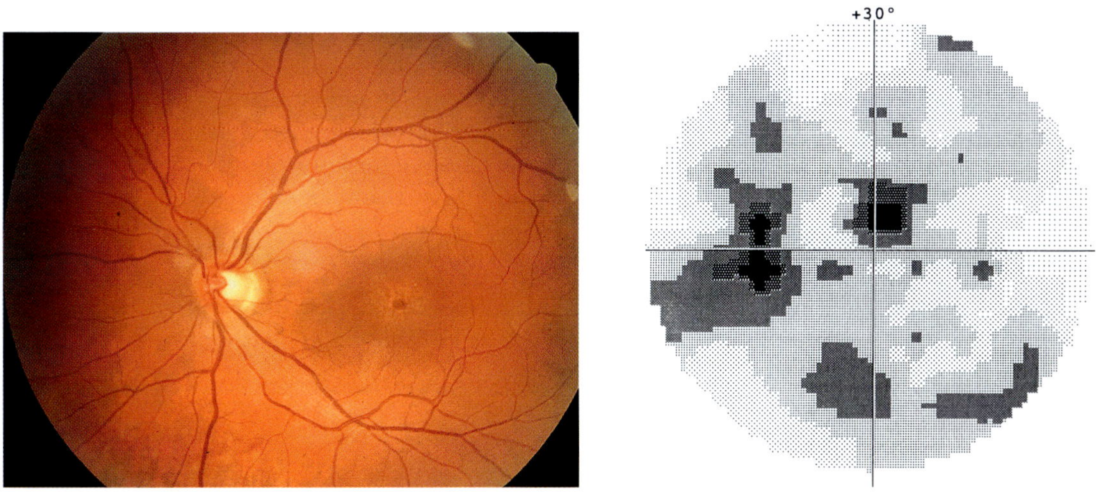

3.5N

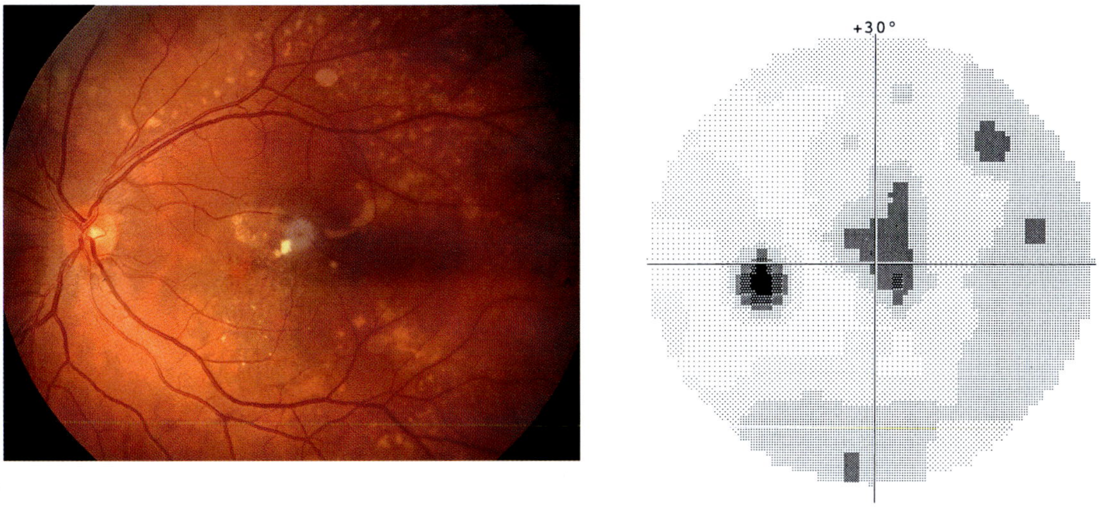

3.5P

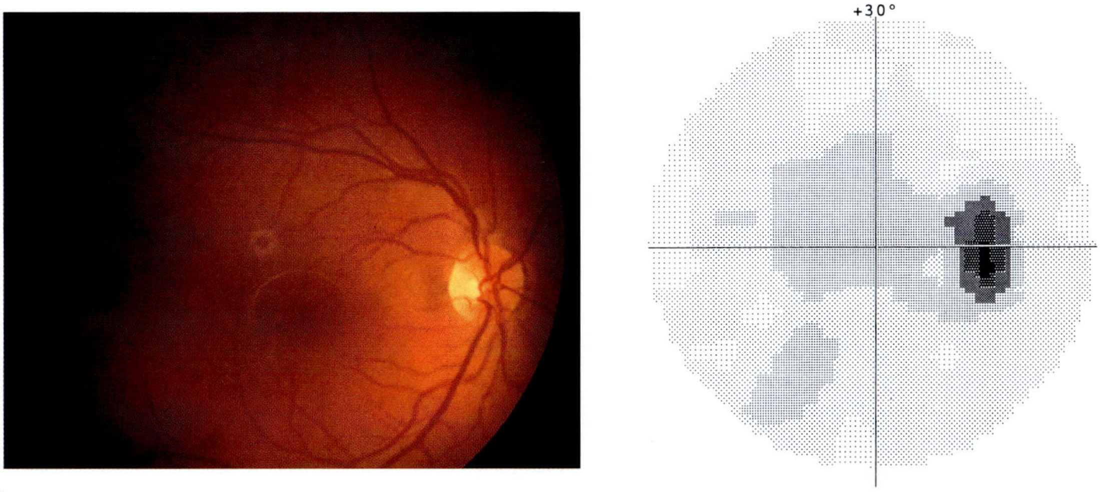

3.5Q

Senile Macular Degeneration

Degenerative alterations of the pigment cause spotty, relative visual field defects in the center. Progression to the exudative stage is accompanied by a large central scotoma. Its shape resembles that of the exudative abnormality, and it is very deep or absolute (Fig. 3.5R). Perimetry serves as a baseline for laser photocoagulation and helps provide advice to the patient about low-vision aids.

Macular Hole

Macular holes cause a relative perimetric defect in the very center of the visual field. The defect is rarely measurable outside of 1° of eccentricity. The loss of visual acuity is more striking than the field alterations (Fig. 3.5S).

Figure 3.5R. Senile macular degeneration in the right eye of a 74-year-old man with visual acuity of 10/200. The 10° field shows an absolute scotoma with sloping margins which has just reached the fixation point (program: HFA 10-2, representation: Peridata norm-related grayscale).

Figure 3.5S. Macular hole in the left eye of a 64-year-old patient with visual acuity of 20/100. Fundus photograph and visual fields (HFA macula program, norm-related grayscale and numerals; HFA profile program with 1° spacing).

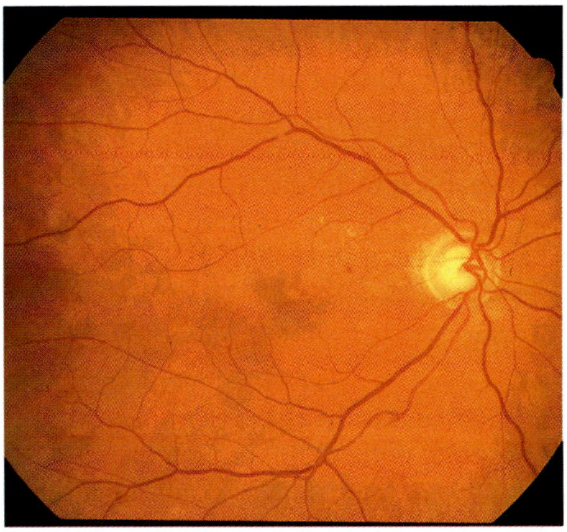

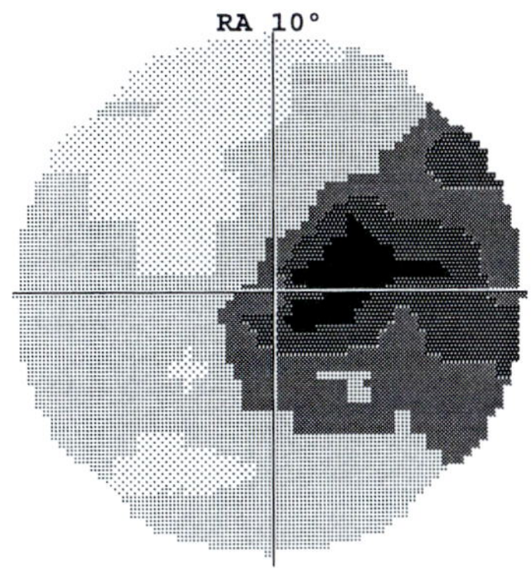
RA 10°

3.5R

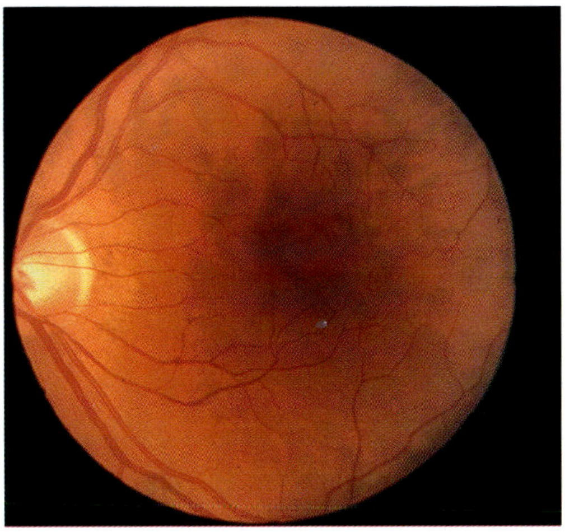

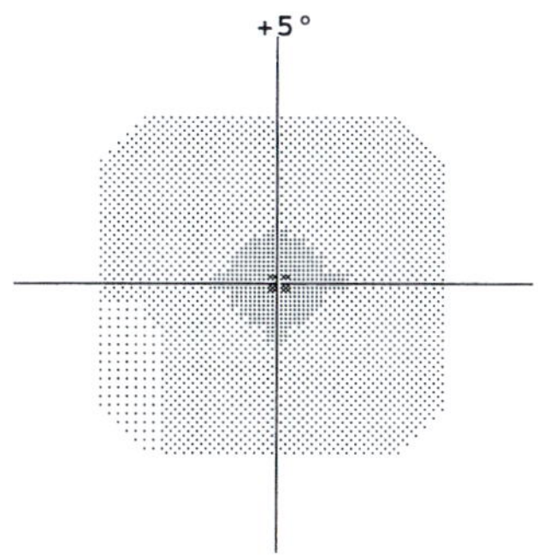
+5°

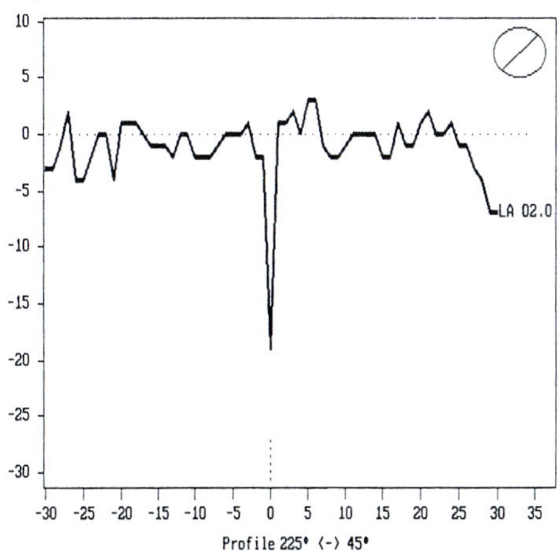
10
5
0
-5
-10
-15
-20
-25
-30
LA 02.0
-30 -25 -20 -15 -10 -5 0 5 10 15 20 25 30 35
Profile 225° (-) 45°

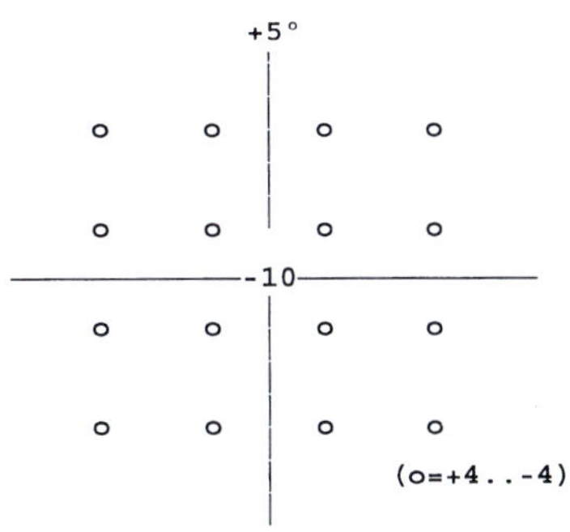
+5°
-10
(o=+4..-4)

3.5S

Toxic Retinopathy

A number of substances may cause toxic retinopathy. One of the most common offenders is chloroquine. On ophthalmoscopy, ring-shaped hypo- and hyperpigmentation of the macula *(bull's-eye retinopathy)* can be seen. The fovea itself remains intact for a long time, and with it the visual acuity. In the visual field is a ring scotoma with a diameter of about 3° (Fig. 3.5T). It is important to perform high-resolution perimetry with a spacing of about 2°. A standard program (with ninefold lower resolution) will miss the defects.

Inflammations

Inflammation of the choroid without (choroiditis) and with (chorioretinitis) involvement of the retina leads to relative or absolute defects, depending on the severity of the tissue damage. With focal inflammation, the damaged areas may be small and assessable only with a dense test point pattern. Acute multifocal placoid pigment epitheliopathy (AMPPE) is an inflammation of the choriocapillaris. In the acute stage, relative visual field defects are found. They are sometimes more pronounced than the retinal appearance may indicate (Fig. 3.5U).

Figure 3.5T. Chloroquine retinopathy after 7 years of therapy for polyarthritis (total dose unknown). The visual acuity is 20/20 in both eyes. Fundus photography shows a typical cocarde shaped pigment pattern (bull's-eye). The smaller rings are reflections of the light source. The high-resolution 10° field shows a ring scotoma. The findings in the other eye were identical (program: HFA 10-2, representation: Peridata norm-related grayscale).

Figure 3.5U. AMPPE in a 23-year-old man. The fundus (center left) shows irregular bright spots, and the fluorescein angiogram (lower left) demonstrates the typical blockage of choroidal fluorescence. With high-dose systemic steroid therapy, the visual acuity increased from 20/30 (July 14, 1989) to 20/20 (July 26, 1989). High-resolution perimetry in the 10° area clearly shows the focal defects and their regression (program: HFA 10-2, representation: Peridata norm-related grayscale).

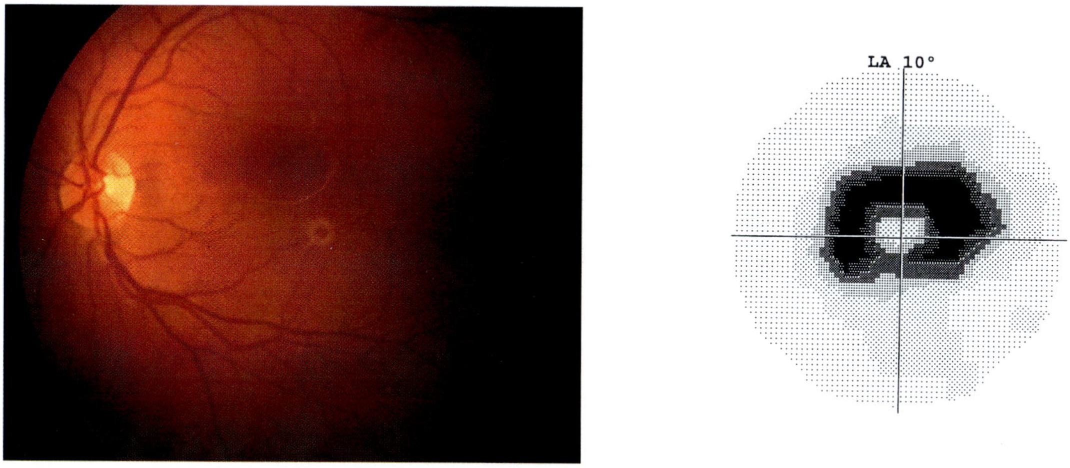

3.5T

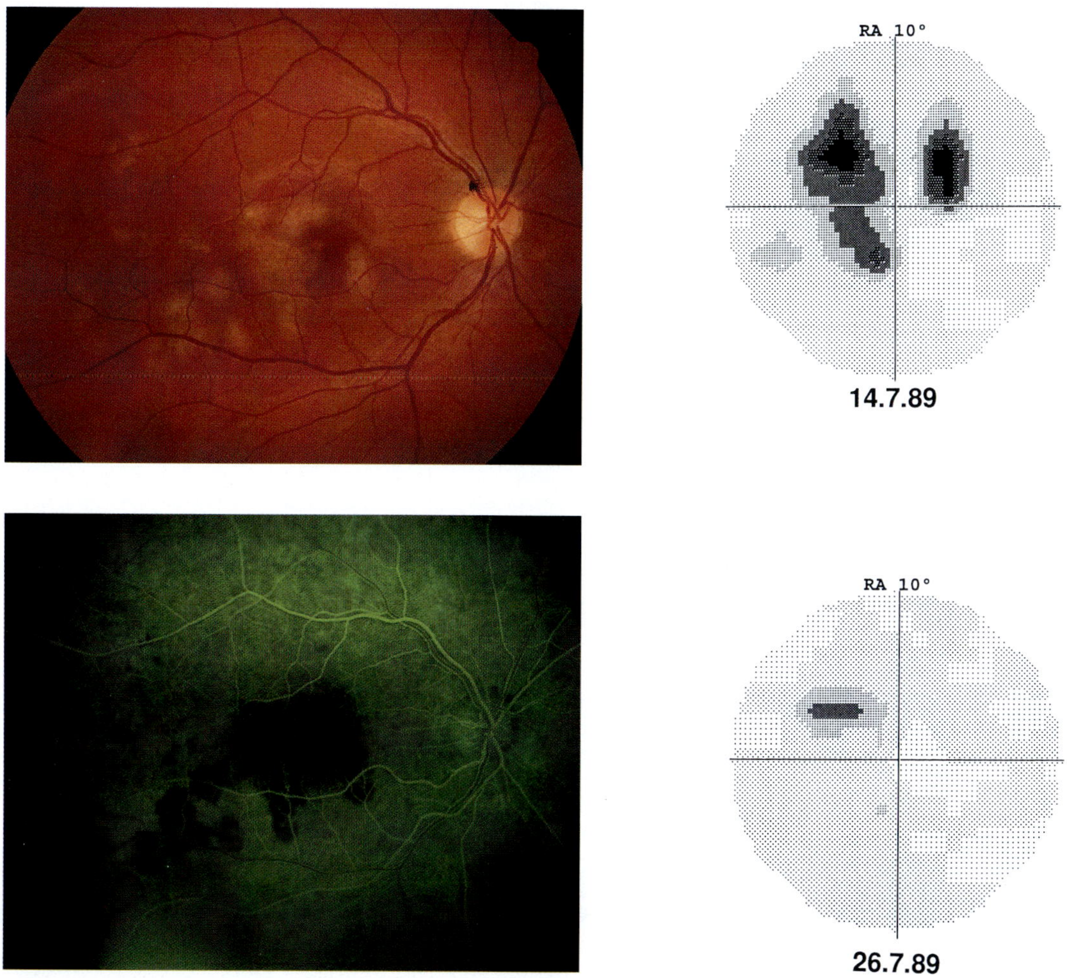

3.5U

3.6 VASCULAR DISEASES OF THE RETINA

Principle

The retinal vessels originate at the optic nerve head from one central artery and one central vein. They run peripherally in an arcuate course. On the way, they split into branches. Their capillaries nourish the inner and middle retinal layers. The major effect of vascular diseases is reduced perfusion to the supplied area and, consequently, alteration in neural function. Damage to vessels also causes leakage, followed by malfunction in the area of intra- and subretinal edema. The visual field defect is a congruent, inverted shadow of the injured area (Fig. 3.6A).

Retinal Veins

The constriction of retinal veins can vary from mild narrowing to complete occlusion and can lead to venous stasis retinopathy. The supplied area suffers from stagnation with capillary hypoperfusion, edema, and bleeding. Hypoperfusion and edema cause relative field defects of varying depth. Intraretinal hemorrhage absorbs light and causes very deep or absolute visual field defects.

Complete or incomplete obstruction of the central vein damages the entire retina and, with it, the entire visual field. In cases of incomplete obstruction there may be regional differences in flow (Fig. 3.6B). Branch vein occlusions involve the related supplied area (Fig. 3.6C), and edema may involve neighboring areas. In branch veins, the edema often affects the macula and reduces visual acuity. The shape of the visual field defect reflects the shape of the damaged vascular area. The depth of the defect depends on the severity of ischemia and the extent of hemorrhage.

Figure 3.6A. Topographical principle of visual field alterations in cases of retinal vascular disease. The visual field loss is a congruent, inverted image of the ischemic retinal area.

Figure 3.6B. Incomplete central vein occlusion. The damage is greatest peripherally and superiorly. The center is only slightly affected. The visual acuity was 0.5 (program: HFA 30-S custom program, representation: Peridata norm-related grayscale).

Figure 3.6C. Complete proximal branch vein occlusion of the temporal superior vein with pronounced hemorrhage. The visual field examined the same day shows relative defects of varying depth. The visual acuity was 0.1 (program: HFA 30-2, representation: Peridata norm-related grayscale).

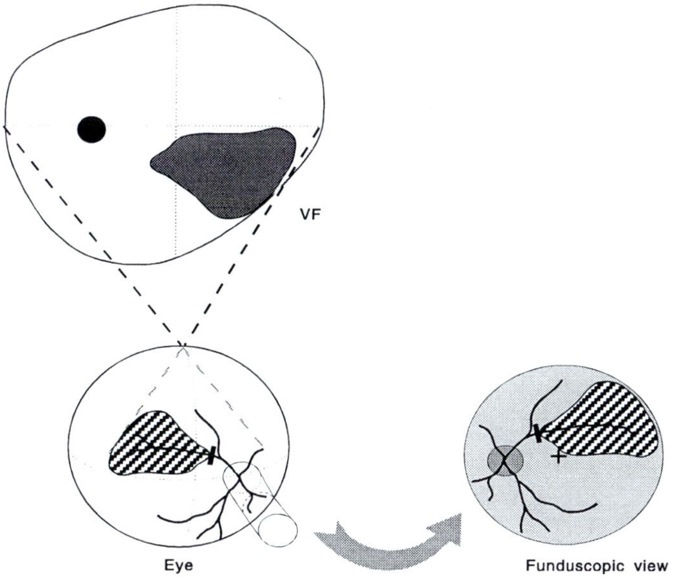

3.6A

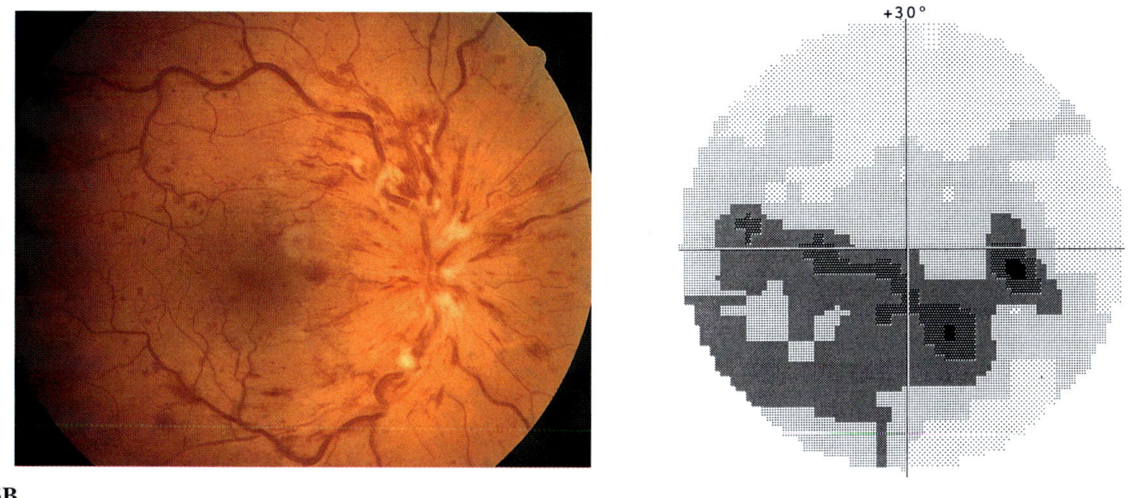

3.6B

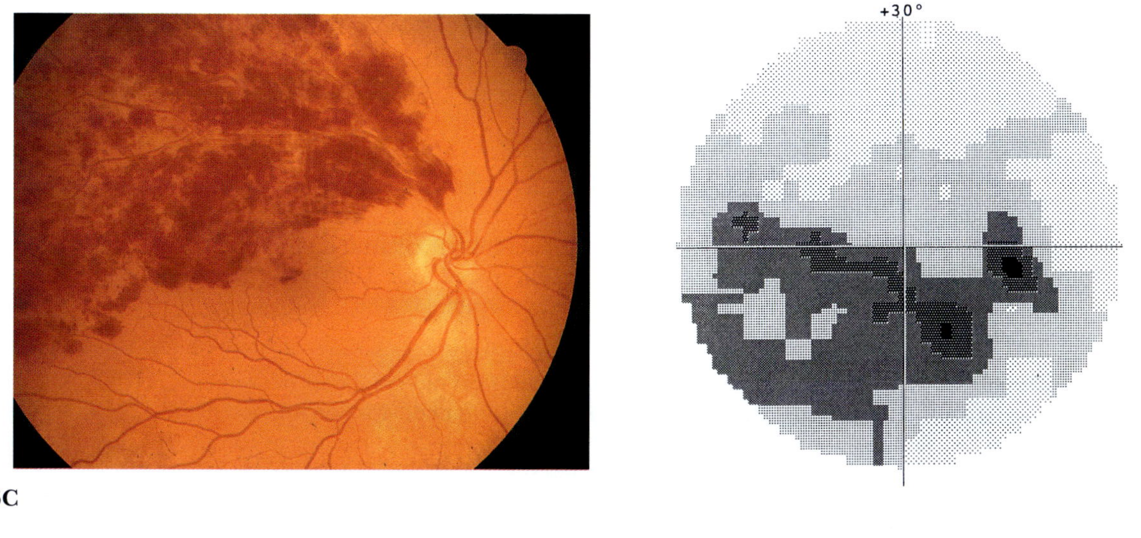

3.6C

Retinal Arteries

Retinal arterial occlusion usually involves minimal perfusion with severe ischemia of the inner retina. Visual function is extinguished, and the field defects are absolute.

Occlusion of the central artery causes rapid ischemia of the entire retina. Visual function is damaged severely and usually does not allow any kind of perimetry. In some cases (about 10%), a cilioretinal artery preserves an island of perfused retina and a small central visual field. The occlusion of branch arteries causes regional ischemia. The shape of the absolute defects reflects the shape of the injured area (Fig. 3.6D).

Diabetic Retinopathy (Microangiopathy)

Diabetic microangiopathy of the retina has several stages, which can be classified differently. From a perimetric point of view, three phases can be distinguished. In the nonproliferative stage there are spot-like relative and absolute defects in regions of capillary destruction, exudates, and laser scars. In the proliferative stage without retinal detachment, shadowing effects from pre- or intraretinal hemorrhage are added. In the stage of traction detachment, the detached regions lose their function too. In every stage, ischemia of the larger vessels can also occur. Ischemia is the most frequent reason for disappointing functional results after successful surgical reattachment of the retina by vitrectomy and internal tamponade.

In the first stage of diabetic retinopathy, the visual field defects start in the midperiphery between 20° and 40° (Fig. 3.6E). With kinetic perimetry, the spotty defects are easily missed and only relative isopter constrictions are apparent. Computerized static perimetry takes a long time due to the large size of the area examined, reducing the contribution of perimetry in patients who become easily fatigued. In the advanced stages of the disease, function is so reduced that only kinetic perimetry with decreased background luminance is possible.

Figure 3.6D. Branch artery occlusion of the inferotemporal retinal artery. The edema involves half of the fovea, producing an incomplete cherry-red spot. The visual field mirrors the defect. The visual acuity is 0.3 (right eye, program: HFA 30-2, representation: Peridata norm-related grayscale).

Figure 3.6E. Preproliferative diabetic retinopathy in a 58-year-old man after panretinal photocoagulation. Little fundus change and moderate isopter constriction are noted on kinetic perimetry, but severe defects in the 60° static field located as close as 10° to fixation in the lower nasal quadrant are evident (left eye, program: HFA 30-2 and 30/60-1, representation: Peridata grayscale of absolute values).

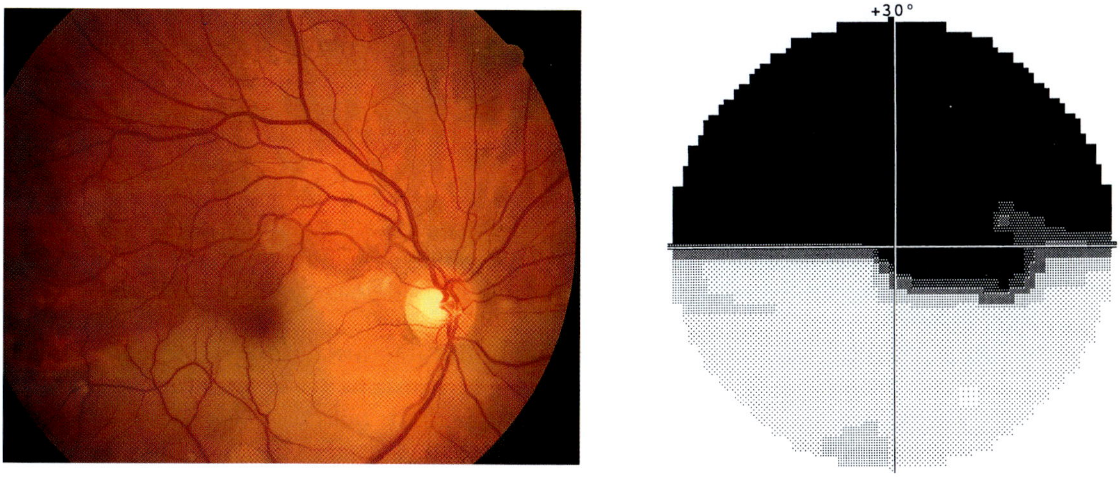

3.6D

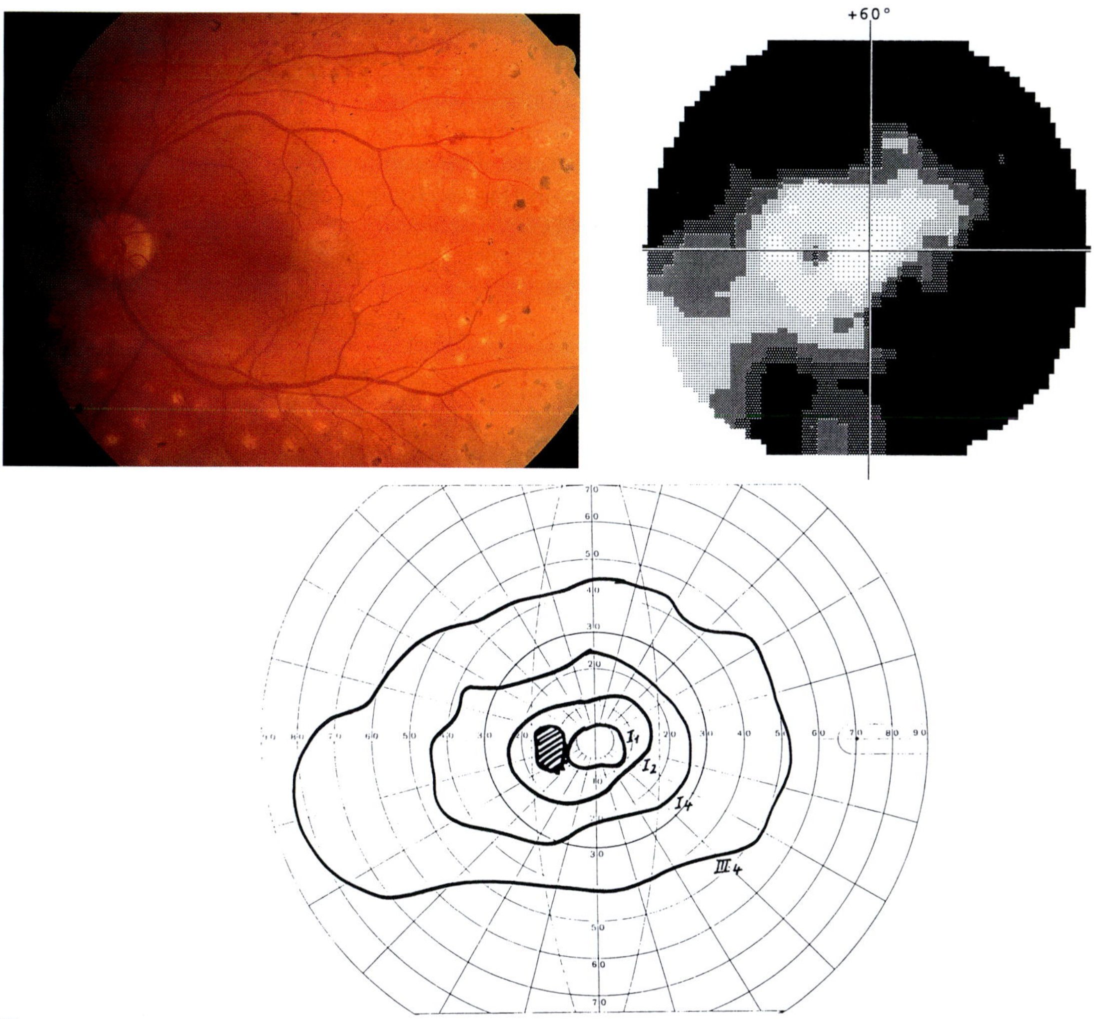

3.6E

3.7 DISEASES OF THE RETINA WITH INVOLVEMENT OF THE NERVE FIBER LAYER

Principle

From the functional point of view, damage of the inner retinal layer has both local and distant effects. The local effect is caused by damage to the local ganglion cells, as well as to the involved receptors and bipolar cells. The topography of the local effect is congruent with the damaged area; the visual field defect is an inverted shadow of the damaged area. This is similar in damage to the intermediate and outer layers.

The distal effect is caused by interruption of transmission through the nerve fiber layer and involves all traversing axons. The entire area peripheral to the damage (with respect to the optic disc) is dysfunctional. The margins of the affected area correspond to the course of the retinal nerve fibers (Fig. 3.7A).

In comparing the retinal image and the visual field, it is crucial to remember that the visual field usually is represented from the patient's point of view but the fundus is represented from the doctor's point of view. Thus, in a direct comparison, the fundus and the visual field are mirror images about the horizontal axis.

Retinochoroiditis Juxtapapillaris (Jensen)

In 1908, Jensen noted that retinal inflammation near the optic disk causes typical arcuate visual field defects. The main cause of these defects is toxoplasmosis. In the acute stage, the retina has a white infiltrate. The visibility of the retina is often blurred by the adjacent vitreal infiltration (Fig. 3.7B). The appearance of a scotoma in the visual field is typical (Fig. 3.7C).

Figure 3.7A. Topographical principle of full-thickness retinal diseases. The visual field defect involves not only the site of damage, but also all traversing nerve fibers and the dependent retinal area.

Figure 3.7B. Acute juxtapapillary retinochoroiditis in the left eye of a 58-year-old man. There is complete loss of the upper half of the field with horizontal splitting of the fixation point. The visual acuity is 0.4 (program: HFA 30-S custom program combined with 10-2, representation: Peridata norm-related grayscale).

Figure 3.7C. Full-thickness scar of the retina and choroid after retinochoroiditis juxtapapillaris (Jensen) in a 19-year-old woman. The visual field defect precisely reflects the topography of the retinal nerve fiber bundles. The gap between the blind spot and fixation is relatively small and is therefore bridged by the grayscale interpolation. The visual acuity is 1.0 (right eye, program: HFA 30-S custom program, representation: Peridata norm-related grayscale).

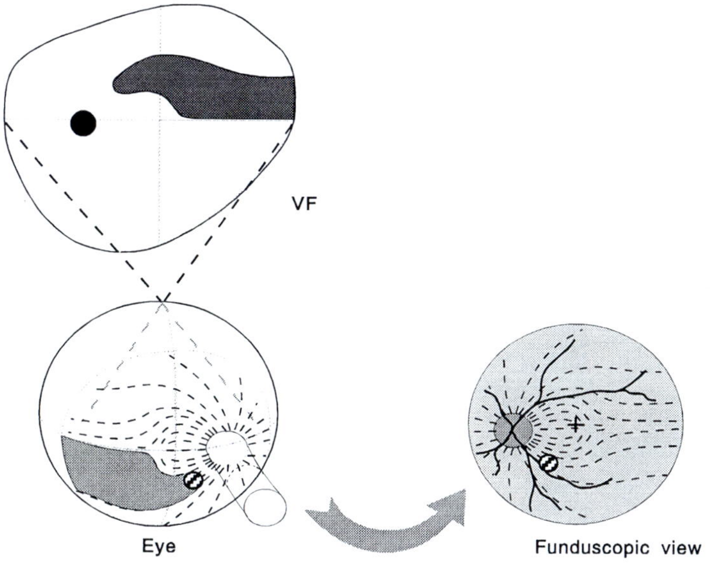

3.7A

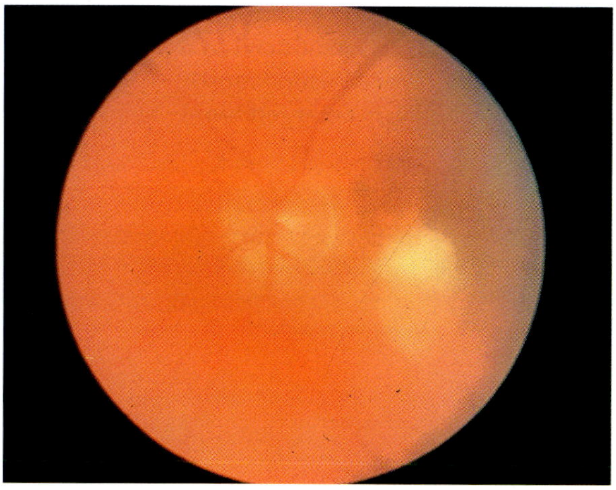

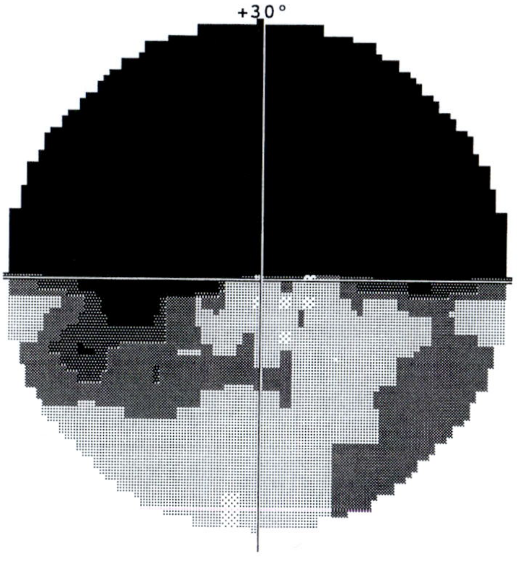

3.7B

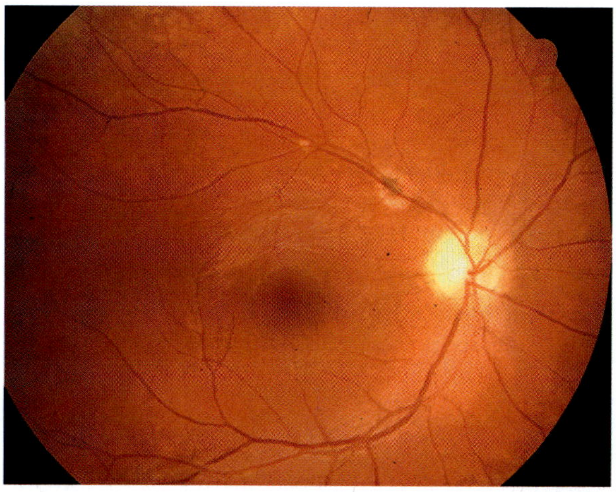

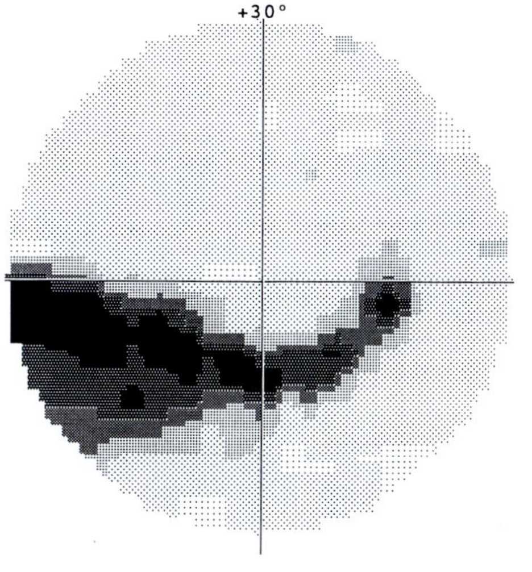

3.7C

Central Retinochoroiditis

Central retinochoroiditis differs from the juxtapapillary type mainly in terms of the area affected. There is also a local effect, and traversing nerve fibers are interrupted (Fig. 3.7D). Toxoplasmosis, which produces an intense white infiltrate in the acute stage and a hyperpigmented margin in the cicatricial stage, is one type of infection. Other macular infections (e.g., histoplasmosis) must be considered in the differential diagnosis.

Necrotizing Retinitis

Necrotizing retinitis (e.g., herpes zoster, cytomegalovirus) totally destroys the outer retinal layers and the nerve fiber layer. The advancing line of retinal destruction is usually irregular, with corresponding functional damage. The disease usually starts in the peripheral retina (Fig. 3.7E).

Medulated-Nerve Fibers

In medulated-nerve fibers, myelinated nerve fibers involve the nerve fiber layer but do not disturb axonal function. In contrast to the other diseases in this category, there are no nerve fiber bundle defects, only local defects produced by a shadow effect over the photoreceptors. Because these defects are located mostly at the optic disk, the usual perimetric equivalent is an irregularly enlarged blind spot (Fig. 3.7F).

Figure 3.7D. Acute central toxoplasmosis retinitis in a 23-year-old woman. There is an absolute visual field defect in the inflamed area and nasally in the region of the damaged nerve fiber bundle. Visual acuity was 0.1 (right eye, program: HFA 30-2, representation: Peridata norm-related grayscale).

Figure 3.7E. Acute herpes retinitis. There is severe destruction of all retinal layers. Progressive constriction from the periphery to the center is apparent. Central visual acuity was 0.4 (right eye, program: HFA 30-2, representation: Peridata norm-related grayscale).

Figure 3.7F. Myelinated nerve fibers. The blind spot is enlarged, but no remote nerve fiber bundle defects are seen (left eye, program: HFA 30-S custom program, representation: Peridata norm-related grayscale).

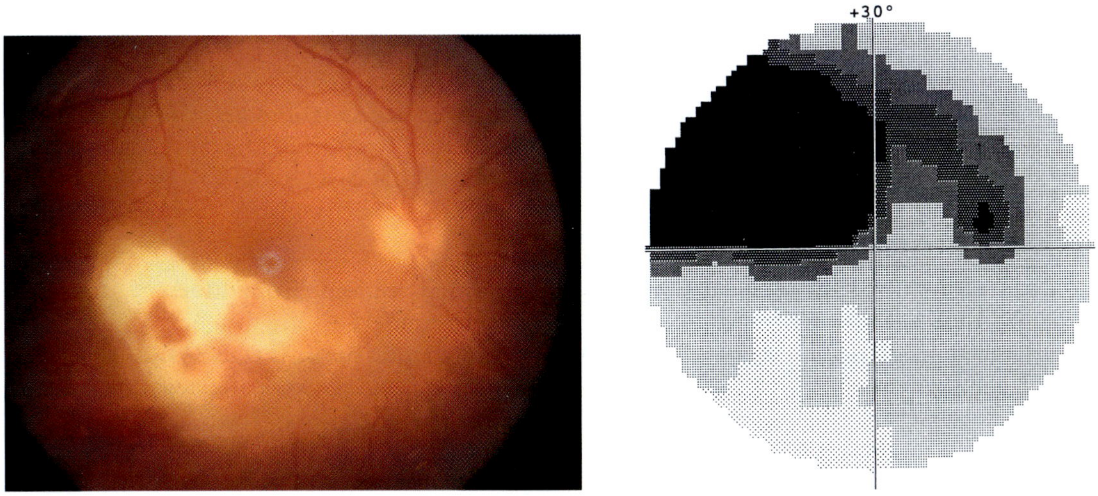

3.7D

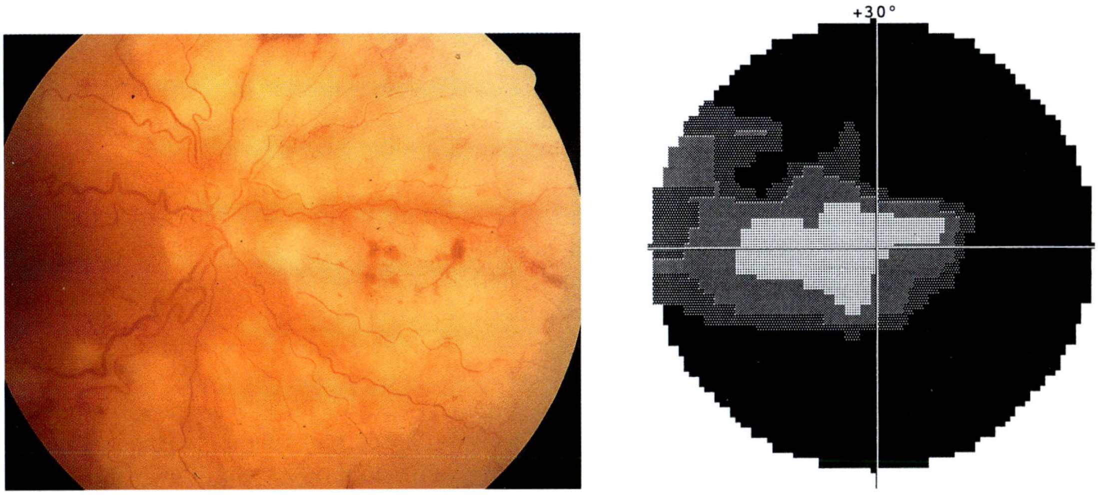

3.7E

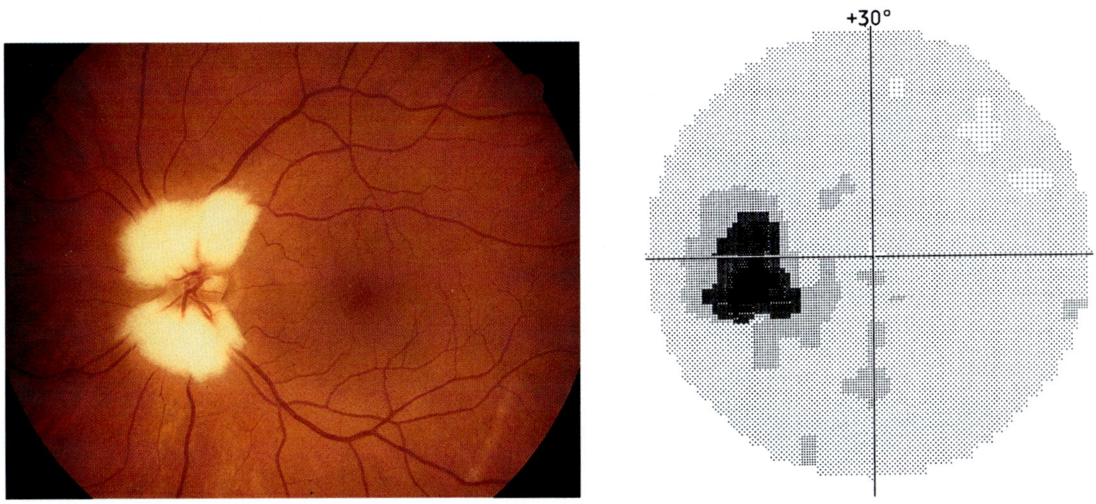

3.7F

3.8 FOCAL OPTIC DISK DISORDERS (OTHER THAN GLAUCOMA)

In this perimetric system, focal optic disk damage regularly leads to limited damage at the optic nerve head and corresponding typical visual field defects. Glaucoma, which falls into this category, is described in Section 3.9 because of its importance and the special role perimetry plays in its care.

Principle

Focal disk damage involves bundles of nerve fibers which originate from distant retinal areas but take a common course in the inner retina, cross the disk border together, and occupy a discrete area in the anterior optic nerve (Fig. 3.8A). Visual perception is abnormal in the entire retinal area belonging to the affected nerve fiber bundle. The shape of the visual field defect can be deduced from the topography of the retinal nerve fiber course. Depending on the site of the bundles, four general shapes are evident (Fig. 3.8B): (1) The temporal nerve fiber bundle defect is sector-shaped. (2) The arcuate scotoma connects the blind spot and the periphery in the shape of a comet. (3) The short arcuate scotoma is similar, but is located closer to the fixation point and ends at the nasal horizontal axis (equivalent of the median retinal neural raphe). (4) The centrocecal scotoma connects the fixation point and the blind spot in an oblong shape.

Additional variations in the shape of papillary nerve fiber bundle defects arise when the bundles are not completely damaged. The resulting visual field defects resemble the nerve fiber layer topography only in the periphery. Centrally, they become flatter and "fade away" before reaching the blind spot (Fig. 3.8C). Often complete defects are flanked by incomplete peripheral defects. Such scotomas have borders that converge toward the disc more than is expected from the nerve fiber layer topography. This type of defect is more marked peripherally. Depending on their position, peripheral nerve fiber bundle defects can have special shapes. One of them is the nasal quadrant defect representing an incomplete arcuate scotoma. Another is the nasal wedge-shaped defect (which is the reason for the nasal step of Ronne), a peripheral nerve fiber bundle defect. The oblique central border is due to the different lengths of the nerve fiber bundles. Bundles closer to the horizontal axis have a more curved course than more distant ones. Points of equal nerve fiber length form an oblique line.

Figure 3.8A. Topographical principle of visual field alteration of focal disk processes. The field defect involves the entire retinal area related to the damaged nerve fiber bundles. The shape arises from the retinal nerve fiber topography.

Figure 3.8B. The four shapes of complete nerve fiber bundle defects.

Figure 3.8C. Variations in nerve fiber bundle defects in cases of incomplete damage.

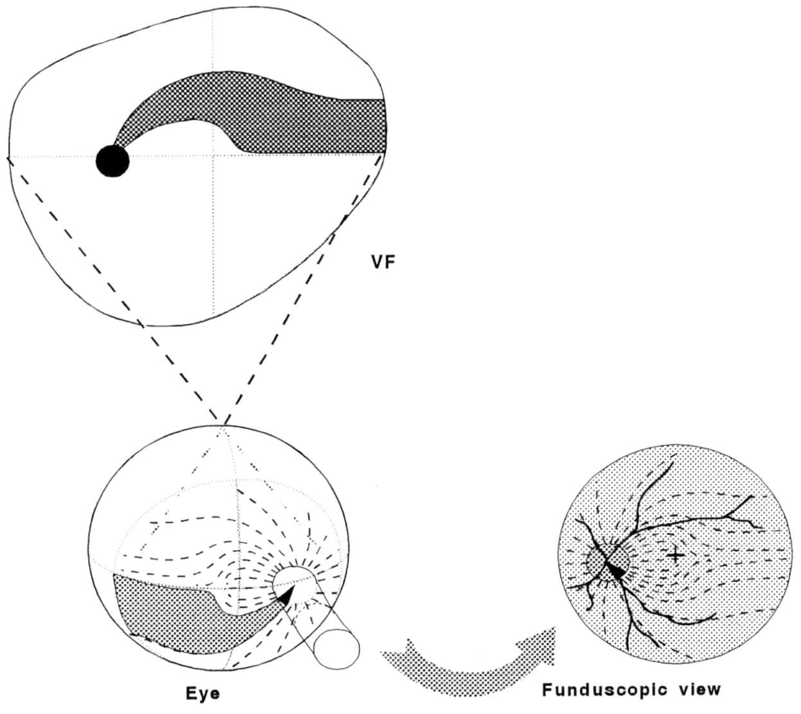
VF
Eye
Funduscopic view

3.8A

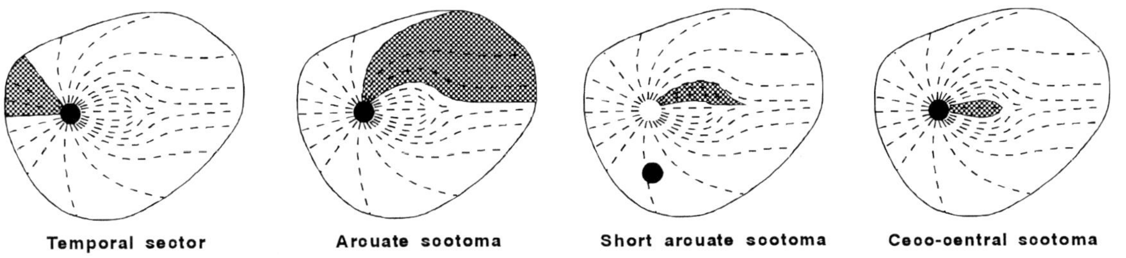
Temporal seotor
Arouate sootoma
Short arouate sootoma
Ceoo-oentral sootoma

3.8B

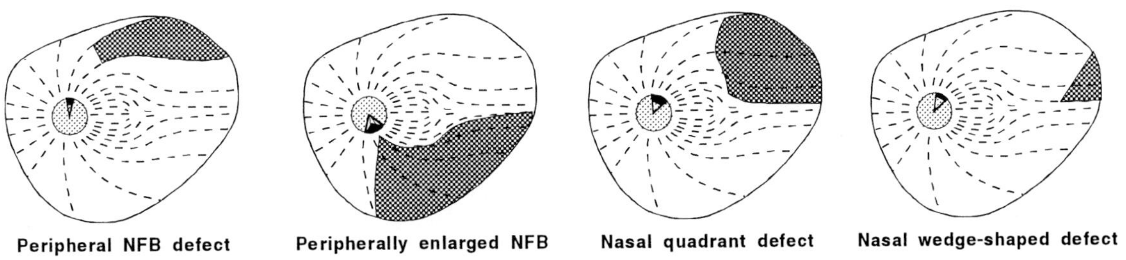
Peripheral NFB defect
Peripherally enlarged NFB
Nasal quadrant defect
Nasal wedge-shaped defect

3.8C

Coloboma of the Disk (Disk Pit)

Coloboma of the optic nerve head can range from a mild congenital disk pit to a "morning glory" disk. The latter are not usually subject to perimetry because of their poor visual function. In cases of disk pit, absolute nerve fiber bundle scotomas can be found (Fig. 3.8D,E).

Tilted Disk

Tilting of the disk is often the result of a staphyloma. Depending on the location of the staphyloma, a temporal conus, inferior conus, superior conus, or nasal conus can be seen on ophthalmoscopy. The frequent posterior staphyloma with a typical temporal conus was treated in the subsection "Myopic Alterations of the Retina and Choroid." Staphylomas and coni are frequently located inferiorly (Fig. 3.8F). The field alterations are a mixture of relative defects adjacent to the blind spot caused by local dysfunction of the retina and choroid and peripheral nerve fiber bundle defects due to damaged nerve fibers traversing the area. The sector in the optic disc related to the nerve fiber bundle damage may not correspond to the site of the staphyloma.

Figure 3.8D. Optic disk pit in the right eye. Short arcuate scotoma inferiorly and visual acuity of 1.0 (right eye, program: HFA 30-S custom store program, representation: Peridata norm-related grayscale).

Figure 3.8E. Crater-like optic disk pit in the right eye. Short superior arcuate scotoma and peripheral defects in nearby nerve fiber bundles, with visual acuity of 1.0 (right eye, program: HFA 30-2, representation: Peridata norm-related grayscale).

Figure 3.8F. Tilted disk with inferior conus and adjacent staphyloma with choroidal thinning inferiorly. The visual field shows a depression in the upper temporal quadrant due to choroidal alterations and a peripheral nerve fiber bundle defect inferonasally. Visual acuity is 20/30 (left eye, program: HFA 30-S custom program, representation: Peridata norm-related grayscale).

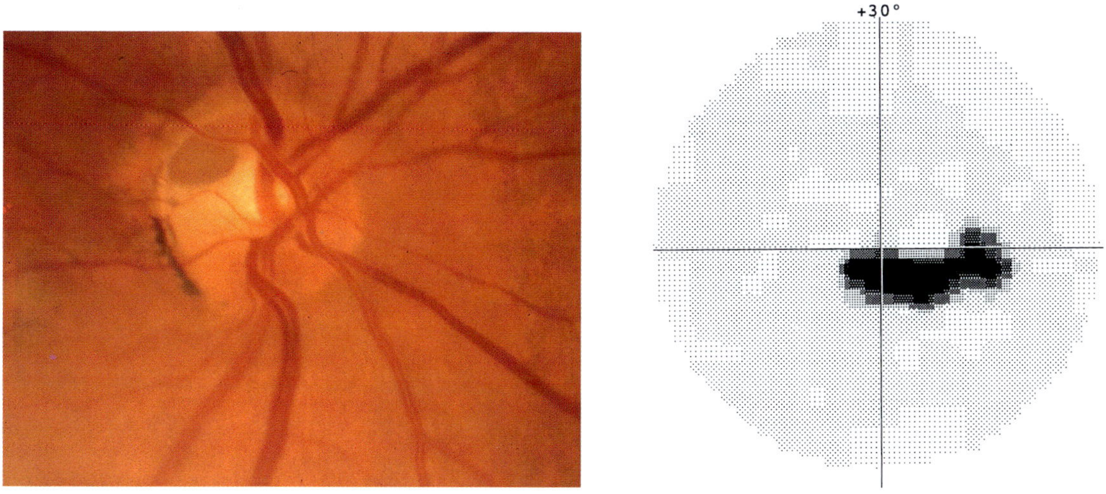

3.8D

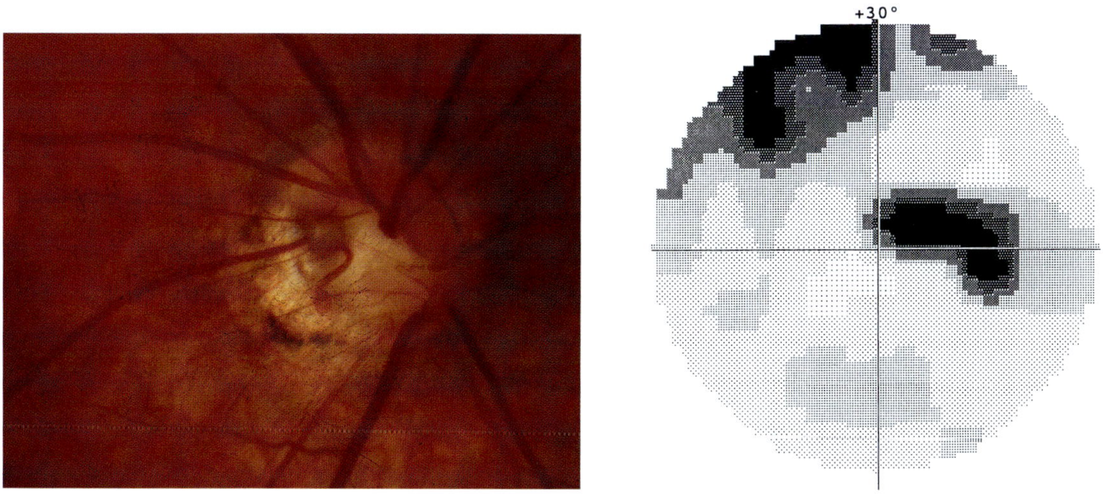

3.8E

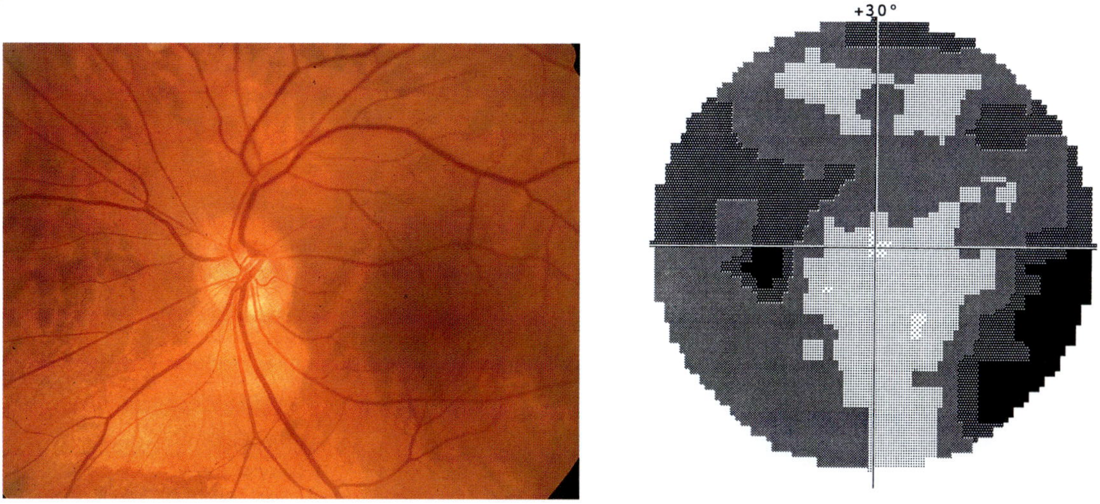

3.8F

Drusen of the Disk

Drusen of the disk are situated in the periphery of the optic nerve and therefore usually impair long nerve fibers. The visual field shows peripherally stressed nerve fiber bundle defects (Fig. 3.8G). Often these defects extend well beyond 30° (Fig. 3.8H).

Unlike other focal optic nerve diseases, the location of the field defects cannot be derived from the appearance of the fundus.

Figure 3.8G. Drusen of the disk in the left eye of an 18-year-old man. The superonasal quadrant defect is a peripheral arcuate scotoma. In the lower half the scotoma is more visible, but it is not connected to the blind spot. The other regions show marked reduction in sensitivity (program: HFA 30-2, representation: Peridata norm-related grayscale).

Figure 3.8H. Fundus photograph of a 30-year-old man with mild drusen of the disk. The left 30° field shows only shallow nasal defects. Perimetry of the 65° field reveals serious peripheral defects. Visual acuity is 1.0 (program: HFA 30-S combined with 30/60-2, representation: Peridata norm-related grayscale).

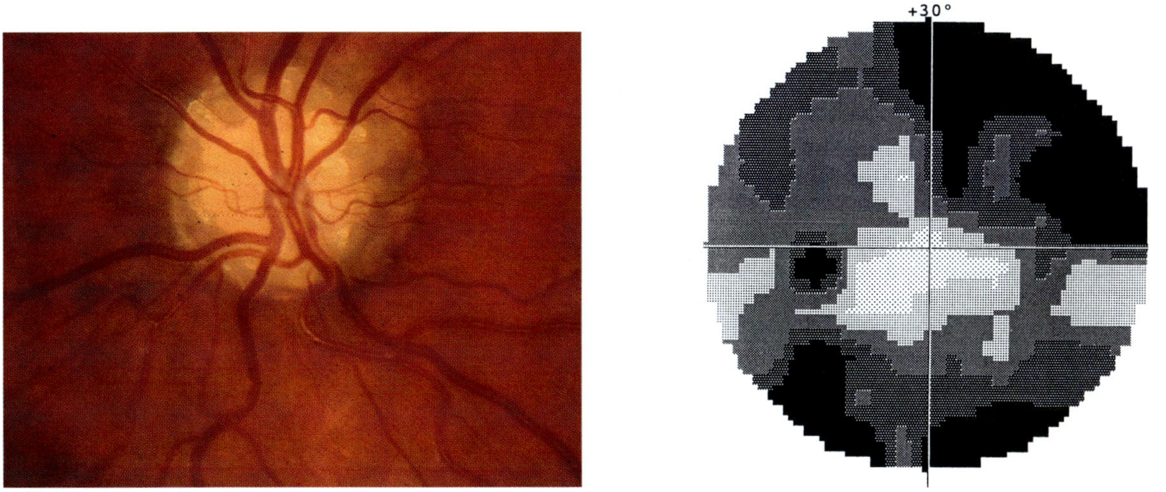

3.8G

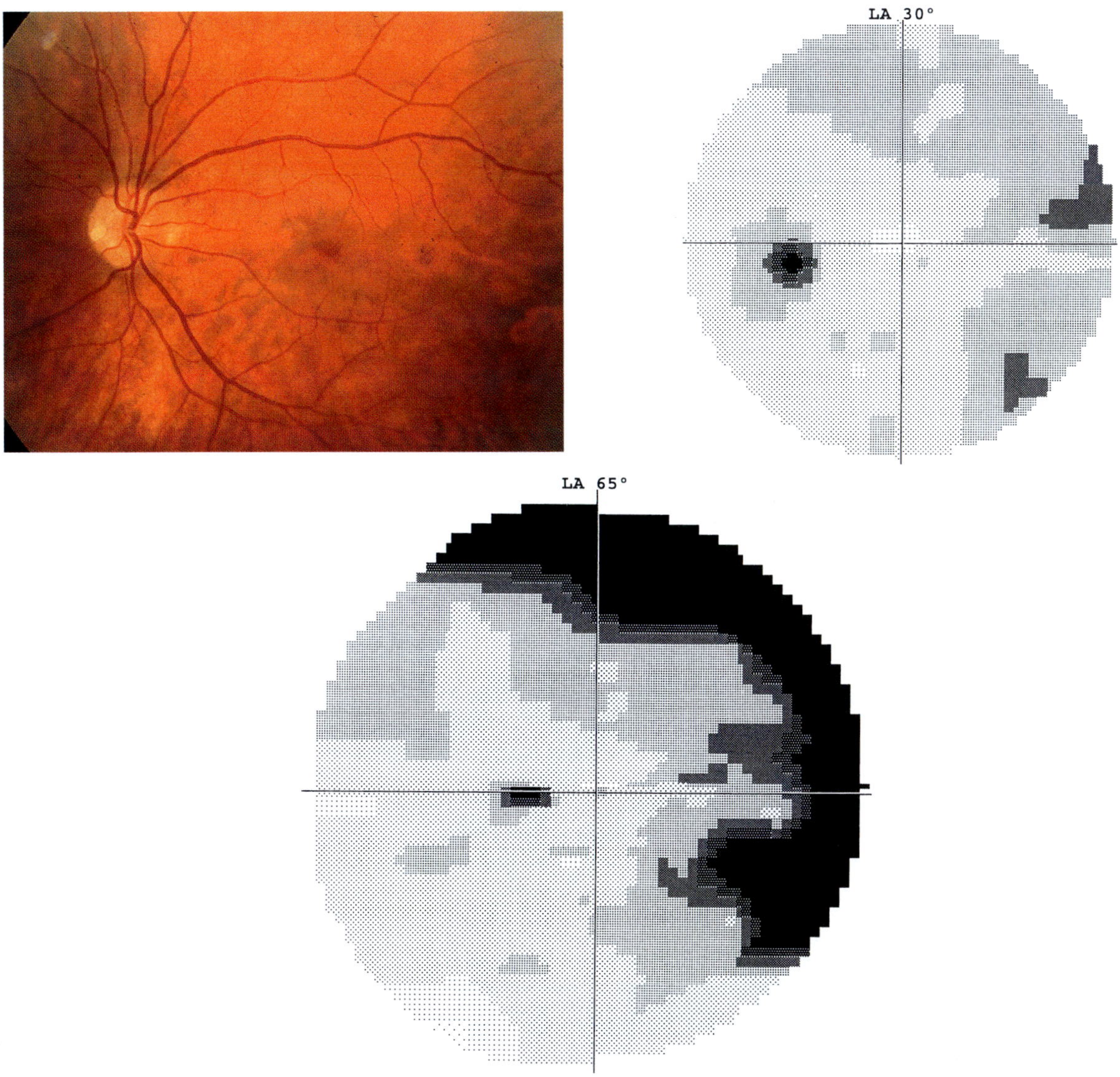

3.8H

Anterior Ischemic Optic Neuropathy (AION)

AION is occlusion of the arteries which supply the anterior part of the optic nerve. On ophthalmoscopy, edema of the disk is evident; it may be sector-shaped. Flame-shaped hemorrhages can be found within the edema. Interruption of neural transmission is complete, and visual field defects are absolute. The location of complete nerve fiber bundle defects depend on the vessel architecture and the involved branch. Most frequent are inferior defects which usually split fixation (Fig. 3.8J). Involvement of an entire hemifield and splitting of fixation is called an *altitudinal defect.* Superior arcuate scotomas (Fig. 3.8K) and even centrocecal scotomas (Fig. 3.8L) can also be detected.

Figure 3.8J. Typical AION with an inferior altitudinal visual field defect. The edema is most pronounced at the upper margin of the optic disk. Visual acuity is 0.8 (program: HFA 30-2, representation: Peridata norm-related grayscale).

Figure 3.8K. AION with a superior arcuate scotoma. The cecocentral region is intact. Visual acuity is 0.5 (program: HFA 30-1 and 30-2 combined, representation: Peridata norm-related grayscale).

Figure 3.8L. Ischemic defect of the maculopapular bundle in the right eye of a 69-year-old man. The 10° field shows a small cecocentral scotoma. The visual acuity was 0.5 (program: HFA 10-2, representation: Peridata norm-related grayscale).

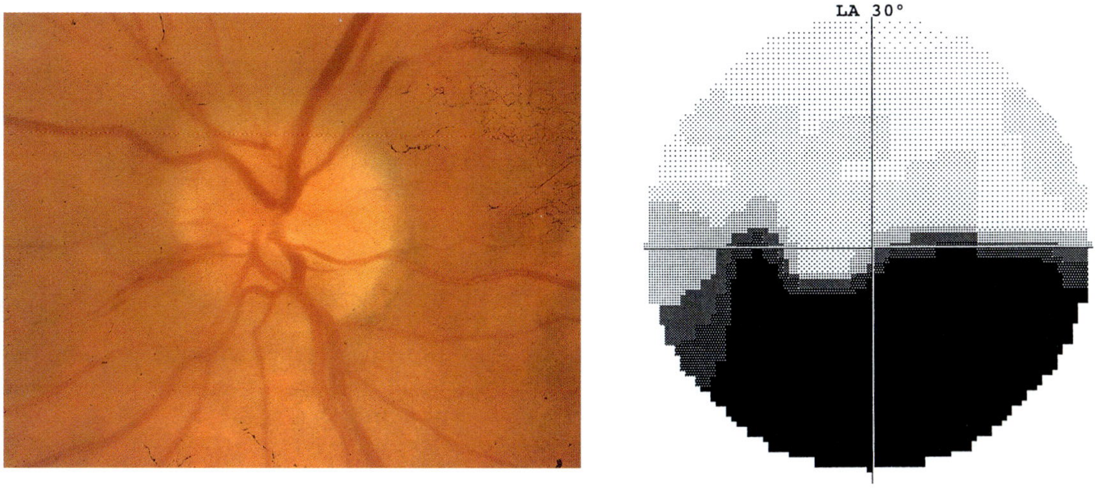

3.8J

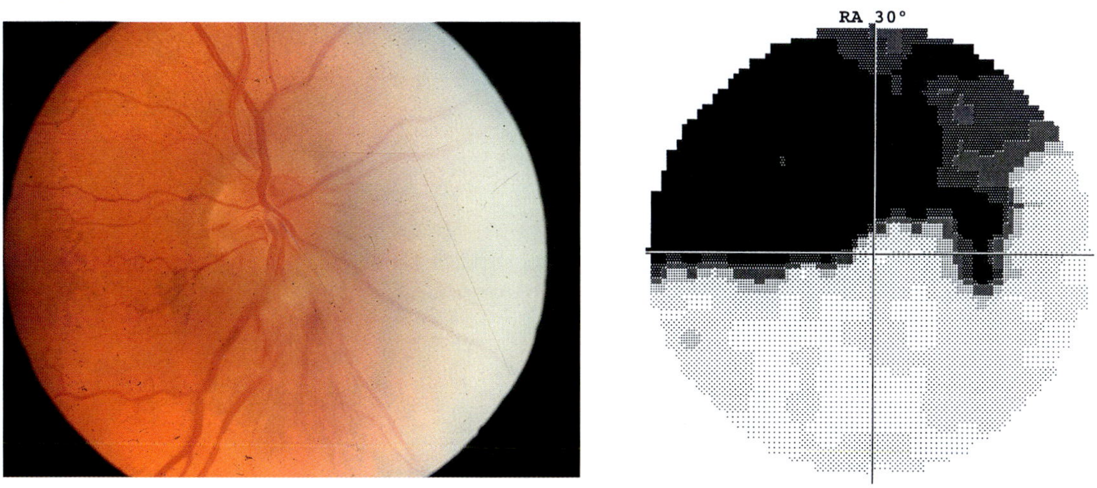

3.8K

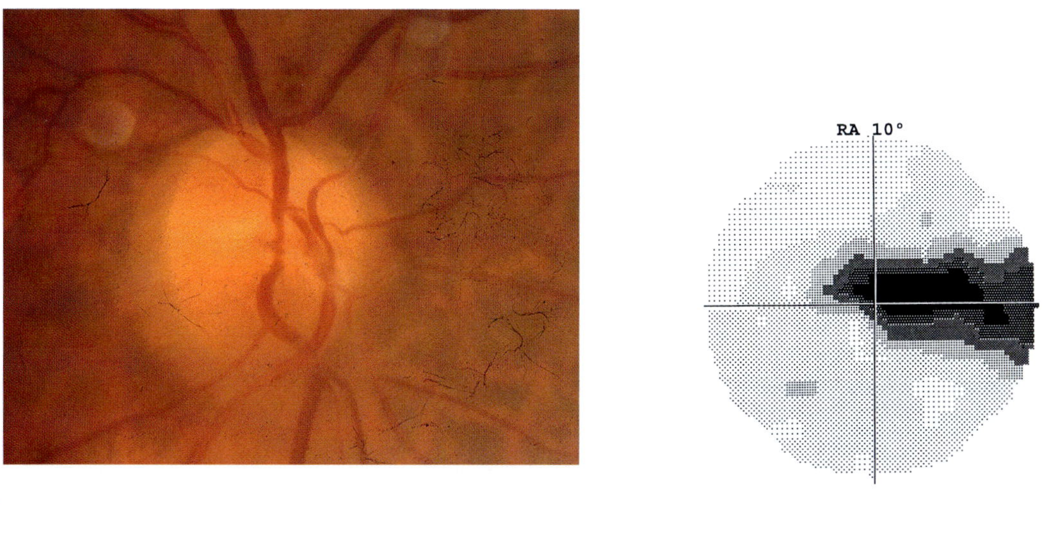

3.8L

Papilledema

Papilledema has two effects on the visual field. First, the blind spot is enlarged by the large peripapillary zone of edema. Second, peripheral nerve fiber bundle defects are caused by damage to the long axons which lie near the dural sheath. The latter defects tend to be inferior arcuate scotomas (Fig. 3.8M).

A rare variant is hemorrhagic papilledema in cases of traumatic bleeding into the cerebrospinal fluid (CSF) space (Fig. 3.8N). The visual field defects are similar to those described above. The ophthalmoscopic image must be distinguished from Terson's syndrome, in which sudden hemorrhage into the CSF space causes a secondary pressure increase in the retinal vasculature with scattered intraretinal hemorrhages, which are seen as multiple blood levels trapped between the nerve fiber layer and internal limiting membrane or, in case of a rupture of the posterior limiting membrane, as vitreous hemorrhages.

In cerebral tumors, papilledema and lesions of the visual pathways caused by the neoplasm may coexist. Field defects are caused by both mechanisms (Fig. 3.8P).

Figure 3.8M. Papilledema of unknown origin; suspected pseudotumor cerebri. The blind spot is enlarged, and there is a peripheral nerve fiber bundle defect in the inferior nasal quadrant (right eye, program: HFA 30-2, representation: Peridata norm-related grayscale).

Figure 3.8N. Hemorrhagic papilledema after cerebral contusion with bleeding into the CSF space in the right eye of a 47-year-old man. Visual acuity was 20/20 (program: HFA 30-2, representation: Peridata norm-related grayscale).

Figure 3.8P. Combination of an enlarged blind spot and a quadrantic defect in a 36-year old man after surgical removal of an astrocytoma in the parietal lobe. Visual acuity was 0.8 (program: HFA 30-2, representation: Peridata norm-related grayscale).

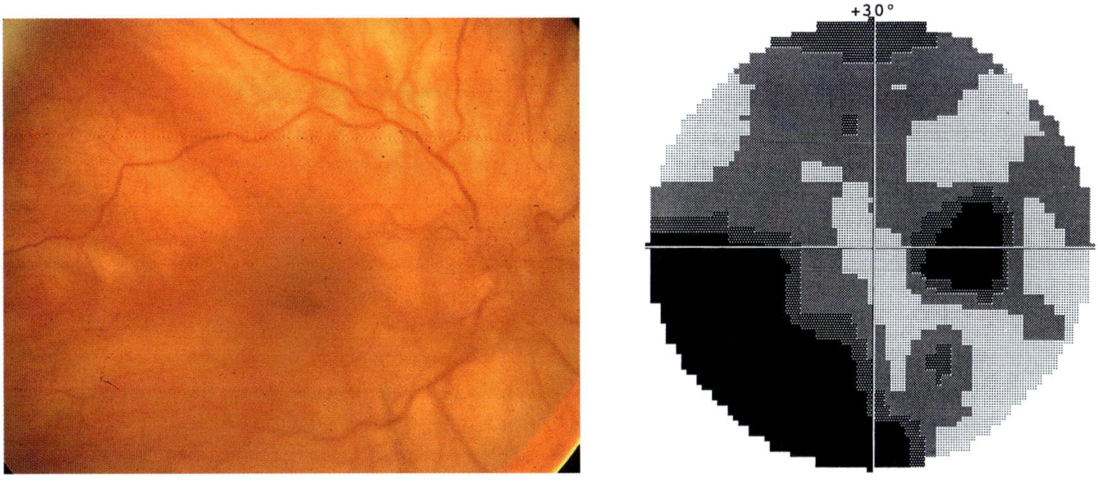

3.8M

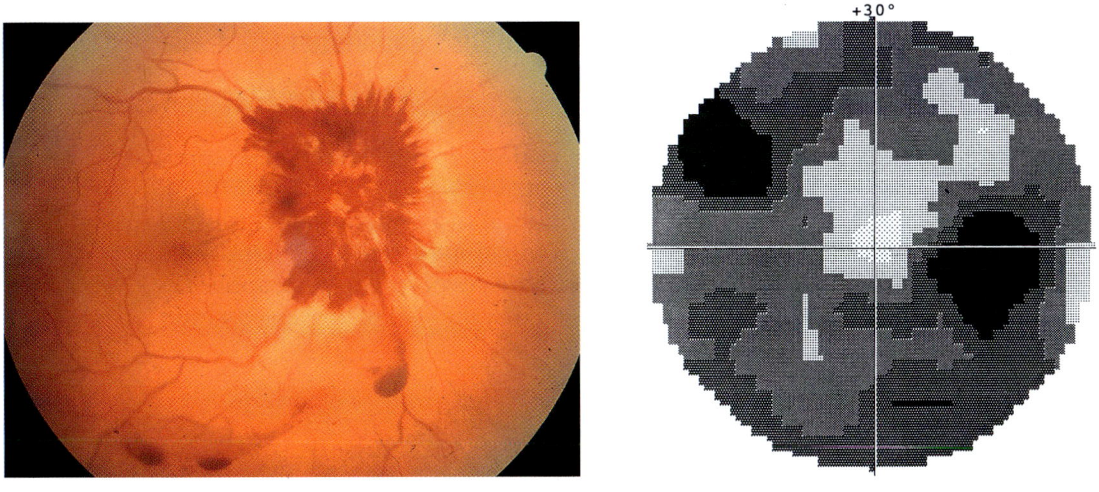

3.8N

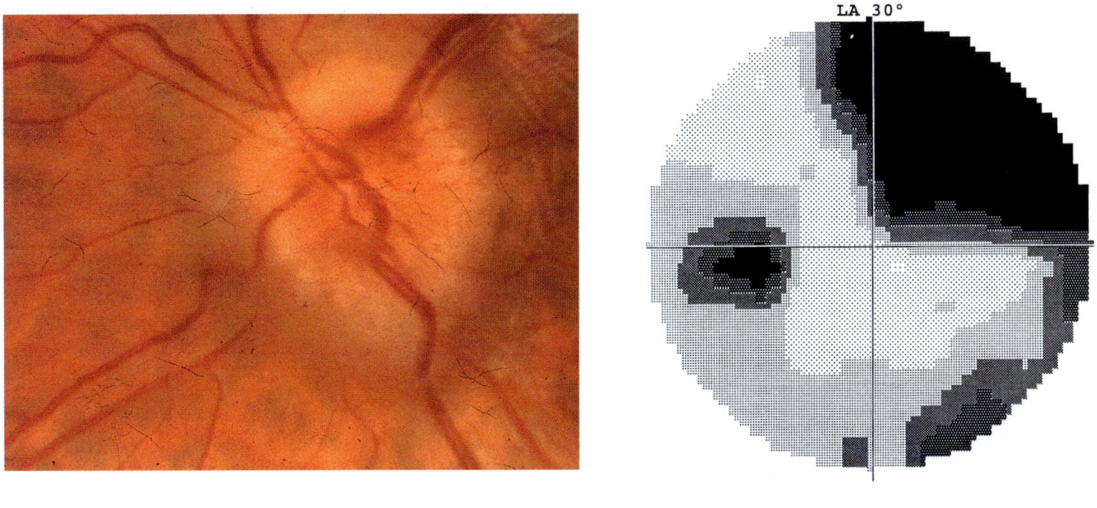

3.8P

3.9 GLAUCOMA

Principle

In glaucoma, the lamina cribrosa is often displaced posteriorly and collapses. Concurrently, the number of axons, glial cells, and capillaries decreases. Both processes, tissue displacement and tissue loss, cause a visible excavation of the surface of the optic nerve head, the glaucomatous cupping of the disk. Most of our knowledge about the topography of the tissue damage is based on these phenomena. In glaucoma, the optic disk cup often enlarges in all directions but not at the same rate. Although the tissue damage is generalized, it is usually more pronounced in certain locations. Inferotemporal and superotemporal sectors show relatively greater loss, and the cup is vertically elongated. In summary, tissue damage in glaucoma is usually generalized but with focal components (Fig. 3.9A).

The visual field defects are analogous; they are generalized, with focal components. The relative focal defects are nerve fiber bundle defects. Because focal tissue damage occurs most frequently in the upper and lower poles of the disk, field defects are mostly long arcuate defects.

Topographical Relationships Between Optic Disk and Visual Field

The optical rules of the eye and the given course of the retinal nerve fiber bundles lead to a constant relationship between the site of structural damage and the location of the functional damage. This relationship is obvious for the upper and lower areas of the disk (Fig. 3.9B). The disk has been mapped for these sectors (Fig. 3.9C). The thinning of the temporal disc rim, however, is often homogeneous, although the cecocentral visual field shows a marked bundle defect. No spatial relationship has been found for this region. The same applies to the nasal region, where evaluation is complicated by the root of the vessels within the nerve head.

Figure 3.9A. Principle of the visual field damage in glaucoma: peripheral nerve fiber bundle defects, which originate most frequently from the inferior and superior sectors of the disk.

Figure 3.9B. Disk and visual field in a patient with focal thinning of the neuroretinal rim inferotemporally and the corresponding focal visual field loss (right eye, program: HFA 10-2 combined with the 30-S custom program, representation: Peridata norm-related grayscale).

Figure 3.9C. Topographical relationship between the disk and the field. The visual field was divided into 21 nerve fiber bundle regions, based on the work of Weber and Ulrich (Int Ophthalmol 15:193–200, 1991). The map of the disk shows the equivalent locations of nerve fiber damage, as far as they could be determined. The figures relate to a right eye. The correlation in the left eye is a mirror image (after Weber et al., Acta Ophthalmol 68:568–574, 1990).

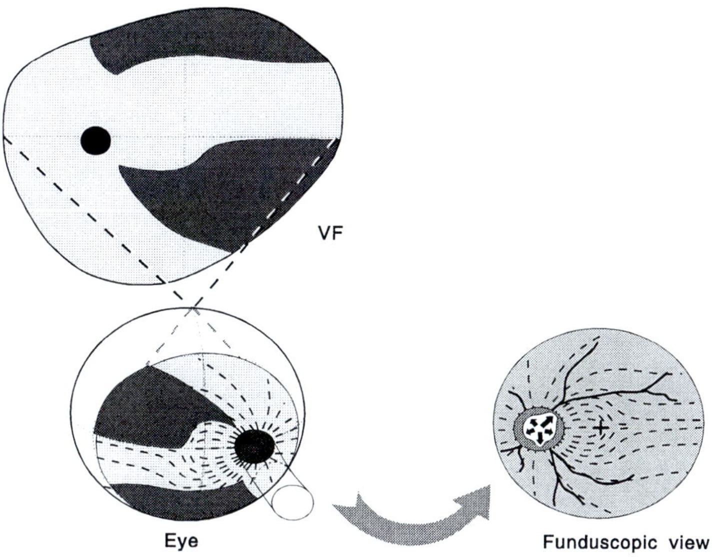
VF
Eye
Funduscopic view

3.9A

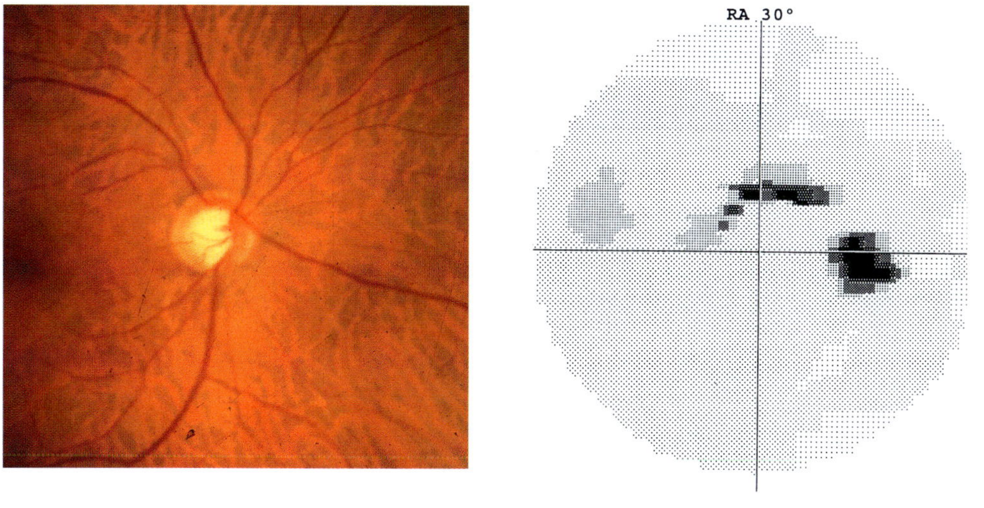
RA 30°

3.9B

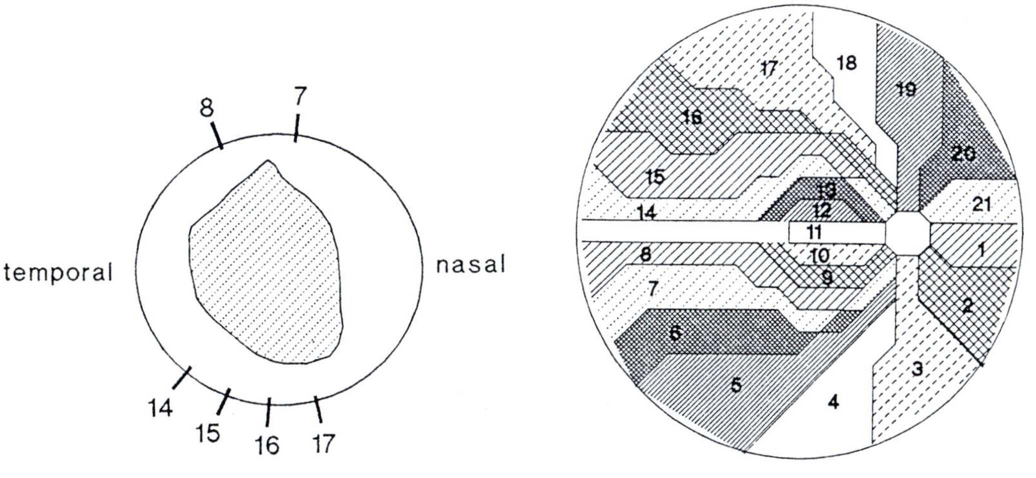
8
7
temporal
nasal
14
15
16
17
+30
17
18
19
16
20
15
13
12
21
14
11
1
8
10
9
7
2
6
3
5
4

3.9C

Superior Arcuate Scotomas

The most frequent type of visual field defect in chronic glaucoma is the long superior arcuate scotoma. The shape varies, depending on which nerve fiber bundles are involved (Fig. 3.9D). Defects of regions 17, 18, and 19, according to the perimetric nerve fiber bundles (PNFB) (after Weber and Ulrich), tend to be peripheral. Therefore, the margins of the scotomas are nearly horizontal. They may be scattered among nonglaucomatous defects, but they can usually be distinguished. Compared to lens artifacts, the shape of the scotoma is not exactly geometrical and the margin is smooth. Ptosis of the brow and dermatochalasis can be excluded by inspection, as can blepharoptosis, which causes more diffuse field damage than expected. A rare but important differential diagnosis is inferior retinal detachment, which may produce similar field defects and progress slowly.

Arcuate scotomas of regions 14 through 17 may be peripheral. The defect may be shaped like a quadrant. Peripheral damage of regions 14 through 16 leads to a nasal wedge. If region 14 alone is damaged, the wedge can be very small, involving only a single point and giving no clue to the wedge shape.

Figure 3.9D. Superior arcuate scotomas: principle and examples of complete and incomplete peripheral nerve fiber bundle defects. All examples are taken from patients with primary chronic open-angle glaucoma (program: HFA 30-S custom program, 129 locations, central resolution 3°; representation: Peridata norm-related grayscale, 30° field).

PNFB = perimetric nerve fiber bundle regions after Weber and Ulrich.

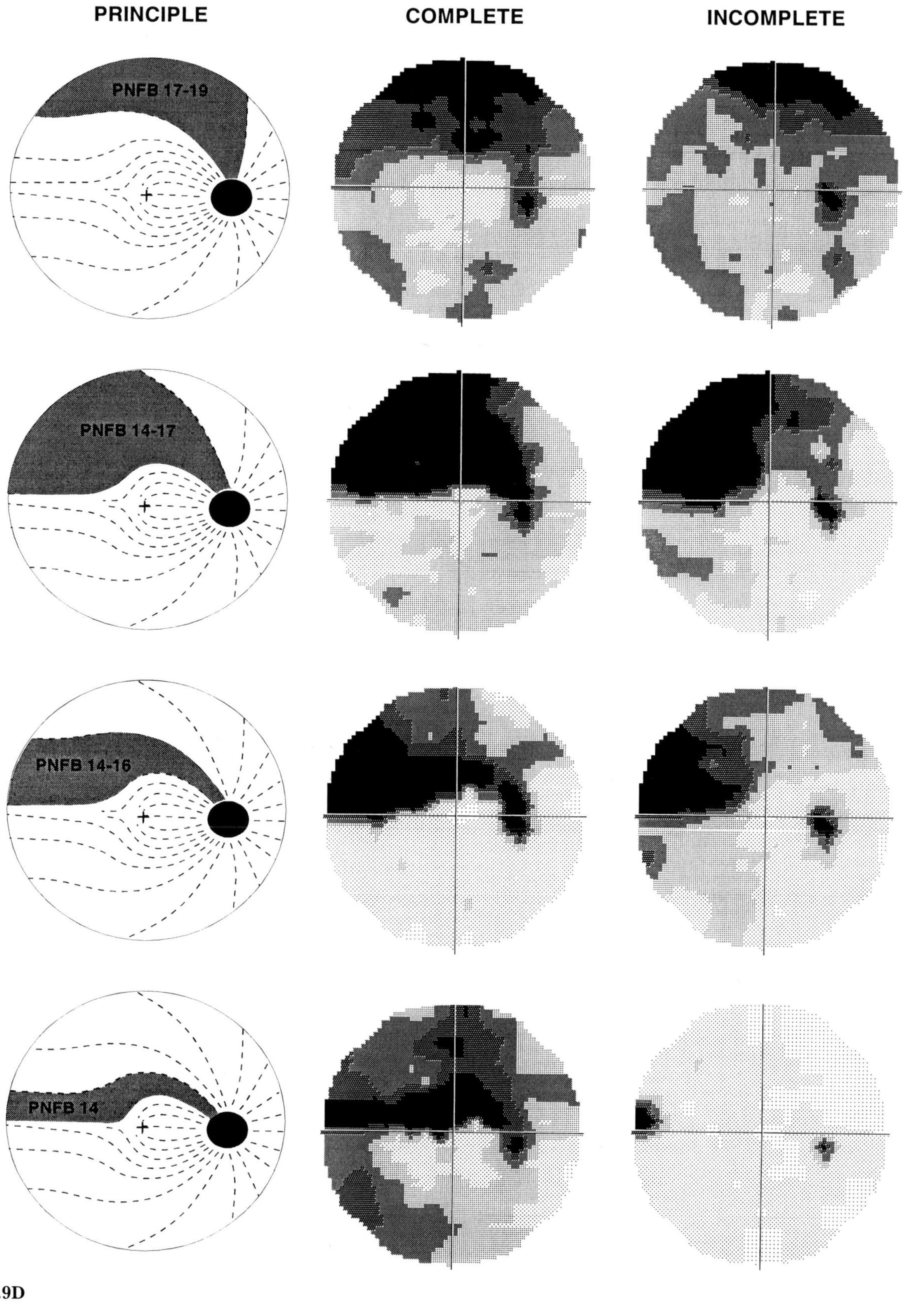
PRINCIPLE
COMPLETE
INCOMPLETE
PNFB 17-19
PNFB 14-17
PNFB 14-16
PNFB 14

3.9D

Short Superior Arcuate Scotomas

Short arcuate scotomas do not break through to the periphery but end nasally at the neural raphe. Thus, they are considerably shorter than the long arcuate scotomas. Detection and assessment require high resolution in the center of the field, with spacing of 3–4° or less. The widely used standard programs 32 (Octopus) and 30-2 (HFA) are not suitable for this purpose. Glaucoma-specific programs with higher central resolution are preferable.

Of all the short arcuate scotomas, the superior ones are most frequent. They are related to the perimetric nerve fiber bundle region 13 (Fig. 3.9E).

Centrocecal Scotomas

Centrocecal defects are small scotomas between fixation and the blind spot (PNFB regions 10, 11, and 12). Isolated centrocecal defects are very rare in glaucoma. They can be assessed only if several test locations lie near or on the horizontal axis. The patient in Figure 3.9F was examined with the custom program 30-S with a central resolution of 3°. We did not find any centrocecal defects, even with this special program, in more than 1000 glaucomatous eyes.

Short Inferior Arcuate Scotomas

Inferior paracentral arcuate scotomas are often combined with other defects. The PNFB region involved is number 9 (Fig. 3.9G).

Figure 3.9E. Short superior arcuate scotomas: principle and examples of complete and incomplete nerve fiber bundle defects.

Figure 3.9F. Cecocentral defects: principle and example.

Figure 3.9G. Short inferior arcuate scotomas: principle and example.

All examples on this page are taken from patients with primary chronic open-angle glaucoma (program: HFA 30-S custom program, 129 locations, central resolution 3°; representation: Peridata norm-related grayscale, 30° field).

PNFB = perimetric nerve fiber bundle regions after Weber and Ulrich.

PRINCIPLE COMPLETE INCOMPLETE

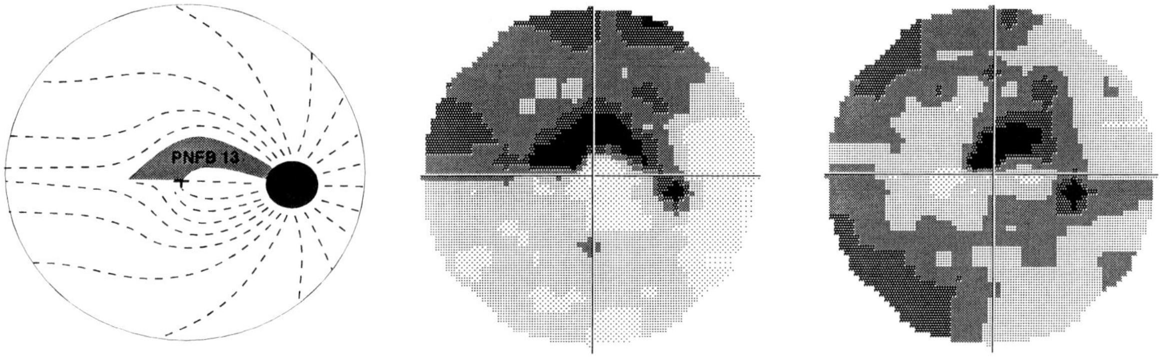

3.9E

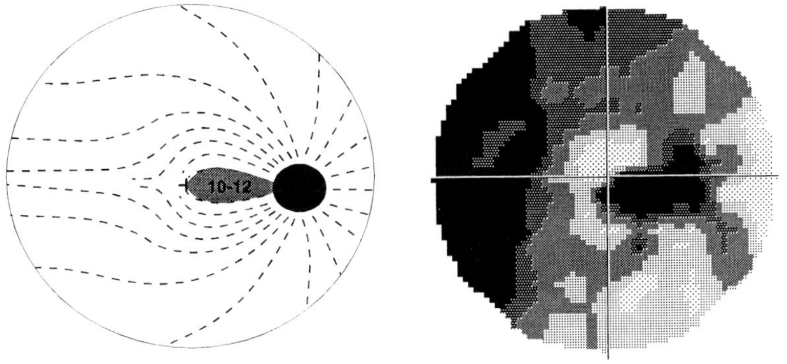

3.9F

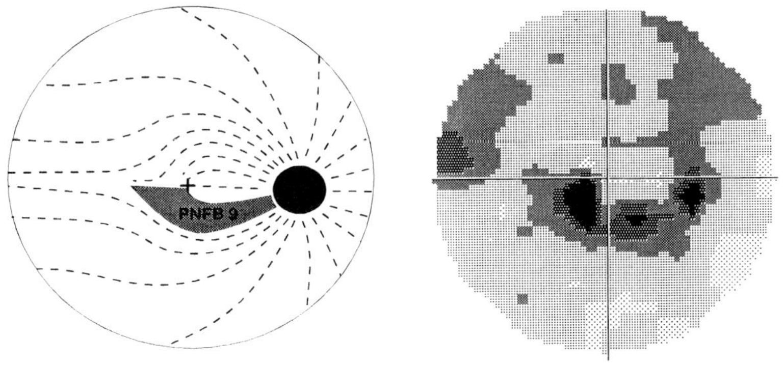

3.9G

Inferior Arcuate Scotomas

Inferior arcuate scotomas (Fig. 3.9H) are less frequent than the superior kind. Lean defects (region 8 isolated) are rare. They tend to involve several regions and to be peripherally stressed. Damage of the long fibers in regions 5 through 8 may result in a nasal quadrant defect.

Temporal Sector (Sector-Shaped) Defects

Temporal sector defects (regions 1,2, 20, and 21; Fig. 3.9J) are infrequent. These eyes are often myopic. Using routine programs which are restricted to 30°, only part of the temporal sector defect can be defined. Therefore, any statement about the completeness or incompleteness of these defects must be interpreted carefully. Many incomplete temporal sector defects are probably missed in routine perimetry.

Figure 3.9H. Inferior arcuate scotomas: principle and examples of complete and incomplete nerve fiber bundle defects.

Figure 3.9J. Temporal sector defects: principle and example.

Both of the examples on this page are taken from patients with primary chronic open-angle glaucoma (program: HFA 30-S custom program, 129 locations, central resolution 3°; representation: Peridata norm-related grayscale, 30° field).

PNFB = perimetric nerve fiber bundle regions after Weber and Ulrich.

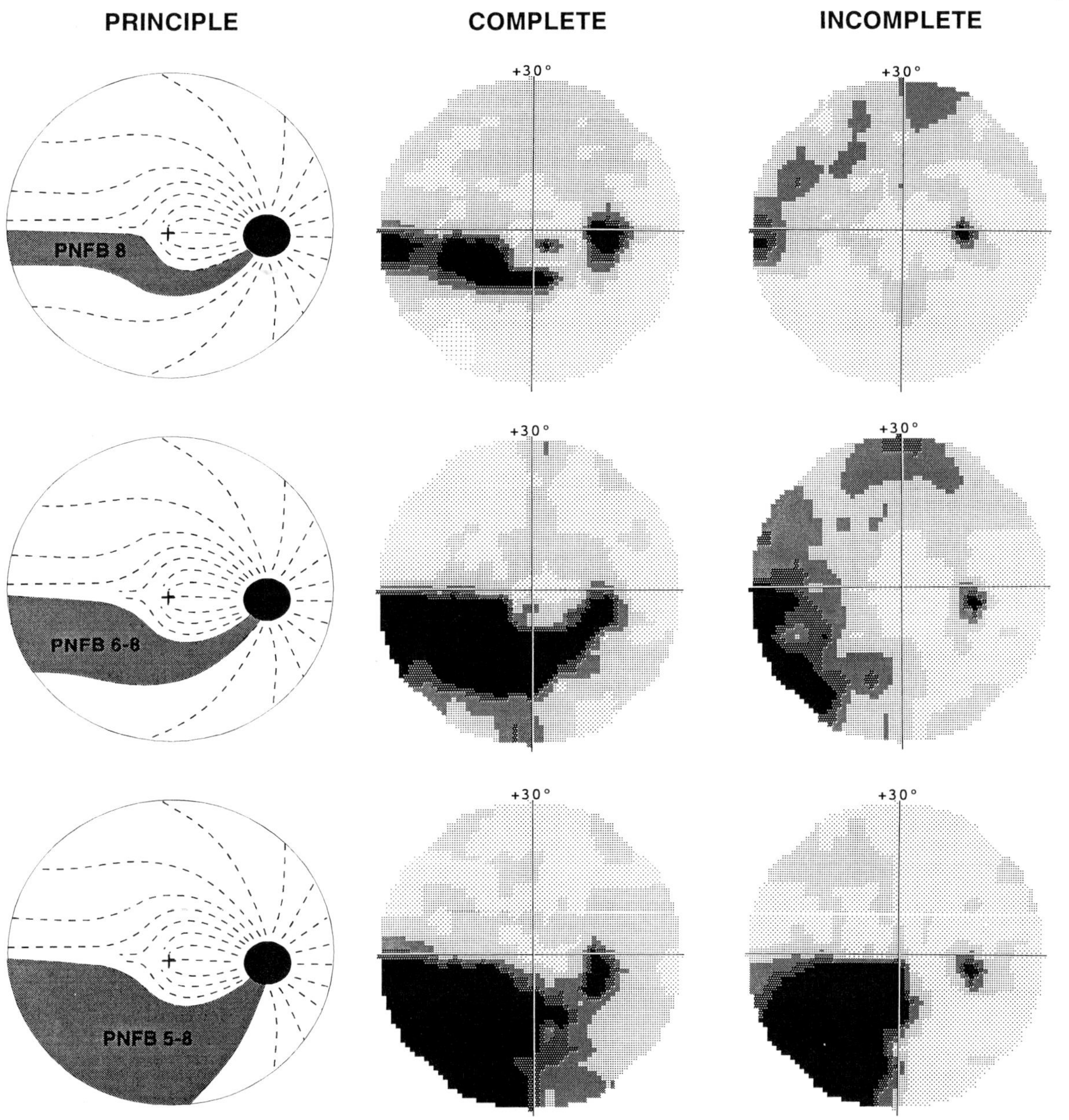
PRINCIPLE
COMPLETE
INCOMPLETE
PNFB 8
+30°
PNFB 6-8
PNFB 5-8

3.9H

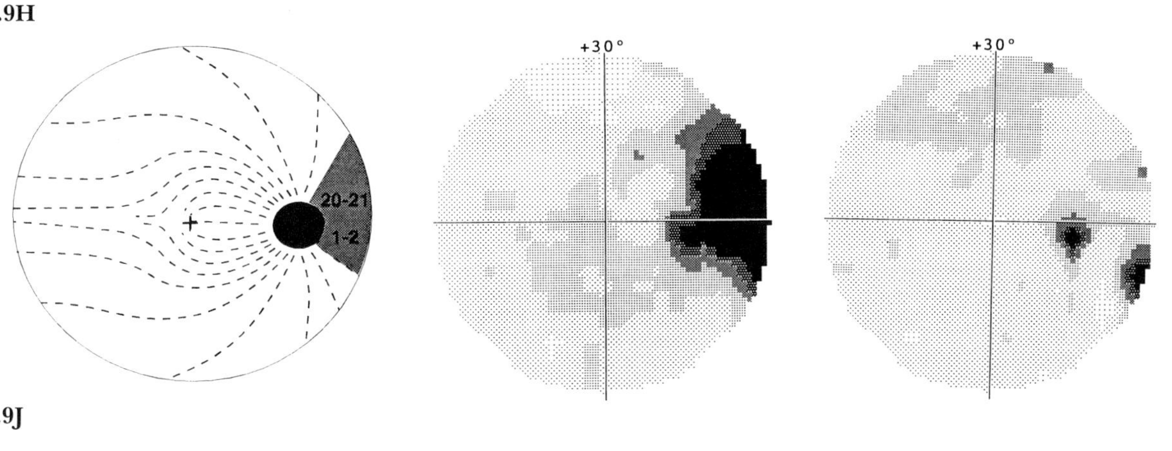
20-21
1-2
+30°

3.9J

Combined Defects

Glaucomatous fields are often a combination of several nerve fiber bundle defects. A typical combination involves two arcuate scotomas in different halves of the visual field (Fig. 3.9K). A combination with temporal defects is less frequent (Fig. 3.9L).

Pseudo–single defects arise if a superior and an inferior nasal defect touch each other and result in a single defect (Fig. 3.9M left). There are two separate loci of tissue damage.

Pseudo–double defects are combinations of short arcuate scotomas and incomplete long arcuate scotomas (Fig. 3.9M right). They can be followed back to a common center of damage. In this example, the damage involves the PNFB region 13 (short arcuate scotomas) and the neighboring regions 14–16 (long arcuate scotomas). A similar phenomenon is found in the inferior half.

Single defects in combination can be complete or incomplete and can involve few or many nerve fiber bundle regions. If upper and lower defects both reach the horizontal axis, the arcs merge nasally and also at the blind spot. The shape is a ring scotoma (Fig. 3.9N). This is the predominant topography of progressive visual field damage. Ronne called it a *split field,* as there is a central island and a temporal crescent.

Figure 3.9K. Combination of upper and lower arcuate scotomas. The lower nerve fiber bundle defects are incomplete and peripheral. The upper arcuate scotomas are incomplete in the left field and complete in the right field.

Figure 3.9L. Left: combination of an upper arcuate scotoma (incomplete, quadrant shape) and a temporal sector defect. Right: Combination of a shallow, inferior arcuate scotoma with a temporal sector defect.

Figure 3.9M. Left: Pseudo–single defect. The defect is a combination of two nasal wedge-shaped defects and also has two centers of damage at the disk. Right: Pseudo–double defect. The defect is a combination of peripheral short and long arcuate scotomas. The anatomical damage involves neighboring nerve fiber bundles and therefore has only one center of damage.

Figure 3.9N. The ring scotoma in glaucoma arises from two arcuate scotomas which merge nasally and at the blind spot. On the left side, the merging is still incomplete; on the right side, it is complete.

All examples on this page are taken from patients with primary chronic open-angle glaucoma (program: HFA 30-S custom program, 129 locations, central resolution 3°; representation: Peridata norm-related grayscale, 30° field).

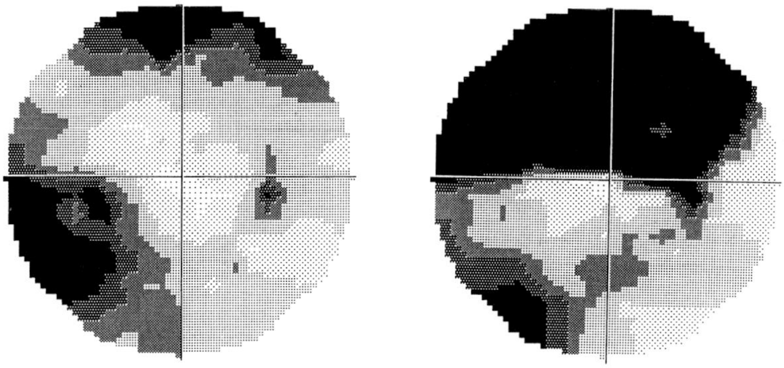

3.9K

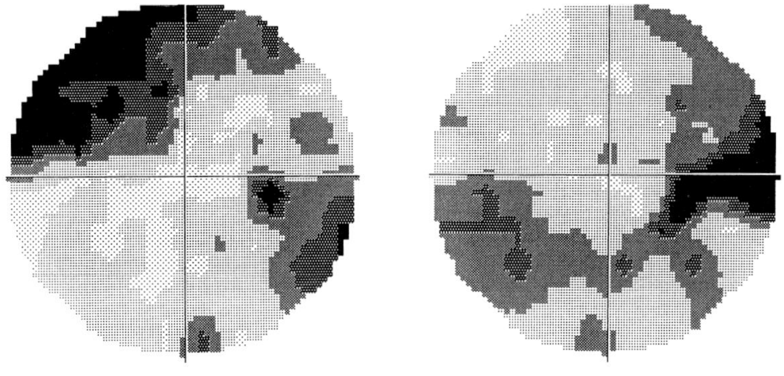

3.9L

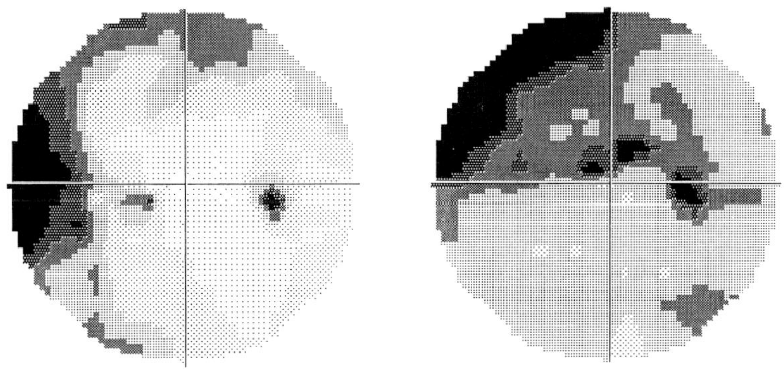

3.9M

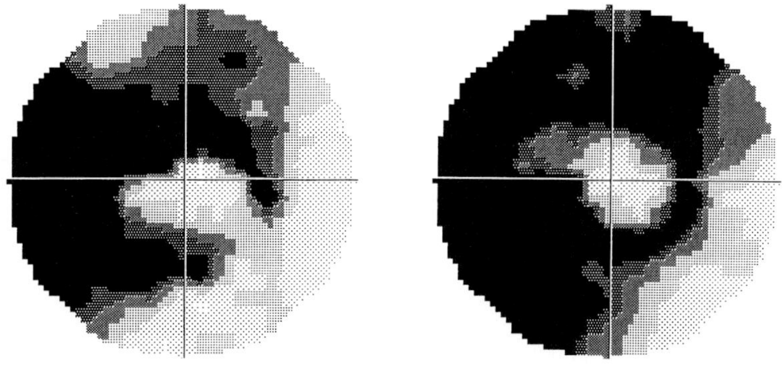

3.9N

Symmetry

Another topographical characteristic of glaucomatous visual field damage is the axial symmetry between the right and left visual fields. The origin of symmetry is the symmetry of tissue damage on both sides. In contrast to the intraindividual symmetry, there is high interindividual variation in the topography of the visual field defects and cupping of the disk. Therefore, intraindividual symmetry is a clue to the symmetric vulnerability of the optic nerve head to glaucomatous damage.

In addition to complete symmetry (Fig. 3.9P), there is topographical symmetry with different degrees of damage (Fig. 3.9Q). Asymmetry is not rare, however (Fig. 3.9R).

Figure 3.9P. Axial symmetry between the right and left visual fields.

Figure 3.9Q. The regions involved are symmetrical, but the extent and depth of the defect (i.e., the degree of damage) are different.

Figure 3.9R. Asymmetric visual fields.

All examples on this page are taken from patients with primary chronic open-angle glaucoma (program: HFA 30-S custom program, 129 locations, central resolution 3°; representation: Peridata norm-related grayscale, 30° field).

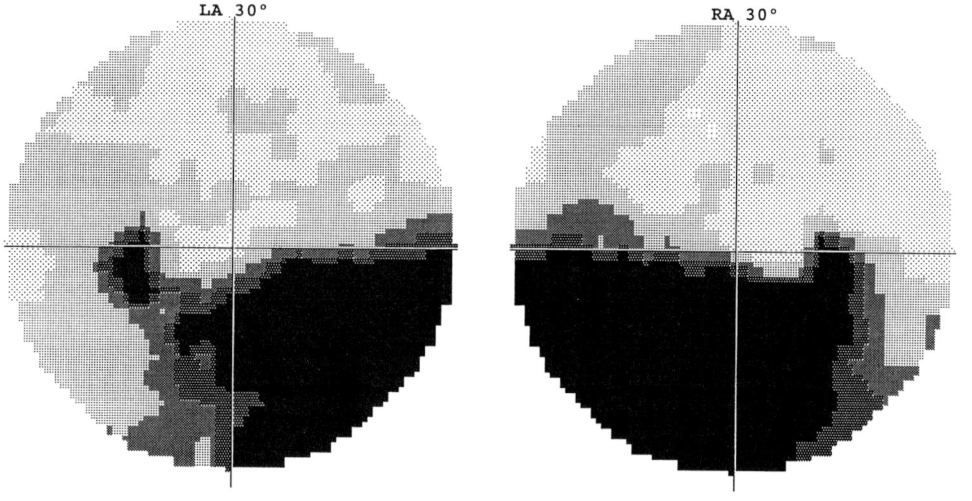

3.9P

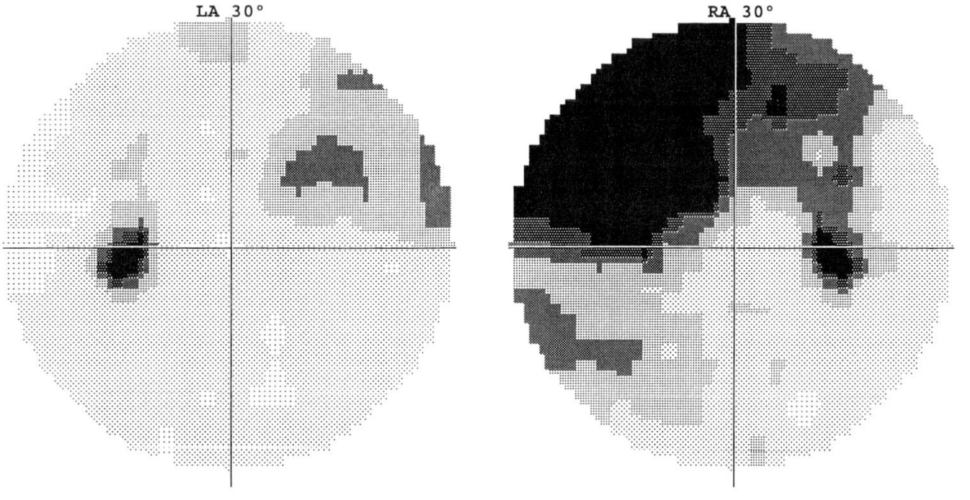

3.9Q

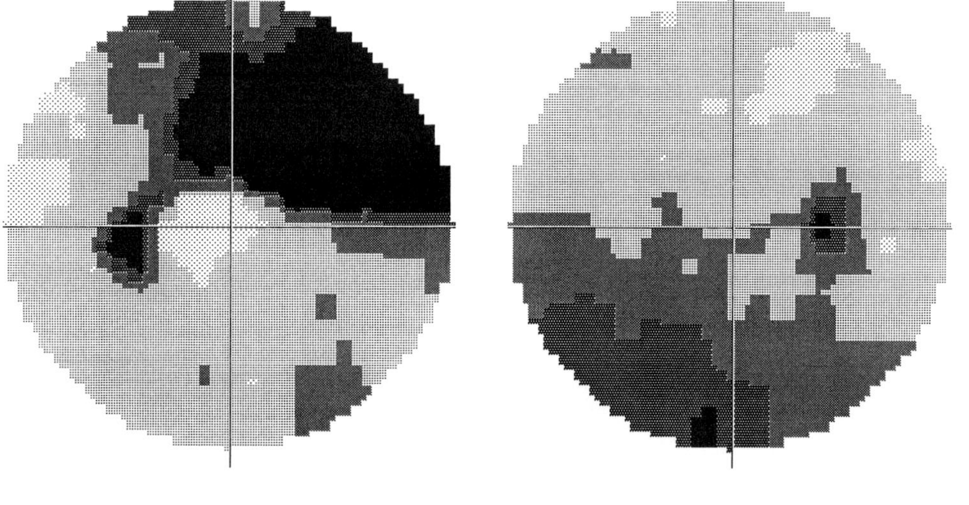

3.9R

Extent of Damage and Secondary Topographical Phenomena

Glaucomatous damage eventually involves the entire visual field and may be generalized; all regions are damaged. However, various regions differ in regard to the degree of damage and how rapidly it progresses. Figure 3.9S illustrates this in a profile cut showing a glaucomatous field in five stages. Visual field 1 is normal. Visual field 2 has mild damage. Regions with rapid progression (vulnerable regions) show defects which are deep enough to exceed the normal range. Other regions may appear normal, although a clear trend toward reduction in sensitivity is present. A pointwise approach to interpretation may mask the damage. In visual field 3, almost the whole area except the center is abnormal. In fields 4 and 5, parts of the visual field defect are so deep that their sensitivity is below the measurement range (absolute scotoma). By using larger stimulus sizes which provide a larger measurement range (relative to the normal values), these scotomas can be made relative again in some regions.

If the visual field is viewed only in a topographical, pointwise fashion, some secondary phenomena arise which may be misleading. For example, "new" defects usually have been present before detection, but were still inside normal range. With progression, they exceed the normal range and "appear" (Fig. 3.9T). "Enlargement" of scotomas may also be part of a generalized depression.

Enlargement of scotomas can lead to changes in shape, depending on the shape of the sensitivity in the border zone. In very mild damage, for example, scotomas are variable because the sensitivity is borderline and crossing of the border is random. Next, larger scotomas with "holes" appear. With progression, they become more consistent and typical. With increasing damage, scotomas approach fixation and constrict the central island.

For assessment of minimal depressions, visual field analysis should include the cumulative defect curve. In glaucoma, both generalized and focal defects can be detected, though purely diffuse depression due to glaucoma is readily rare (Fig. 3.9U).

Figure 3.9S. Progression of the glaucomatous visual field in a profile cut. The damage is widespread, but the rate of progression shows regional differences.

Figure 3.9T. Secondary phenomena of progression. "New" defects and "enlargement" are only outcomes of the generalized depression.

Figure 3.9U. Cumulativė defect curve in glaucoma: generalized depression, with a higher rate of progression on the right side.

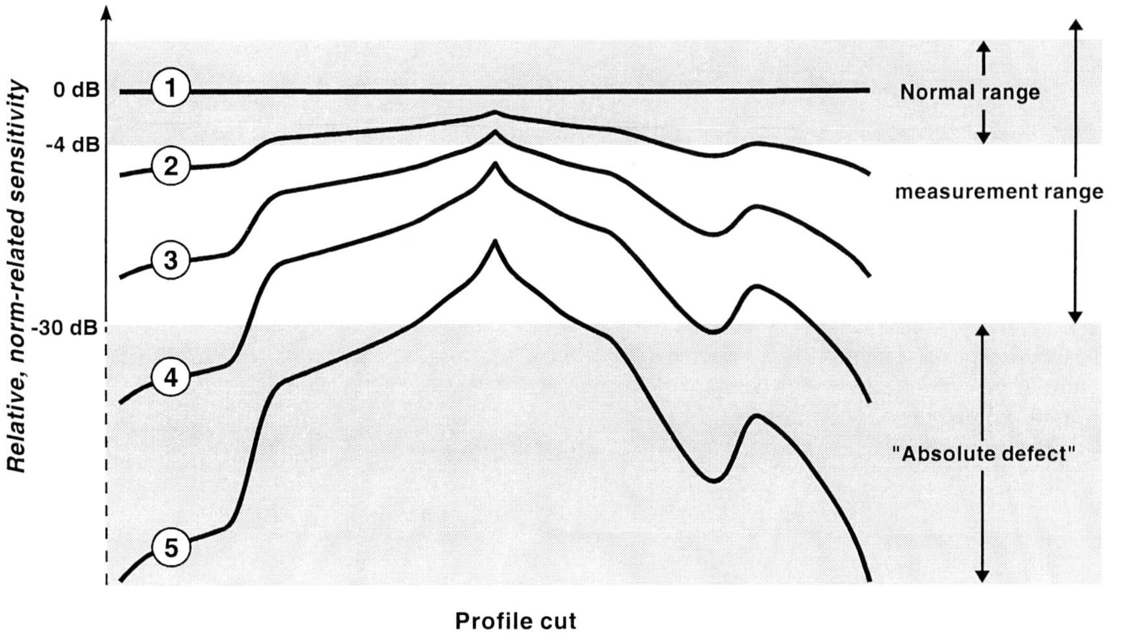
Relative, norm-related sensitivity
0 dB
-4 dB
-30 dB
1
2
3
4
5
Normal range
measurement range
"Absolute defect"
Profile cut

3.9S

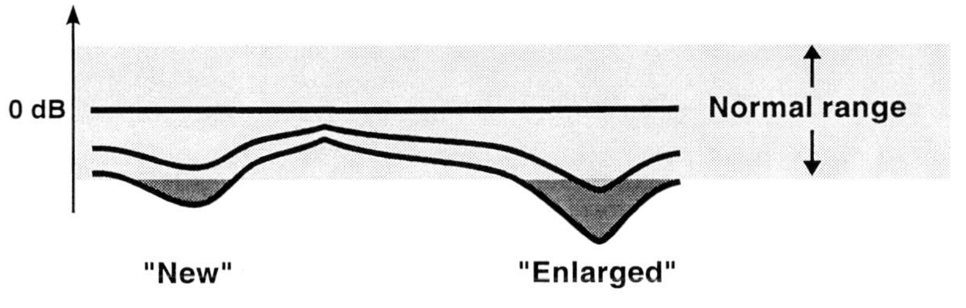
0 dB
Normal range
"New"
"Enlarged"

3.9T

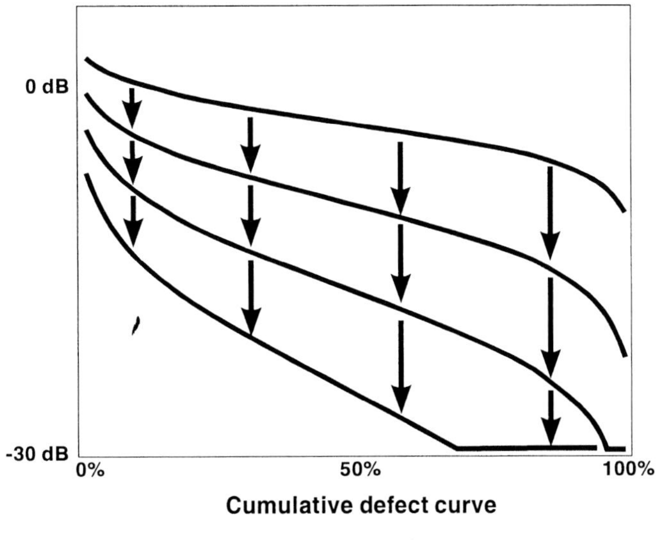
0 dB
-30 dB
0%
50%
100%
Cumulative defect curve

3.9U

Mild and Moderate Damage

Very mild visual field alterations cannot be distinguished easily from normal fields. Scattered defects of –9 dB (see, Fig. 3.9V, top) can also seen in normal eyes. A generalized sensitivity loss where the global mean value (MD) is –0.4 dB is within the normal range, which extends down to –2 dB. The cumulative defect curve is well within the dotted lines indicating normal limits.

When overall depression progresses and abnormal depressions involve several neighboring points, the suspicion of glaucoma is reasonable (Fig. 3.9V, second field from the top). The global MD exceeds the lower normal limit, and the cumulative defect curve touches the limit line or crosses it. The topography, however, is not yet typical, but the nasal position of deeper defects in this example is a clue to glaucoma. It can be seen as damage of the long fibers in the arcuate nerve fiber bundles. Other regions may also be involved at this stage.

During progression, defects enlarge while the whole field sinks (Fig. 3.9V, third field from the top). At particular points, absolute defects may occur (Fig. 3.9V, bottom). The cumulative defect curve shifts further downwards. A global mean defect of –5.2 dB indicates moderate damage, since a depression of –6 dB represents a loss of approximately 50% of nerve fiber axons.

Figure 3.9V. Examples of mild and moderate damage in regions with both long arcuate scotomas. The examples are taken from different patients with primary chronic open-angle glaucoma (program: HFA 30-2, representation: Peridata "compressed": norm-related grayscale, numerals [norm-related sensitivity], standard indices, cumulative defect curve).

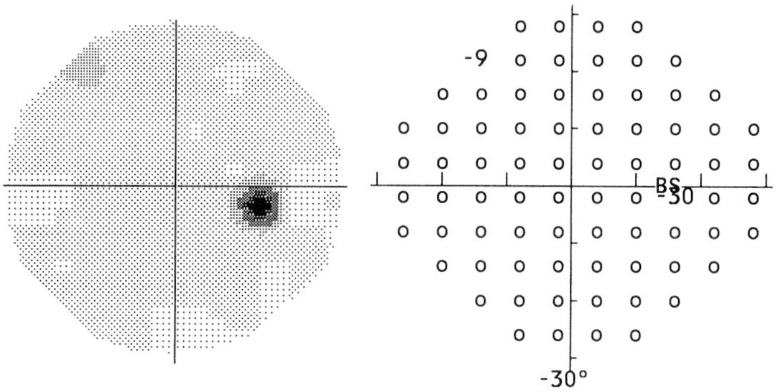

MD	-0.4
LV	2.7
CLV	0.0
PSD	1.6
CPSD	0.0
SF	2.1
N	74.0
MS	28.5
FS	96.7

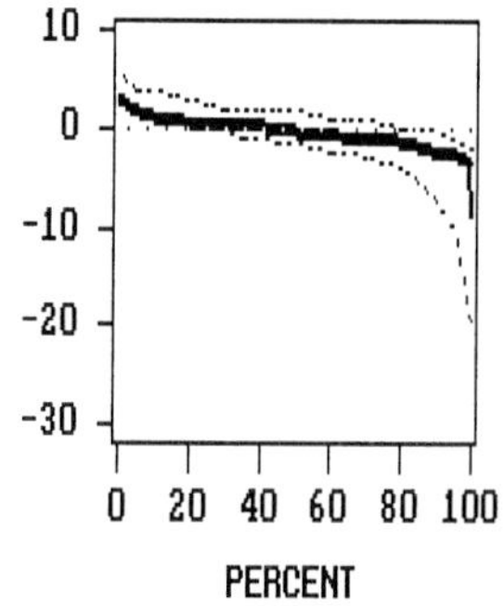

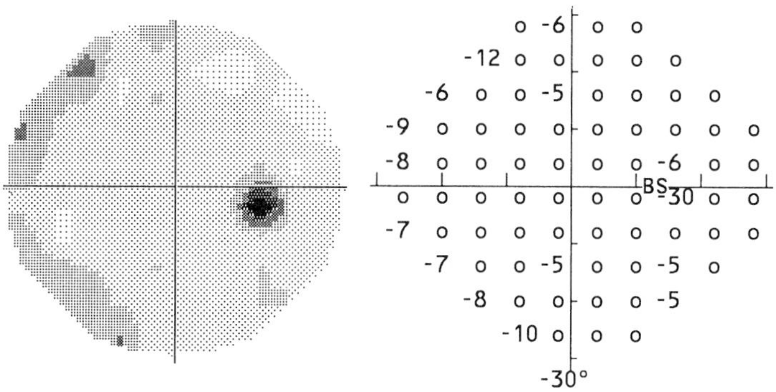

MD	-2.6
LV	7.8
CLV	0.0
PSD	2.8
CPSD	0.0
SF	3.3
N	74.0
MS	25.2
FS	79.3

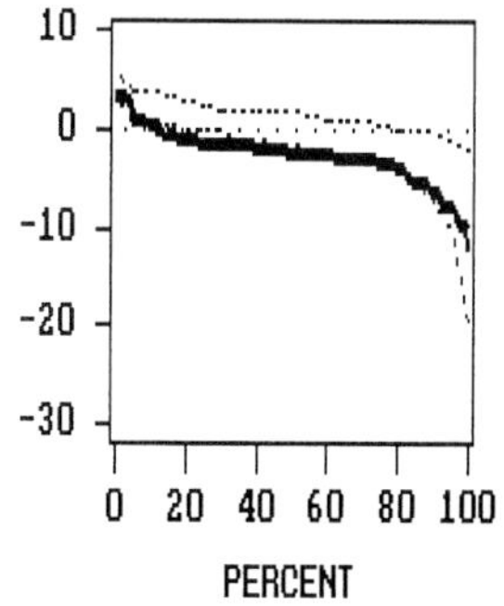

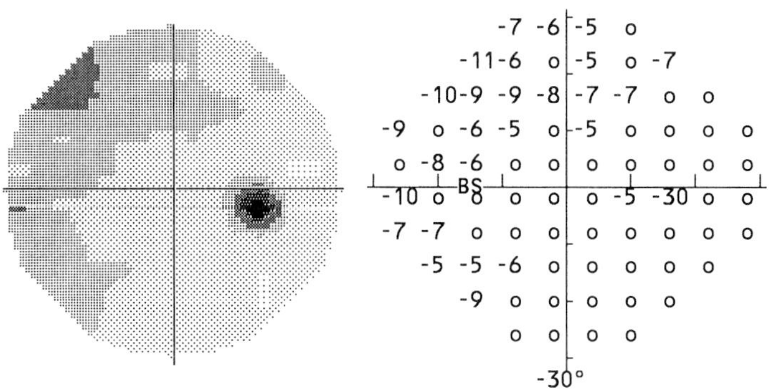

MD	-3.9
LV	8.7
CLV	2.9
PSD	2.9
CPSD	1.7
SF	2.5
N	74.0
MS	25.5
FS	70.8

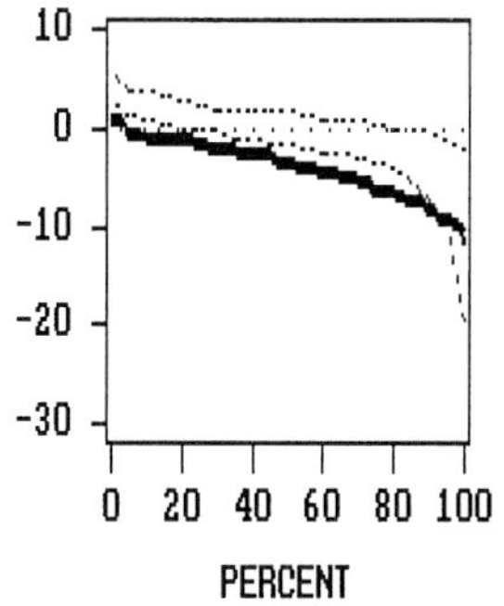

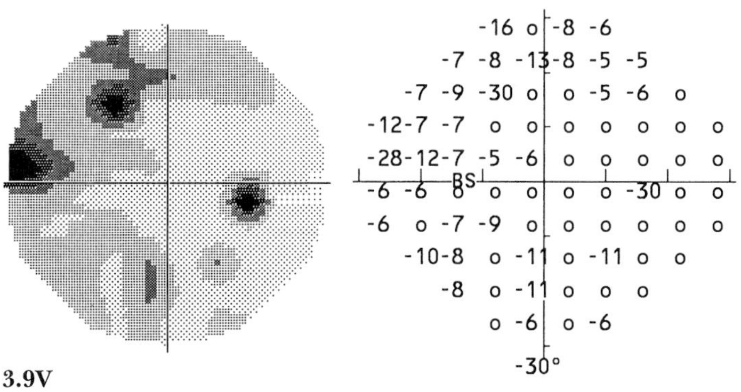

MD	-5.2
LV	29.6
CLV	25.2
PSD	5.4
CPSD	5.0
SF	2.4
N	74.0
MS	24.7
FS	66.1

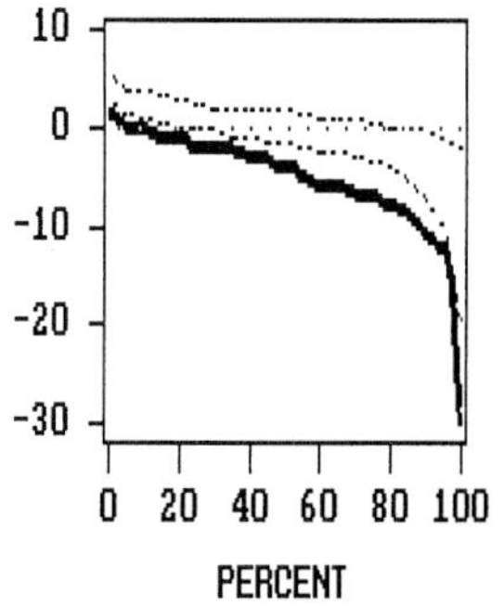

3.9V

Severe Damage

In severely damaged visual fields, absolute defects spread. Areas with defects of different depths and different rates of progression may coalesce. As the defects spread, peripheral defects join with the blind spot (Fig. 3.9W, first to third fields from the top). Defects in the more normal half of the field deepen as well and approach the blind spot (Fig. 3.9W, third field). A ring scotoma may be formed (Fig. 3.9W, bottom), and the central island and temporal field split. The central island represents the region which shows the slowest rate of progressive damage and, therefore, the least damage at all stages.

Figure 3.9W. Continuation of the series from the previous page: examples of severe damage in both regions with long arcuate scotomas. The examples are taken from different patients with primary chronic open-angle glaucoma (program: HFA 30-2, representation: Peridata "compressed": norm-related grayscale, numerals [norm-related sensitivity], standard indices, cumulative defect curve).

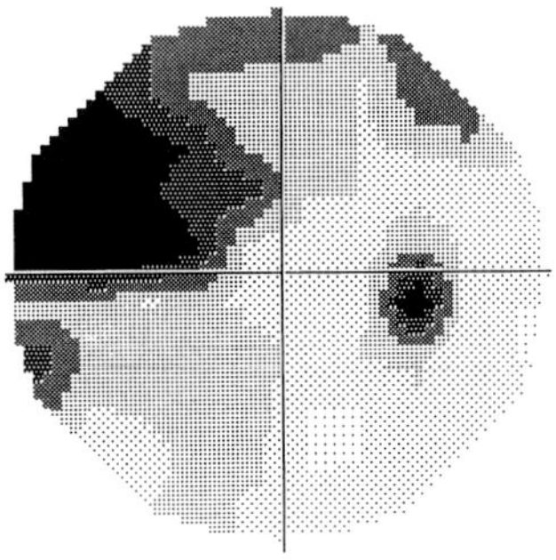

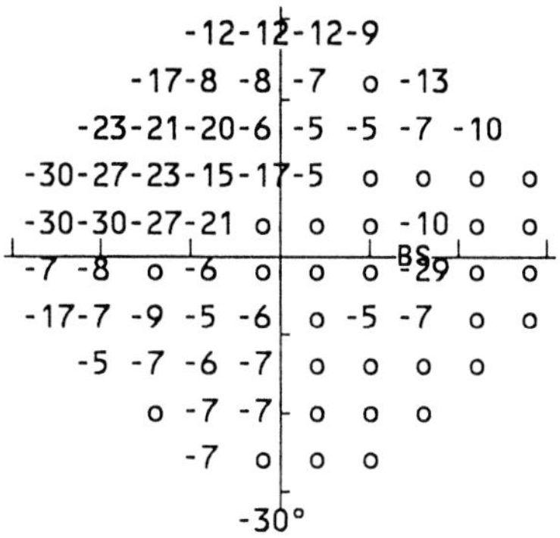

MD	-7.9
LV	66.1
CLV	61.9
PSD	8.1
CPSD	7.9
SF	2.3
N	74.0
MS	19.6
FS	56.5

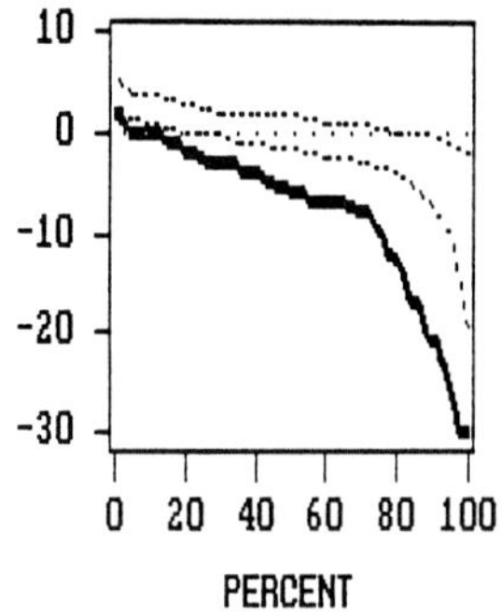

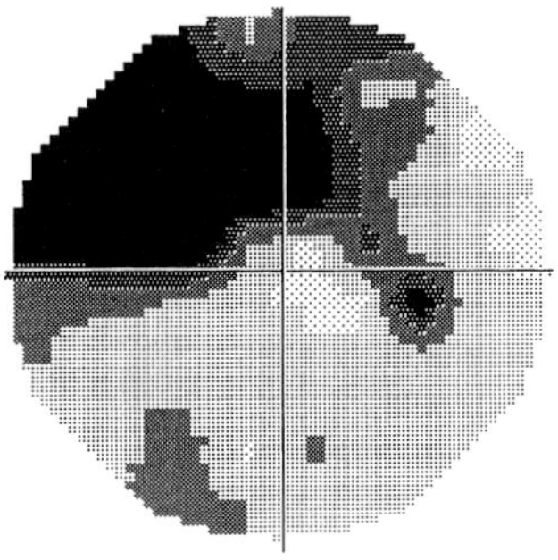

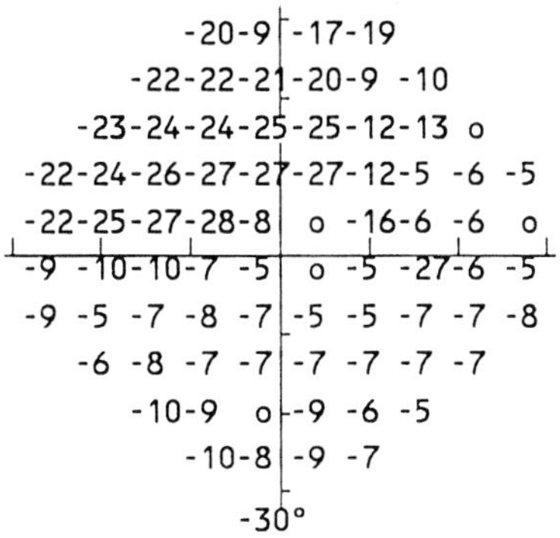

MD	-12.2
LV	62.0
CLV	59.4
PSD	7.9
CPSD	7.7
SF	1.9
N	74.0
MS	15.7
FS	36.1

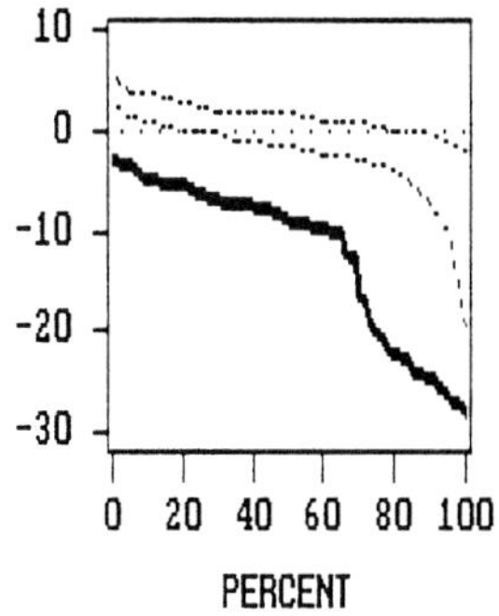

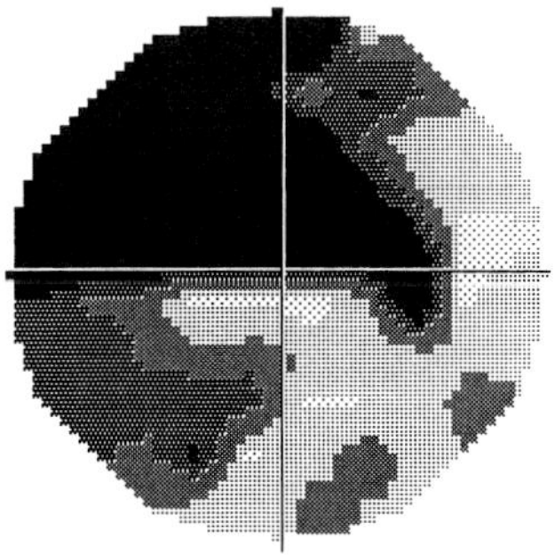

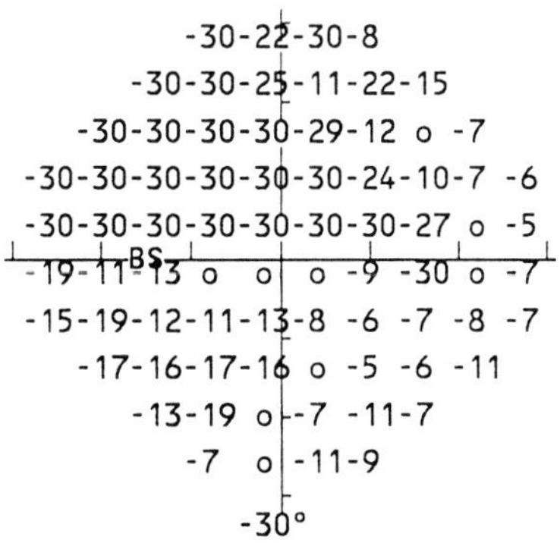

MD	-16.2
LV	104.6
CLV	99.3
PSD	10.2
CPSD	10.0
SF	2.7
N	74.0
MS	12.5
FS	27.8

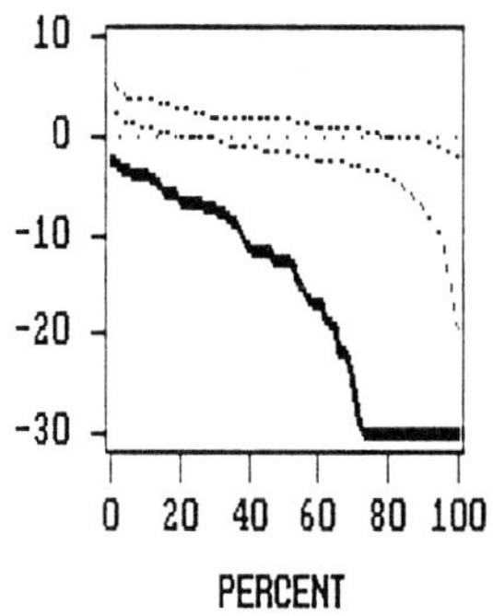

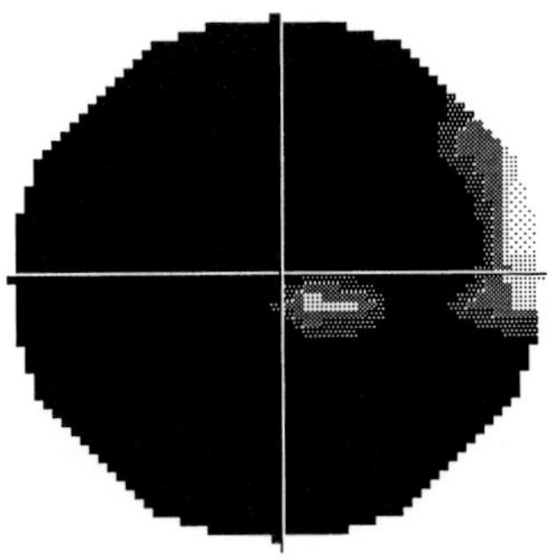

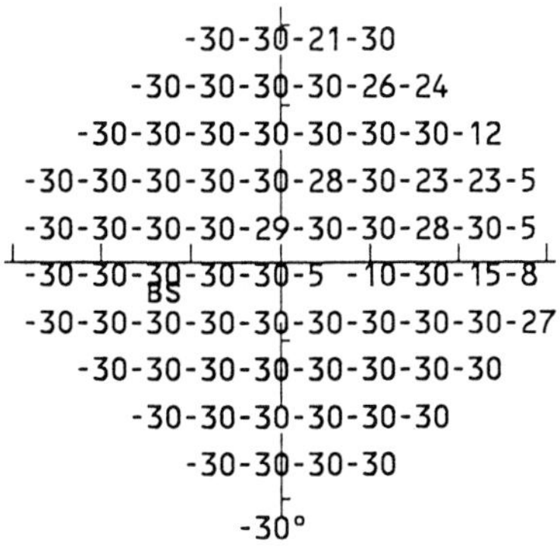

MD	-27.5
LV	41.9
CLV	33.5
PSD	6.5
CPSD	5.8
SF	3.1
N	74.0
MS	0.7
FS	4.3

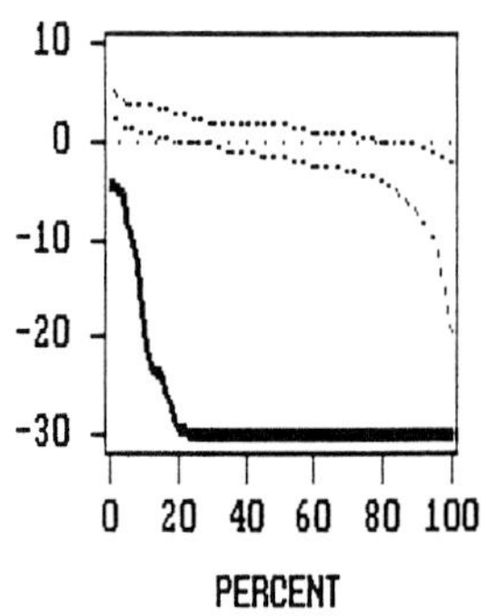

3.9W

3.10 OTHER DISEASES OF THE OPTIC NERVE

Principle

In contrast to focal disk processes (according to the definition in Section 3.8), which are characterized by limited damage to a cross section of fibers within the optic nerve, there is no clearly defined location of the lesion in other diseases of the optic nerve. Instead, functional defects caused by disease diverge from expected retinal nerve fiber topography.

Regardless of the etiology of the disease, central and centrocecal scotomas are frequent. The corresponding optic fibers are located centrally in the optic nerve and temporally at the optic nerve head (Fig. 3.10A). In cases of permanent damage, the temporal sector of the disk often shows pallor. Other types of defects are diffuse, nerve-fiber shaped, hemianopic, and amorphous.

Figure 3.10A. Principle of the cecocentral scotoma in other optic nerve diseases.

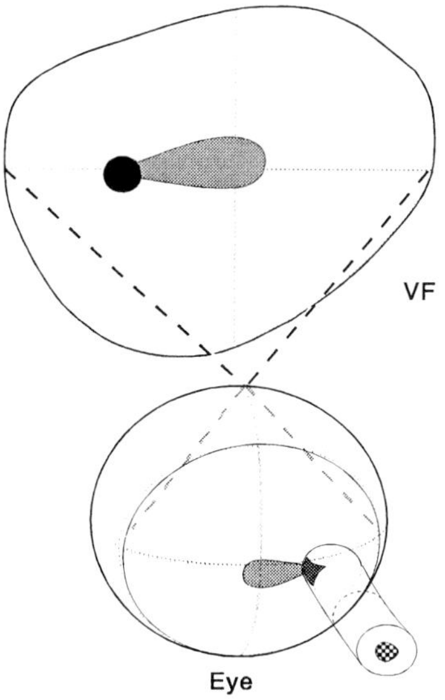

3.10A

Hereditary Optic Nerve Atrophy

In Leber's optic nerve atrophy, a bilateral central scotoma is found, mostly in connection with the blind spot (centrocecal scotoma, Fig. 3.10B). The latter includes the center, in contrast to the centrocecal nerve fiber bundle defect (Section 3.8), which touches the center only with its tip. Therefore, visual acuity drops to about 0.1. Visual field defects in dominant hereditary optic atrophy are similar but not as deep, and visual acuity tends to be better.

Figure 3.10B. Leber's optic atrophy in a 19-year-old man. Visual acuity is 0.4 in the right eye and 0.1 in the left eye. Both disks show temporal pallor (program: HFA 30-2, representation: Peridata norm-related grayscale).

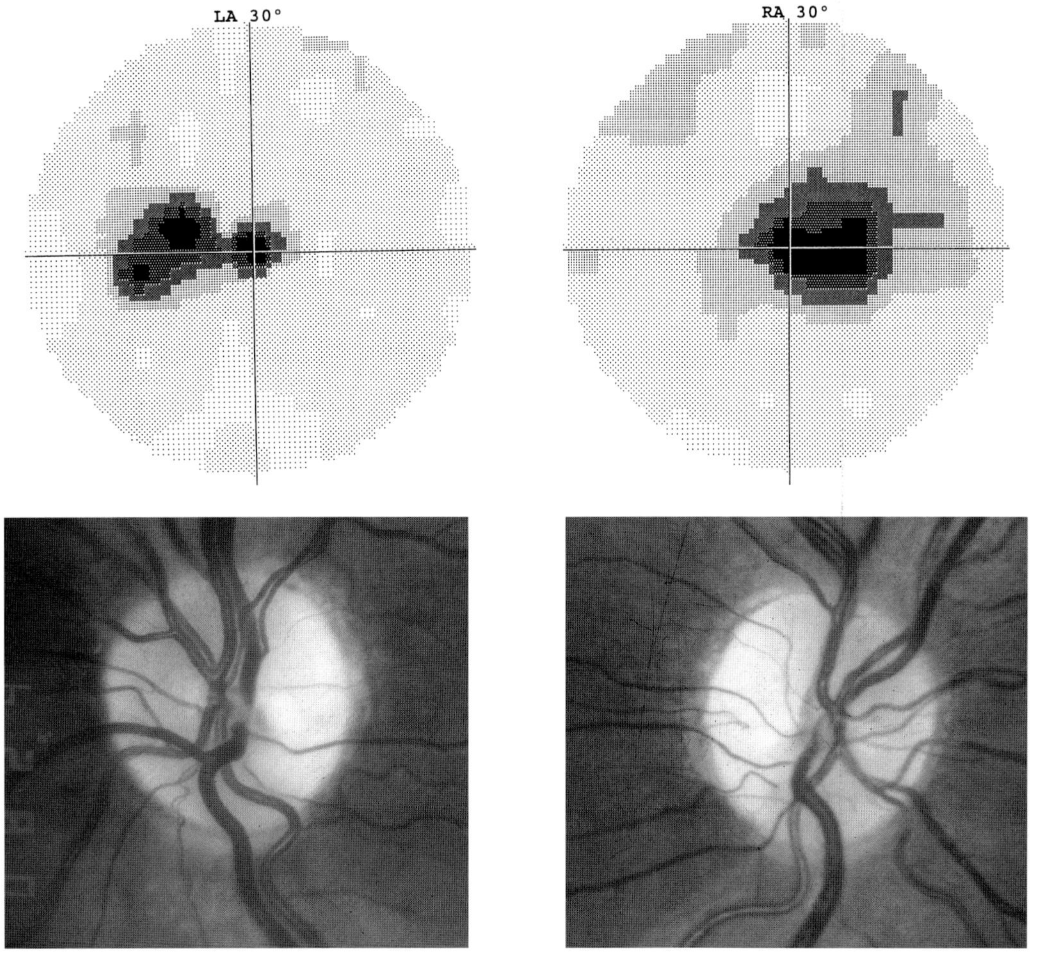

3.10B

Toxic Atrophy (Optic Atrophy)

Toxic damage of the optic nerve leads to central or centrocecal scotomas, with substantial decrease in visual acuity. Several substances are possible causes. Most frequent are tobacco-alcohol amblyopia (Fig. 3.10C), methanol, and ethambutol. Rare substances such as cytarabine should also be considered (Fig. 3.10D). For new medicines, potential neurotoxicity may not yet be observed.

In such cases, it is important to measure the 10° field with high resolution. Even in cases of poor patient fixation, valuable information can be obtained, and involvement of central vision can be identified with reasonable precision (Fig. 3.10E).

Figure 3.10C. Both visual fields of a 64-year-old patient with heavy use of tobacco and alcohol. The visual acuity decreased bilaterally to 0.3 (program: HFA 30-2, representation: Peridata norm-related grayscale).

Figure 3.10D. Both 30° fields of a 13-year-old boy who was treated with cytarabine for acute myelogenous leukemia. Visual acuity was 0.6 in the right eye and 0.7 in the left eye (program: HFA 30-2, representation: Peridata norm-related grayscale).

Figure 3.10E. Same patient as in Figure 3.10D. Despite bad fixation (malfixation index 70% to 100%), the 10° field shows the exact position, size, and shape of the scotoma. With good fixation, the depth of the defect may have been deeper (program: HFA 10-2, representation: Peridata norm-related grayscale).

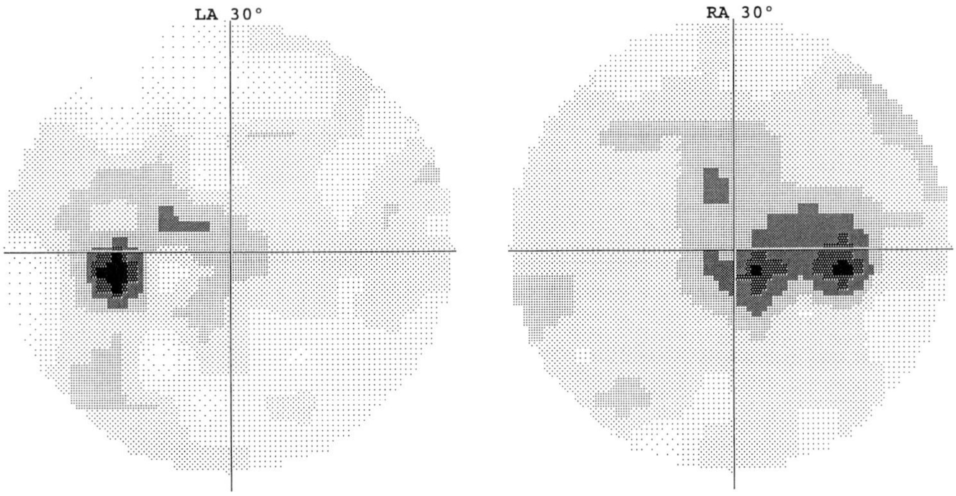

3.10C

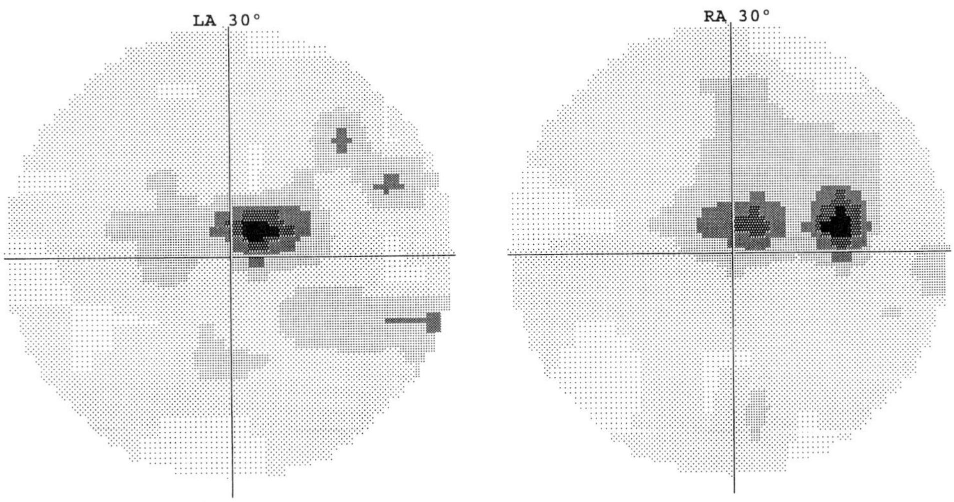

3.10D

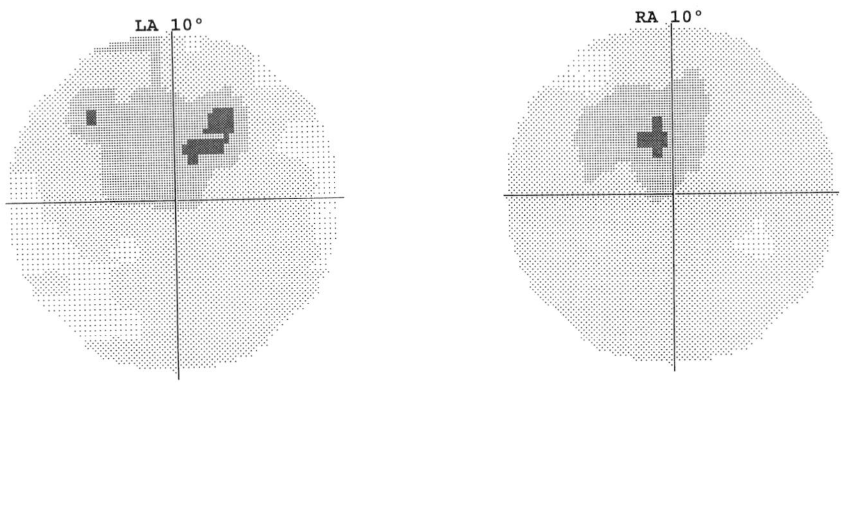

3.10E

Optic Neuritis

Inflammation of the optic nerve typically causes a large centrocecal scotoma in the acute stage. In the natural course of the disease, the functional damage persists longest in the center (Fig. 3.10F).

In addition to the typical cecocentral scotoma, there are functional impairments throughout the whole field which are irregular and not readily assessable with kinetic perimetry. Using static perimetry, the existence of other defect patterns was detected (Fig. 3.10G–M). Pathognomonic signs are involvement of the center, decreased visual acuity, and—excluding the rare syndrome of Devic—unilateral involvement. Young age (15–35 years), acute onset, and a significant afferent pupillary defect are additional signs.

Figure 3.10F. Optic neuritis in a 15-year-old girl. A series of six visual field measurements were made at intervals of 3 to 7 days. Visual acuity improved from 0.05 (first field) to 0.8 (last field). Moderate doses of systemic steroids were common in those days (program: HFA 30-2, representation: Peridata norm-related grayscale).

Figure 3.10G. Diffuse depression in a case of optic neuritis (right eye, program: HFA 30-2, representation: Peridata norm-related grayscale).

Figure 3.10H. Loss of the superior half in a case of optic neuritis (right eye, program: HFA 30-S custom program, representation: Peridata norm-related grayscale).

Figure 3.10J. Nasal hemianopia in a case of optic neuritis (right eye, program: HFA 30-2, representation: Peridata norm-related grayscale).

Figure 3.10K. Nerve fiber bundle defect in a case of optic neuritis (right eye, program: HFA 30-2, representation: Peridata norm-related grayscale).

Figure 3.10L. Temporal nerve fiber bundle defect in a case of optic neuritis (right eye, program: HFA 30-S custom program, representation: Peridata norm-related grayscale).

Figure 3.10M. Combined defect in a case of optic neuritis: cecocentral scotoma, temporal sector, and nasal wedge (right eye, program: HFA 30-2, representation: Peridata norm-related grayscale).

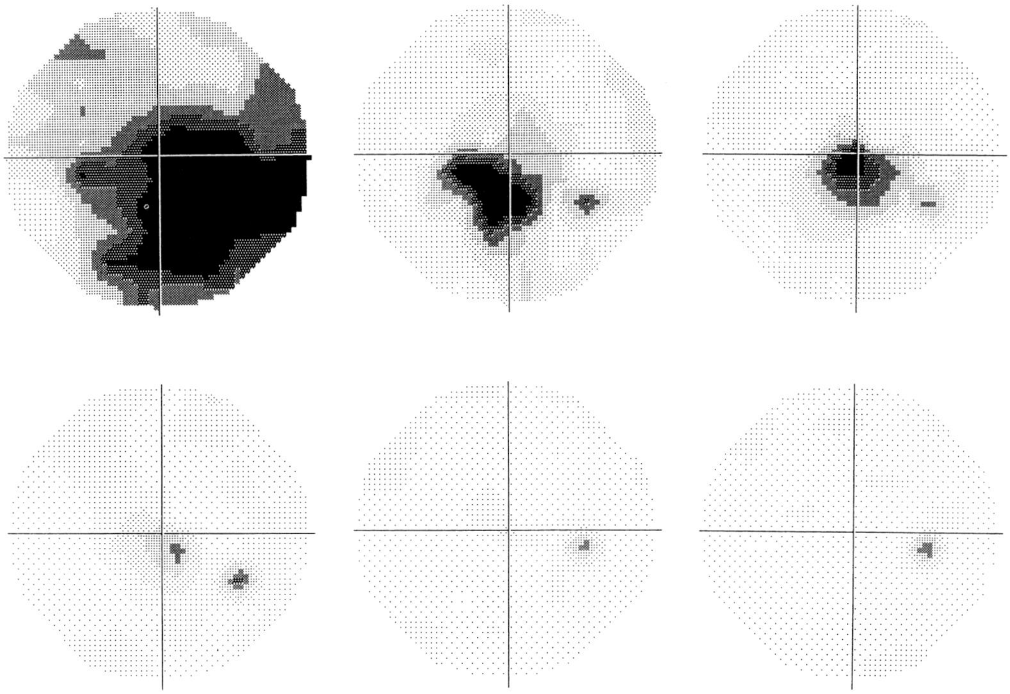

3.10F

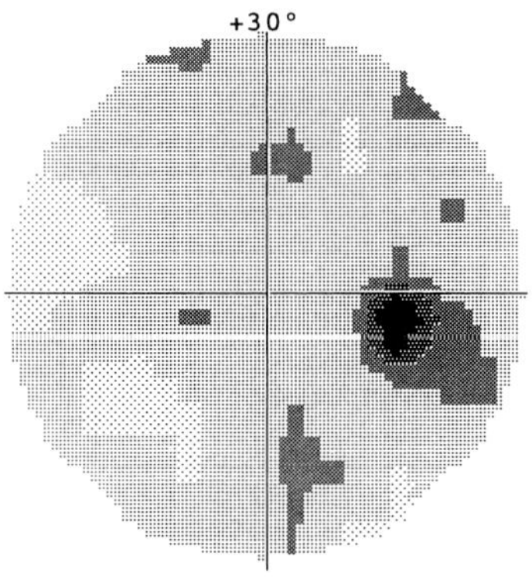

3.10G

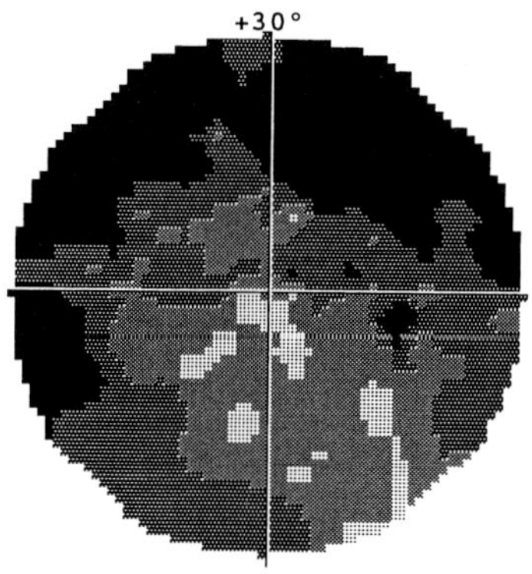

3.10H

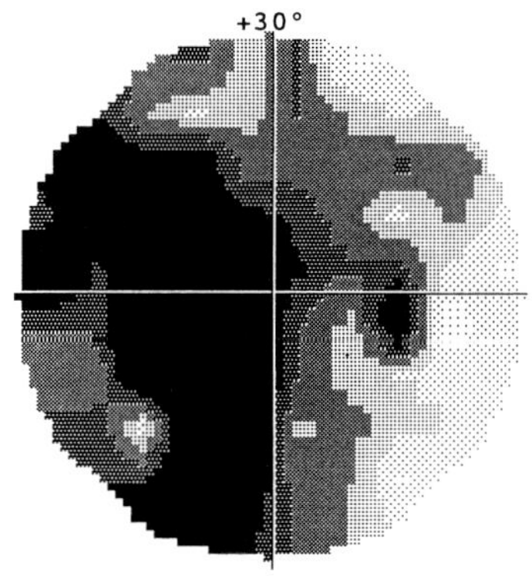

3.10J

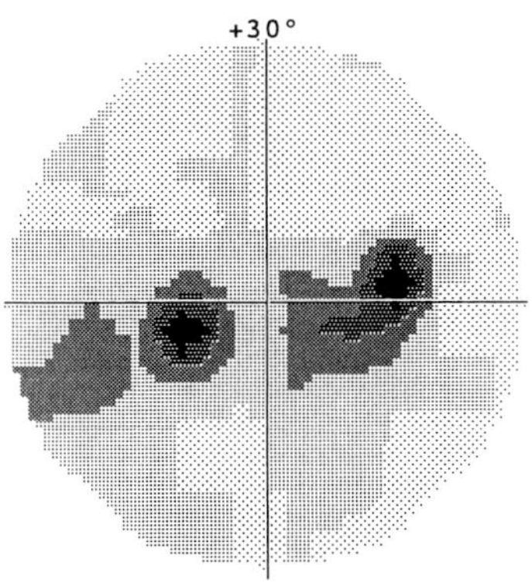

3.10K

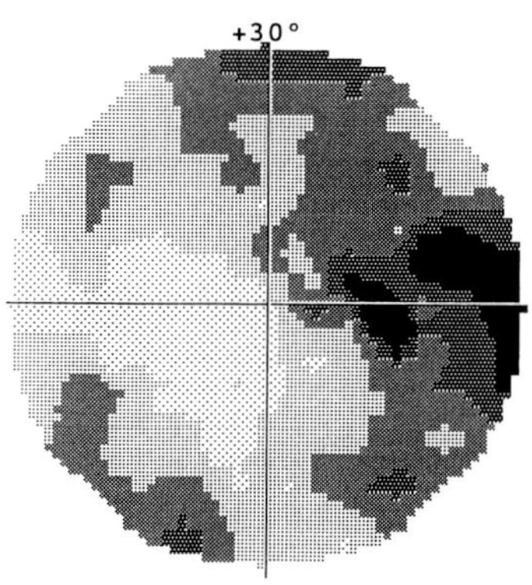

3.10L

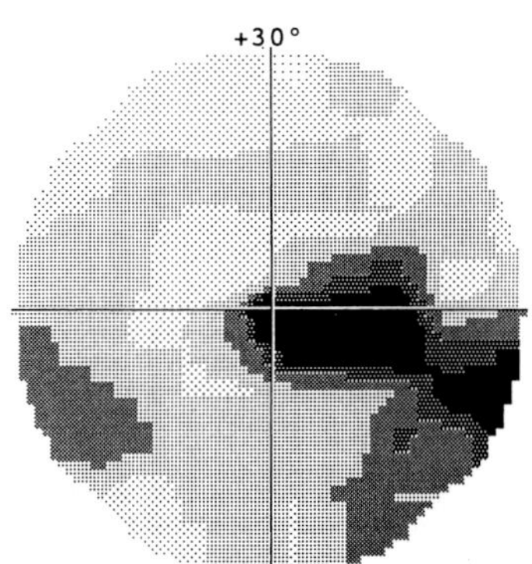

3.10M

3.11 ORBITAL DISORDERS

Principle

Orbital disorders are pathological processes which have their primary origin in the optic nerve sheath or outside the optic nerve. Several mechanisms are responsible for the functional damage. Compression leads to a direct mechanical interference with axonal flux, resulting in sectoral, peripheral, or sometimes diffuse visual field defects. The orbital edema causes relatively severe peripapillary edema and, therefore, a relative or absolute scotoma around the blind spot *(pericecal scotoma)* which is manifested by an enlargement of the blind spot. Stenosis and obliteration of the posterior ciliary arteries may occur, followed by choroidal ischemia with paracentral, spotty field defects. Reduced perfusion of the optic nerve head may cause nerve fiber bundle defects. Exophthalmos may lead to corneal problems, with generalized depression of the field. Figure 3.11A shows the main mechanisms.

Figure 3.11A. Topographical principle of visual field defects due to orbital disorders. Compression leads to a sector-shaped peripheral lesion of the optic nerve, with consecutive nerve fiber bundle defects in the field. With orbital edema, the peripapillary edema causes a pericecal field defect.

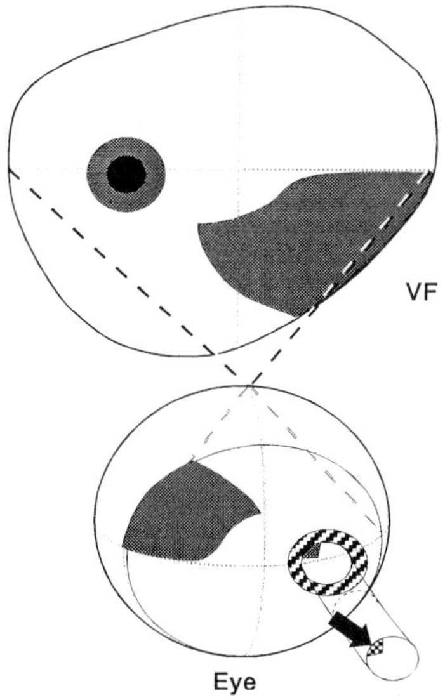

3.11A

Trauma

Accidental and surgical trauma which primarily damages the orbit may secondarily affect the optic nerve by compression due to hemorrhage or edema. Figure 3.11B–C shows an example in which disk edema and peripapillary edema are the main signs. The visual field defect is reminiscent of a refractive scotoma or staphyloma scotoma.

Fig 3.11B. Right visual field of a 30-year-old patient with orbital bleeding on the nasal side after surgical correction of a blowout fracture. Between operations on the fields on the left and right sides, there was a 5-day treatment period with high-dose systemic steroids. Visual acuity was always 1.0 (right eye, program: HFA 30-2, representation: Peridata norm-related grayscale).

Figure 3.11C. Fundus photograph of the patient in Figure 3.11B. Visible, dune-shaped folding of the retina is seen in the lower half.

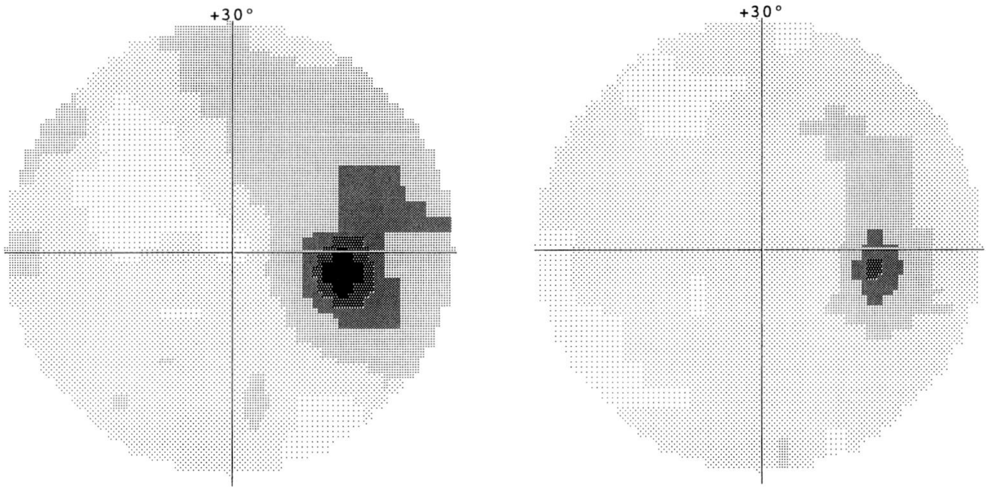

3.11B

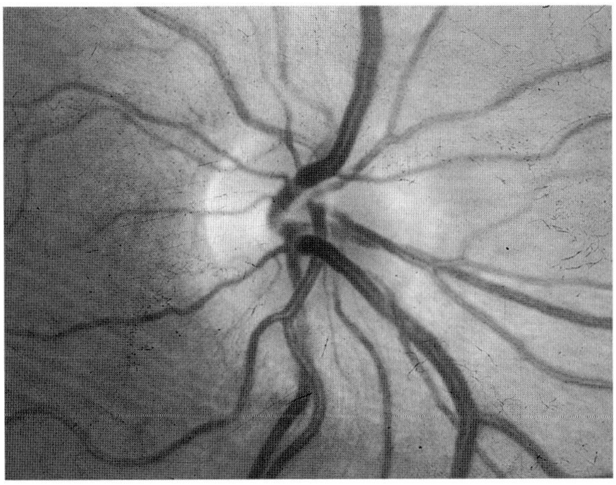

3.11C

Graves' Disease (Thyroid Ophthalmopathy)

In Graves' disease, several factors may be responsible for functional reduction. In mild cases, lid retraction and infrequent blinking can cause dry eyes and diffuse reduction in sensitivity (Fig. 3.11D). In severe cases with disc edema, pericecal scotomas and sectoral defects are found (Fig. 3.11E–F).

Figure 3.11D. Graves' disease in a 46-year-old man. Exophthalmos (proptosis) occurred but no disc edema was found, and full visual acuity was retained. The visual field shows generalized, homogeneous depression (program: HFA 30-2, representation: Peridata norm-related grayscale).

Figure 3.11E. Graves' disease in a 66-year-old man. The left visual field suffers from a lower temporal quadrantanopia, combined with deeper relative defects in the adjacent quadrants. The right visual field has an enlarged blind spot and a peripheral nerve fiber bundle defect. The visual acuity was 0.4 in both eyes (program: HFA 30-S custom program, representation: Peridata norm-related grayscale).

Figure 3.11F. Same patient as in Figure 3.11E, showing disc edema with hemorrhage on both sides.

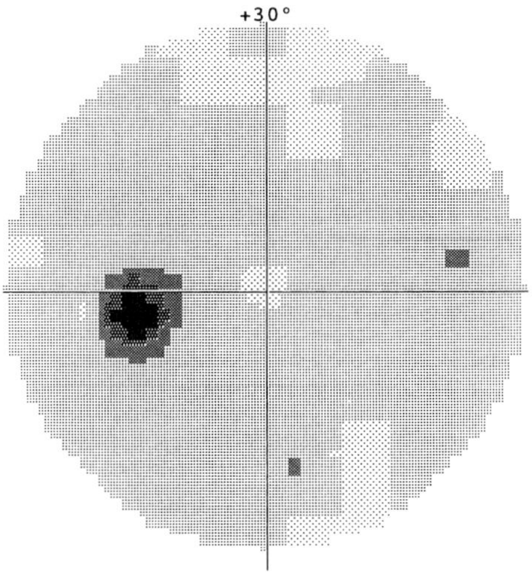

3.11D

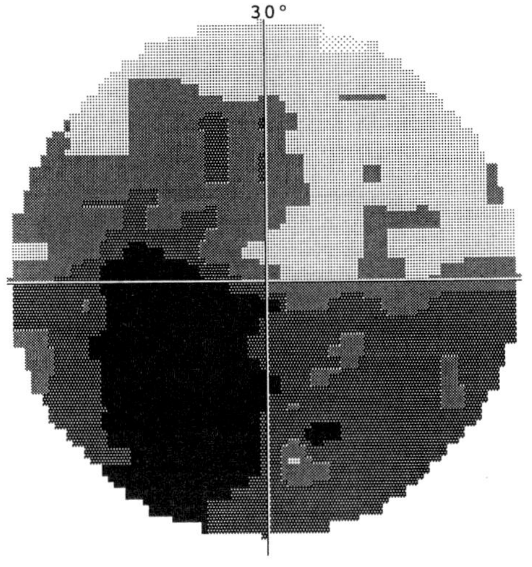

3.11E

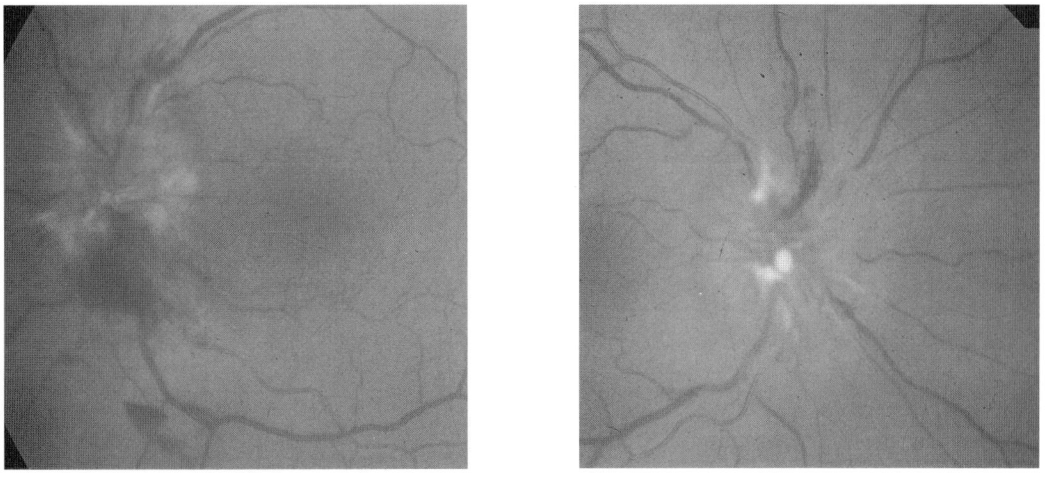

3.11F

Orbital Meningioma

Even a small optic nerve sheath meningioma may cause considerable visual field defects. Modern imaging techniques can usually localize these tumors and follow their changes in size. In Figure 3.11G, the size of the lesion did not change on computed tomography, but the visual field deteriorated slowly (the interval between tests was 1 year). Surgery was not performed since it was more likely to destroy the remaining visual field than to save it.

Orbital apex meningiomas are often associated with altitudinal defects (Fig. 3.11 H–J). Appropriate perimetric resolution shows that the cecocentral region is often preserved; visual acuity is still good at this stage. In more advanced stages, the visual field damage progresses as the optic sheath meningioma grows larger.

Figure 3.11G. Optic nerve sheath meningioma in the right eye of a 61-year-old patient. In this patient, 30° fields, recorded at 1-year intervals, show deterioration of function. Visual acuity decreased from 0.8 to 0.4 over the same period of time (program: HFA 30-S custom program, representation: Peridata norm-related grayscale).

Figure 3.11H. Orbital apex meningioma (left side) in a 62-year-old patient. Right and left 30° fields are shown. Visual acuity was 1.0 in both eyes (program: HFA 30-S custom program, representation: Peridata norm-related grayscale).

Figure 3.11J. Sphenoid ridge meningioma with involvement of the left orbital apex after surgery. Visual acuity was 0.5 in the left eye and 0.7 in the right eye; 30° fields are shown (program: HFA 30-2, representation: Peridata norm-related grayscale).

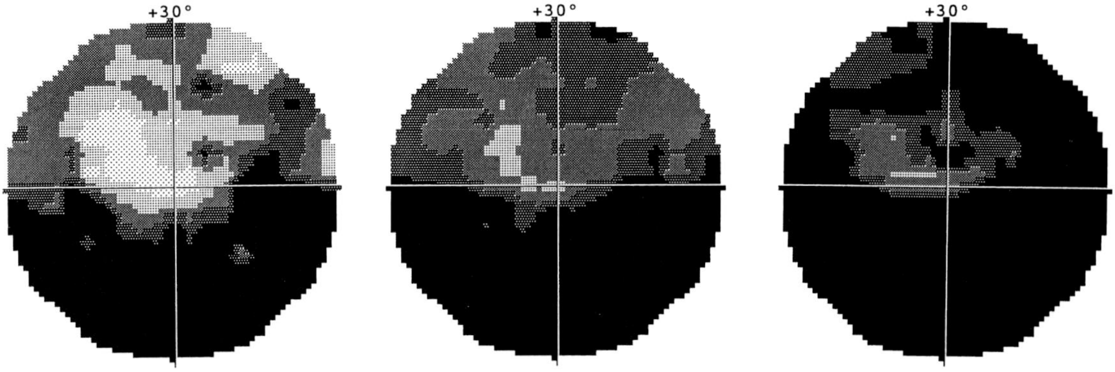

3.11G

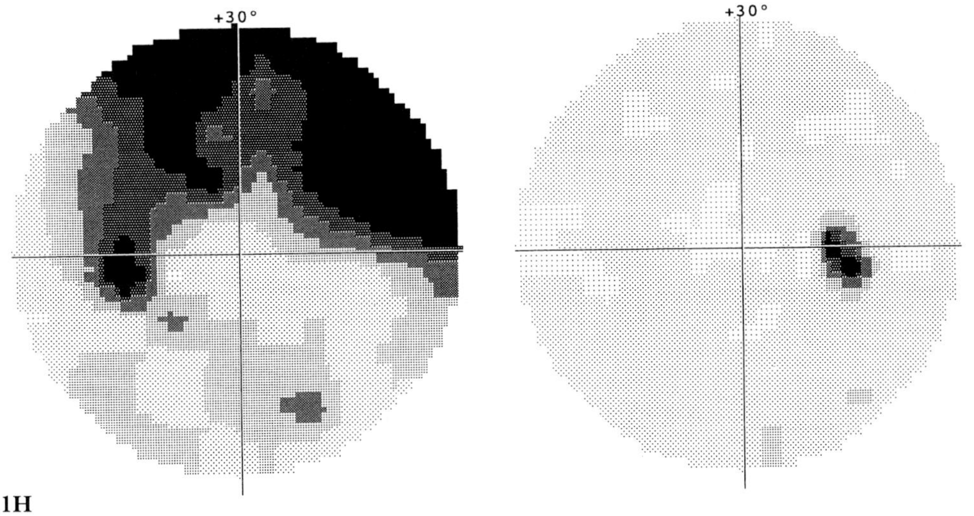

3.11H

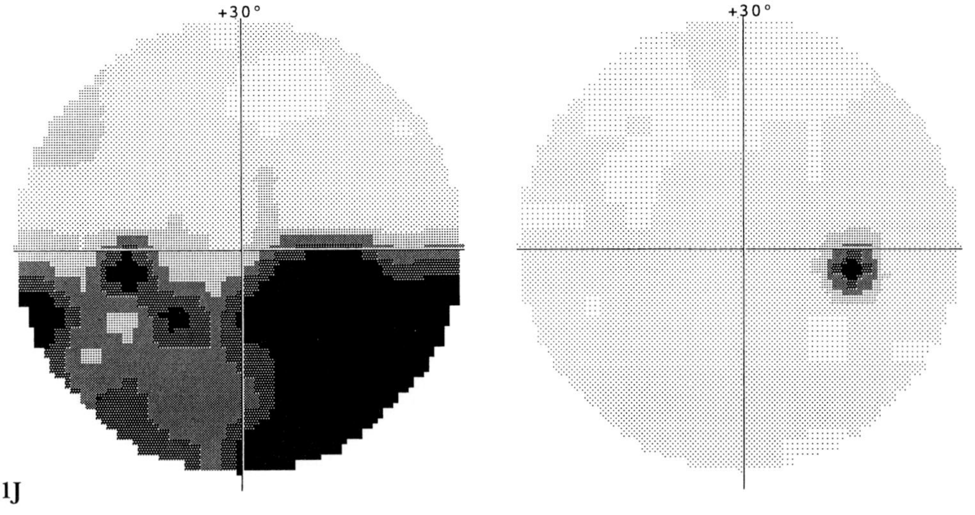

3.11J

3.12 OPTIC CHIASM

General Remarks

The chiasm is an area of substantial, complicated regrouping and crossover of nerve fibers. Topographically, consecutive visual field defects vary widely, but they can be classified into several types. The most frequent lesions involve damage to the anterior crus and the center of the chiasm. Isolated lateral lesions or damage to the posterior crus are rare and will not be discussed in this text.

Principle of Anterior Lesions of the Chiasm

Lesions of one of the anterior branches of the chiasm not only cause ipsilateral damage to the optic nerve but also damage to axons from the contralateral optic nerve. The lower part of axons crossing from the contralateral optic nerve do not run straight into the optic tract but curve into the anterior crus. This anatomical peculiarity, called *Wilbrand's knee,* is named after its discoverer (Fig. 3.12A). The associated visual field defect is an upper quadrantic defect of the contralateral field. The equilateral side has a total or subtotal loss of function. This important clinical combination is also called an *anterior junctional scotoma.*

Sphenoid Ridge Meningioma

The anterior junctional scotoma is often caused by sphenoid ridge meningiomas. Figure 3.12B is a classical example.

Figure 3.12A. Topographical principle of the anterior junctional scotoma. Due to direct optic nerve compression, the equilateral visual field is damaged totally or subtotally. Damage to the fibers in Wilbrand's knee affects the upper temporal quadrant of the contralateral visual field.

Figure 3.12B. Visual fields in a 44-year-old patient with a sphenoidal meningioma on the left side. The left visual field is severely damaged (visual acuity 0.5); the right visual field has an upper temporal quadrantanopia and mild depression in the lower temporal quadrant. Visual acuity is full (program: HFA 30-1, representation: Peridata norm-related grayscale).

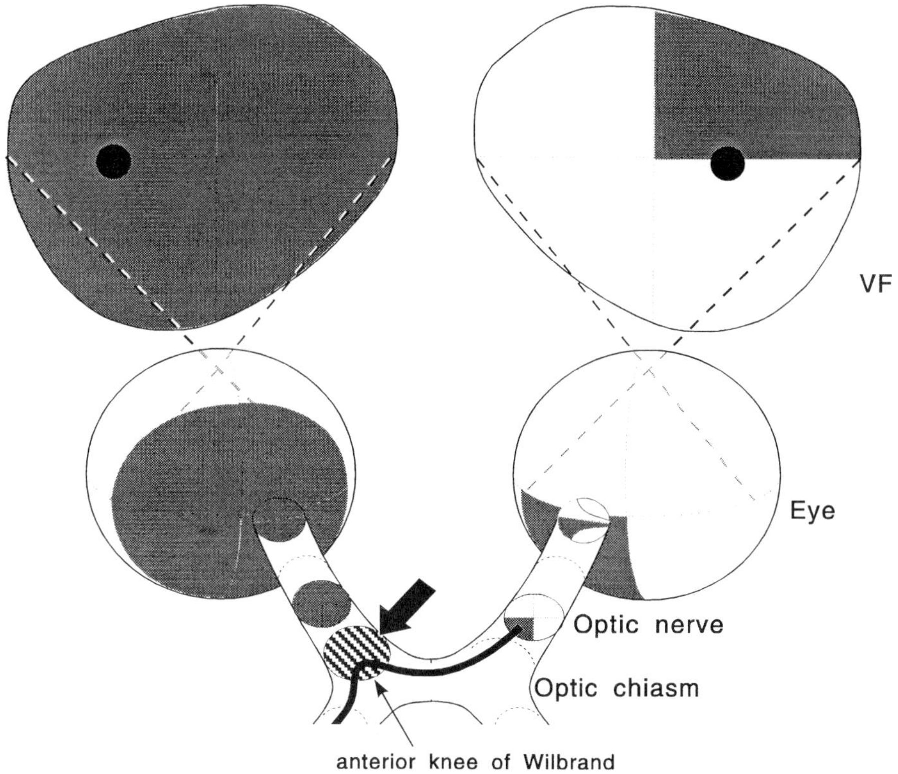
VF
Eye
Optic nerve
Optic chiasm
anterior knee of Wilbrand

3.12A

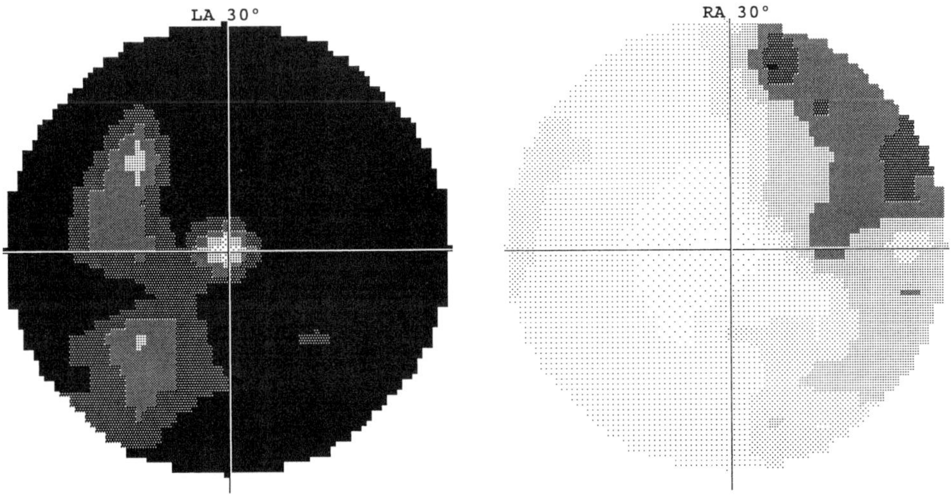
LA 30°
RA 30°

3.12B

Principle of Chiasmal Damage from Below

Damage of the optic chiasm from below is almost always caused by a tumor. A tumor below the chiasm first damages the lower crossing fibers, causing upper temporal quadrant defects in both visual fields (Fig. 3.12C). The next stage is damage to the upper crossing fibers, producing field defects in both lower temporal quadrants. A classic bitemporal hemianopia has then occurred. Progressive tumor growth also damages the lateral, noncrossing fibers. Superior fibers (inferior nasal field quadrant) are damaged first because they run more medially in the posterior part of the chiasm, as indicated in Figure 3.12C. But there are exceptions to this rule. Additional exceptions are found after surgery because of asymmetric, traumatic damage.

First Defects in Pituitary Adenoma

The well-reported early bitemporal defect is seldom found with automated static perimetry. In cases where manual kinetic perimetry shows such a defect, static perimetry usually demonstrates incomplete quadrantic defects. These static defects may be shallow, however. The light gray defects shown in Figure 3.12D have a depth of 5 to 10 dB. They can be assessed only with threshold measurements. Suprathreshold algorithms would miss them because they occur within the tolerance range.

Figure 3.12C. Topographical principle of chiasmal damage from below in chronological order: lower crossing fibers, upper crossing fibers, upper noncrossing fibers, lower noncrossing fibers.

Figure 3.12D. Very mild upper bitemporal quadrant defects in a 24-year-old woman with pituitary adenoma detected because of nonspecific visual disturbances; visual acuity was 1.0 in both eyes. The diagnosis was confirmed at surgery (program: HFA 30-2, representation: Peridata norm-related grayscale).

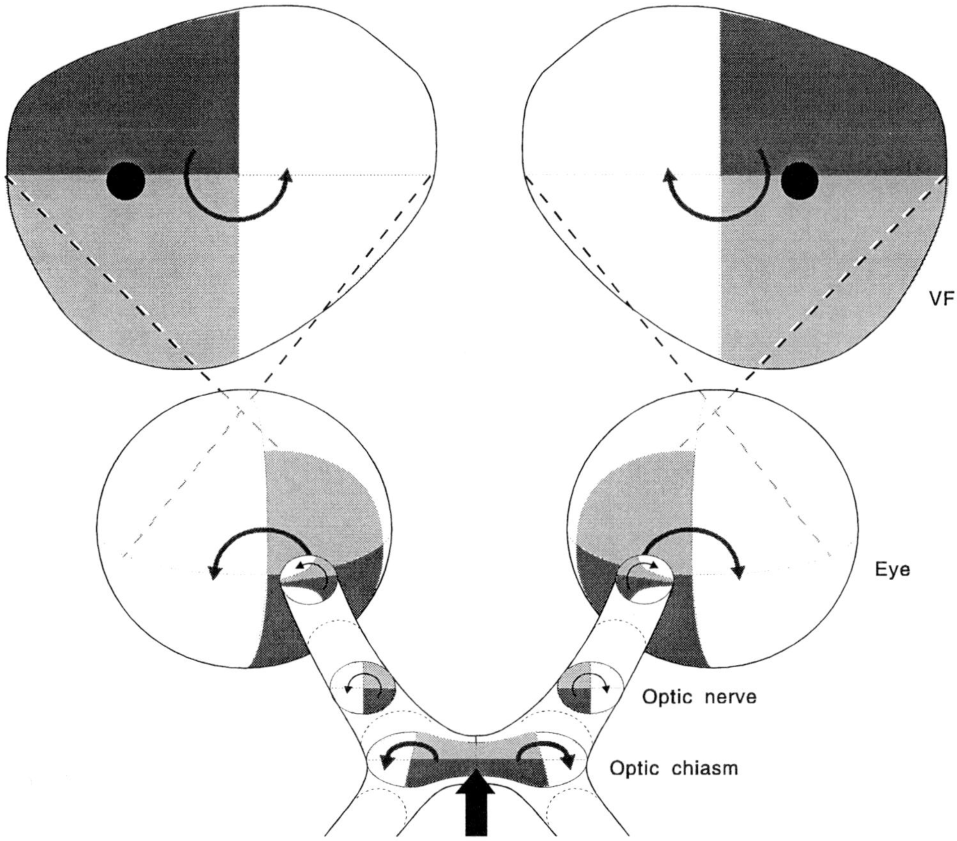

3.12C

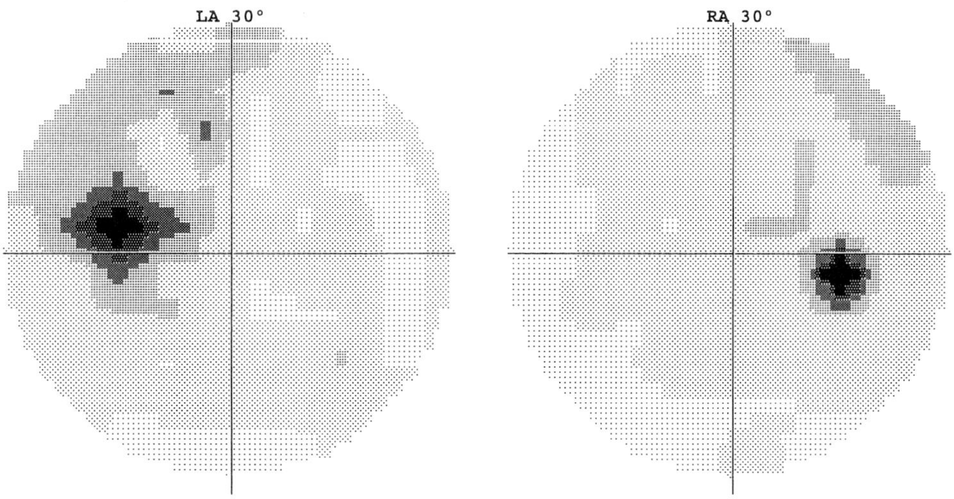

3.12D

Bitemporal Quadrant Defects in Pituitary Adenoma

Quadrantic defects in pituitary adenoma may be shallow (Fig. 3.12E), unilateral (Fig. 3.12F), or complete (Fig. 3.12G). There is always some incongruence between the two fields because the pituitary gland and the chiasm are never aligned exactly at the midline, and the adenoma may not be aligned at the midline.

Figure 3.12E. Relative bitemporal quadrant defect in a 65-year-old man 1 year after surgical removal of a pituitary adenoma. Visual acuity was 0.8 in both eyes (program: HFA 30-2, representation: Peridata norm-related grayscale).

Figure 3.12F. Unilateral quadrantanopia in a pituitary tumor confirmed by computed tomography. The patient was a 56-year-old man with suspected adenoma. Visual acuity was 0.8 in the left eye and 0.2 in the right eye (program: HFA 30-2, representation: Peridata norm-related grayscale).

Figure 3.12G. Typical upper bitemporal quadrant defect in a 55-year-old man. One month later, a pituitary adenoma was removed. Visual acuity was 0.8 in both eyes (program: HFA 30-2, representation: Peridata norm-related grayscale).

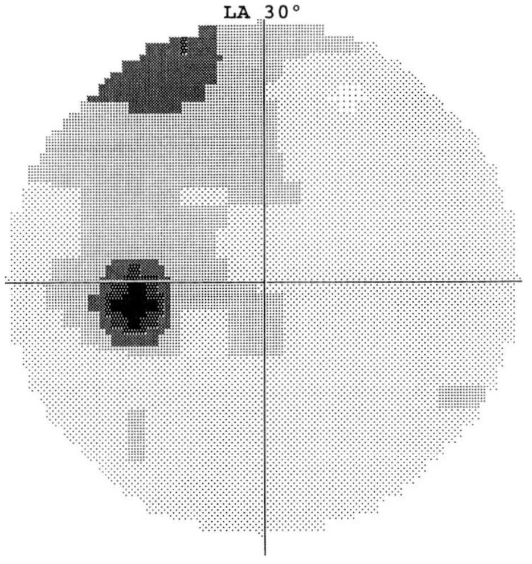

3.12E

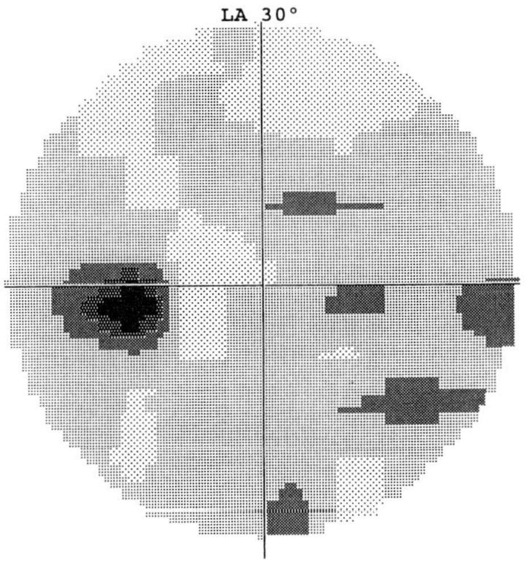

3.12F

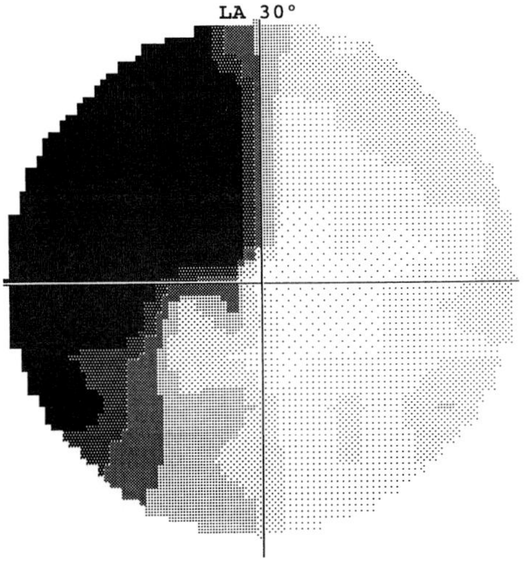

3.12G

Bitemporal Hemianopia in Pituitary Adenoma

Even hemianopic defects are not always congruent. There may be differences in the extent (Fig. 3.12H) and the depth of the defects (Fig. 3.12J). If all crossing fibers are interrupted, the typical congruent hemianopia is found (Fig. 3.12K). However, initial defects in noncrossing fibers may be incongruent. Figure 3.12J shows an inferonasal quadrant defect on the left side; the right nasal quadrants are mainly intact.

Figure 3.12H. Incomplete bitemporal hemianopia in a histologically confirmed pituitary adenoma in a 53-year-old woman. Visual acuity was 0.8 in both eyes (program: HFA 30-2, representation: Peridata norm-related grayscale).

Figure 3.12J. Incongruent bitemporal hemianopia in a 64-year-old woman. Four months later, a pituitary adenoma was surgically removed. Visual acuity was 0.8 in the left eye and 0.5 in the right eye (program: HFA 30-2, representation: Peridata norm-related grayscale).

Figure 3.12K. Complete bitemporal hemianopia in a 57-year-old man with histologically confirmed pituitary adenoma. Visual acuity was 0.8 in the left eye and 0.1 in the right eye (program: HFA 30-2, representation: Peridata norm-related grayscale).

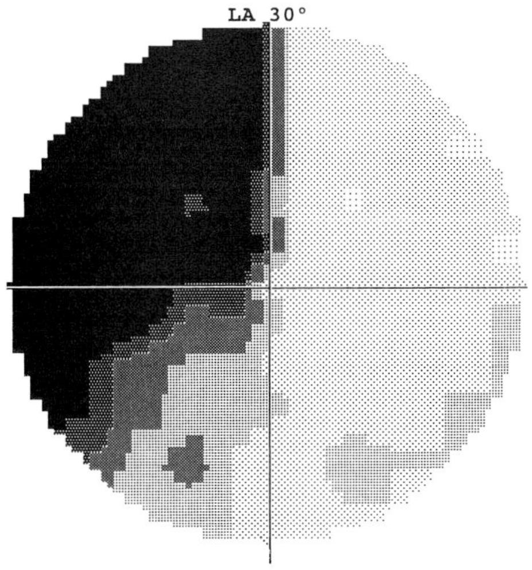

3.12H

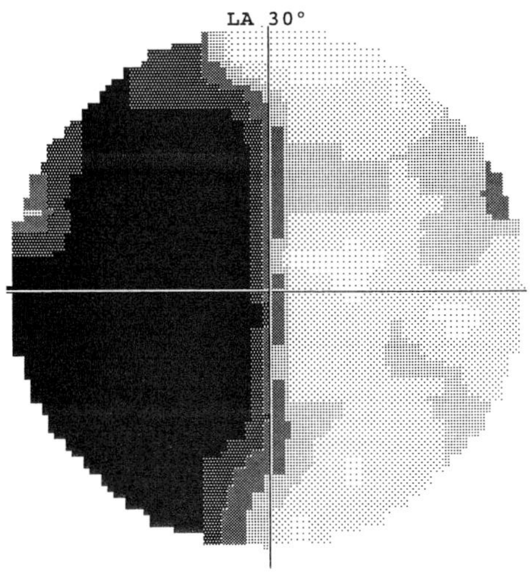

3.12J

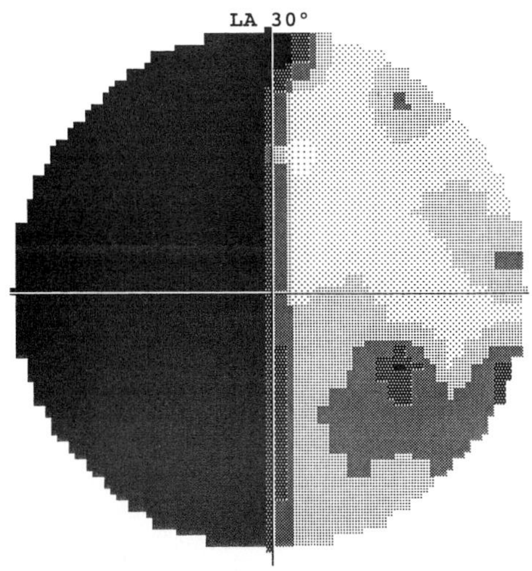

3.12K

Subtotal Defects in Pituitary Adenoma

Even in subtotal defects, the bitemporal pattern is usually detectable (Fig. 3.12L). However, asymmetric damage causes asymmetric field defects even before surgery (Fig. 3.12M–N).

Figure 3.12L. Bitemporal hemianopia with severe damage of the remaining field (*binasal remnant*) in a 61-year-old woman. A few days after perimetry, a chromophobe pituitary adenoma was removed. The visual field recovered considerably. Visual acuity was 0.5 in both eyes (program: HFA 30-2, representation: Peridata norm-related grayscale).

Figure 3.12M. Very large, hormonally active pituitary adenoma in a 53-year-old man treated with a prolactin inhibitor. Incongruent binasal remnants were found. Visual acuity was 1.0 in both eyes (program: HFA 30-2, representation: Peridata norm-related grayscale).

Figure 3.12N. Computed tomogram of the patient in Figure 3.12M. After injection of contrast fluid, the tumor was well visualized.

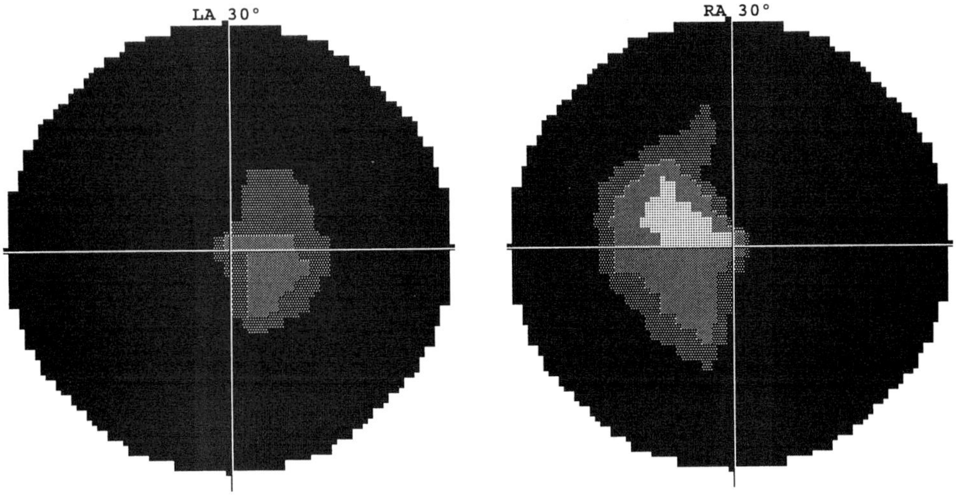

3.12L

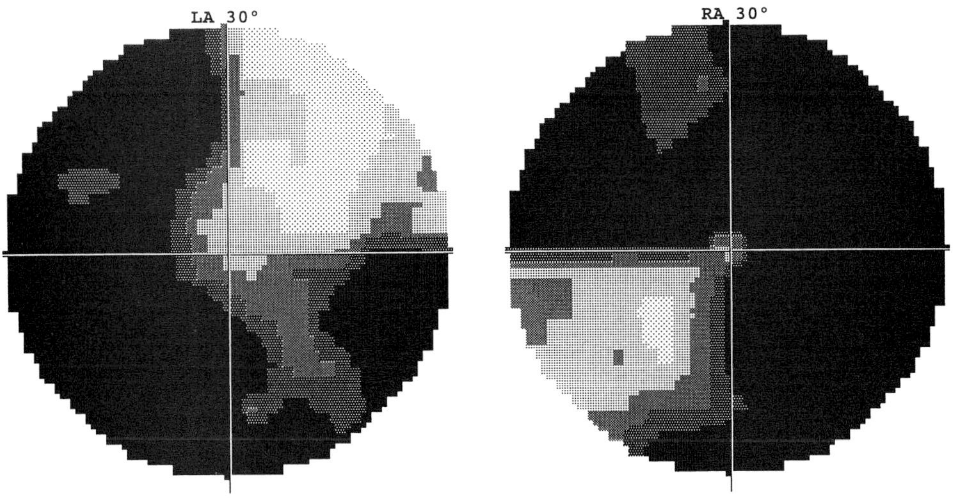

3.12M

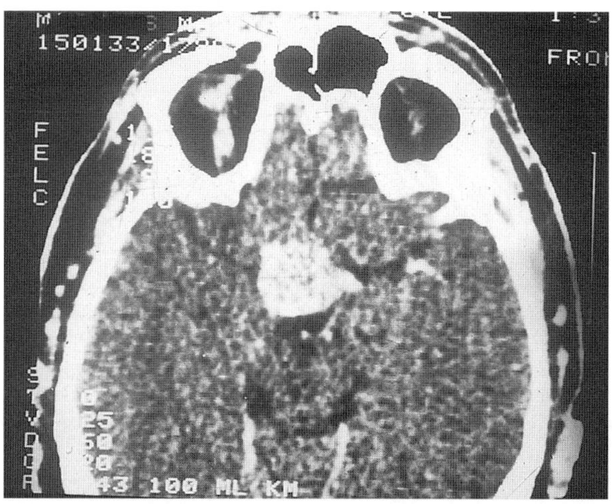

3.12N

Principle of Chiasmal Damage from Above

Tumors which originate from above the chiasm affect the portions of the visual field in the opposite order from that of typical pituitary adenomas. Damage first affects the superior crossing fibers, with a corresponding defect in both lower temporal quadrants (Fig. 3.12P). It is followed by damage to the inferior crossing fibers and, thus, to both upper temporal quadrants. A classical bitemporal hemianopia occurs.

Craniopharyngioma

Craniopharyngioma is the typical cause of a chiasmal lesion from above. Figure 3.12Q shows an example. It should be mentioned that the top position is only one possible, but typical, position of a craniopharyngioma. Other locations are below or lateral to the chiasm, with the corresponding field defects.

Figure 3.12P. Topographical principle of a chiasmal lesion from above in chronological order: first, damage to superior crossing fibers, then damage to inferior crossing fibers.

Figure 3.12Q. Craniopharyngioma in a 49-year-old man confirmed by computed tomography. Visual acuity was 0.6 in both eyes (program: HFA 30-2, representation: Peridata norm-related grayscale).

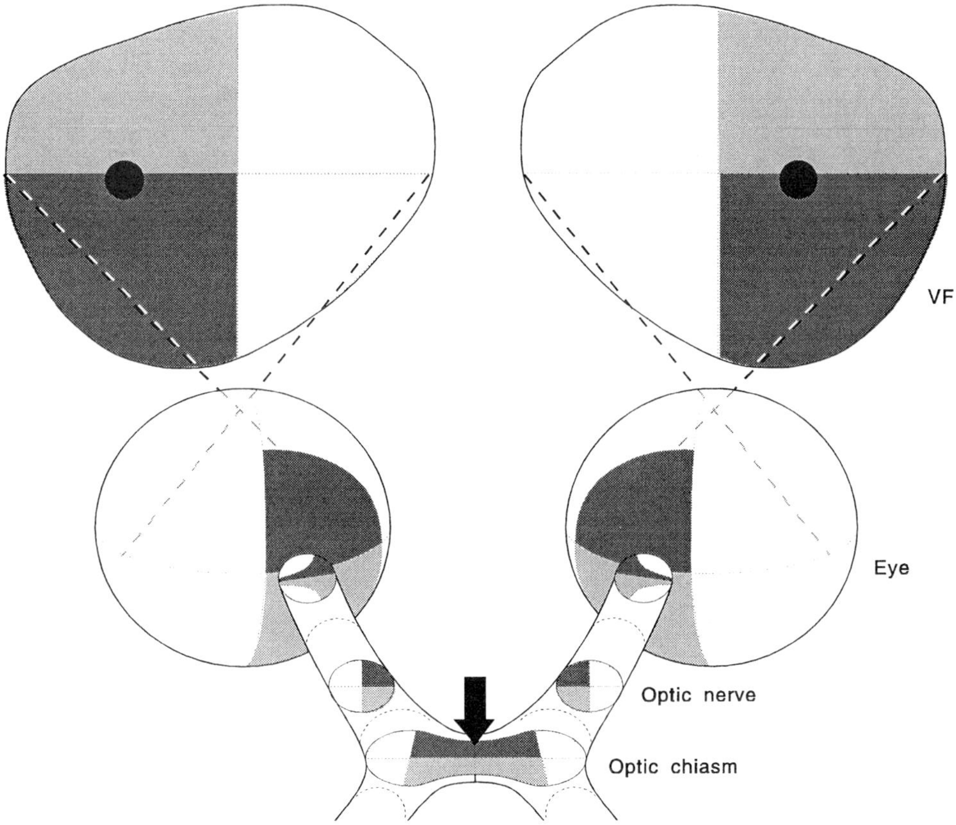

3.12P

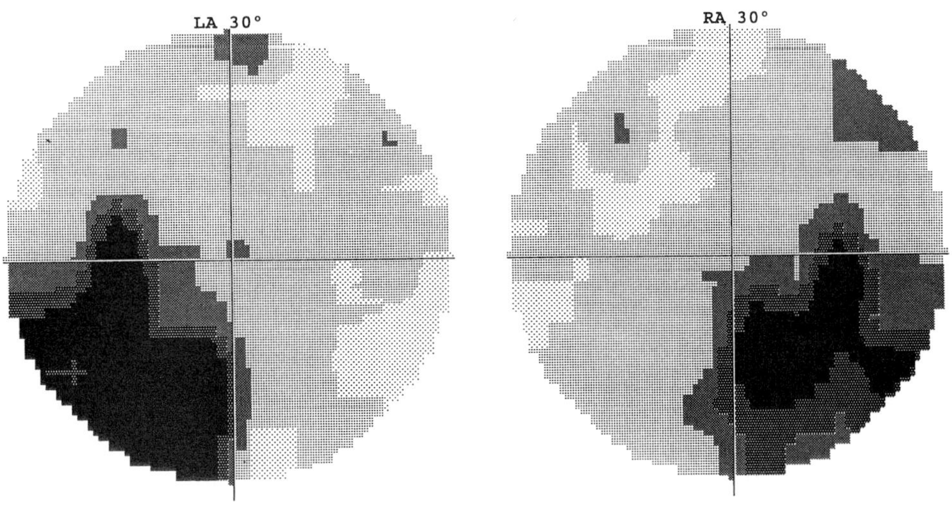

3.12Q

Meningioma with Chiasmal Compression

Midline meningiomas cause bitemporal hemianopias like pituitary adenomas (Fig. 3.12R). With severe damage, the nasal field quadrants are affected in a similar way (Fig. 3.12S). The more frequent type of meningioma shows eccentric growth with blindness on one side and temporal hemianopia (Fig. 3.12T) on the contralateral side. Macular sparing may be more frequent in meningioma than in adenoma.

Figure 3.12R. Suprasellar meningioma in a 57-year-old woman 2 years after her first operation. Visual acuity was 0.8 in both eyes (program: HFA 30-2, representation: Peridata norm-related grayscale).

Figure 3.12S. Pre- and suprasellar meningioma in a 70-year-old woman before surgery. Visual acuity was 0.1 in the left eye and 0.7 in the right eye (program: HFA 30-2, representation: Peridata norm-related grayscale).

Figure 3.12T. Pre- and suprasellar meningioma after multiple surgery in a 48-year-old man. Visual acuity was 0.1 in the left eye, with no light in the right eye (program: HFA 30-2, representation: Peridata norm-related grayscale; the right field was artificially created).

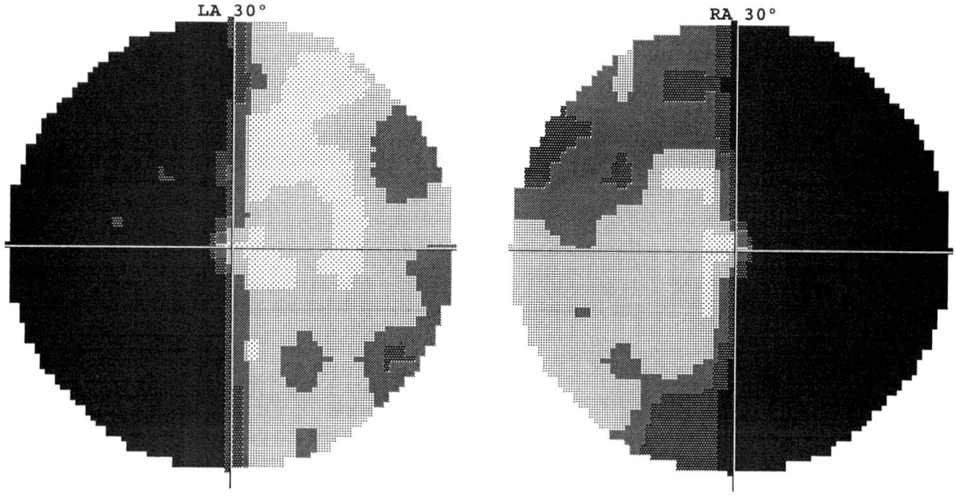

3.12R

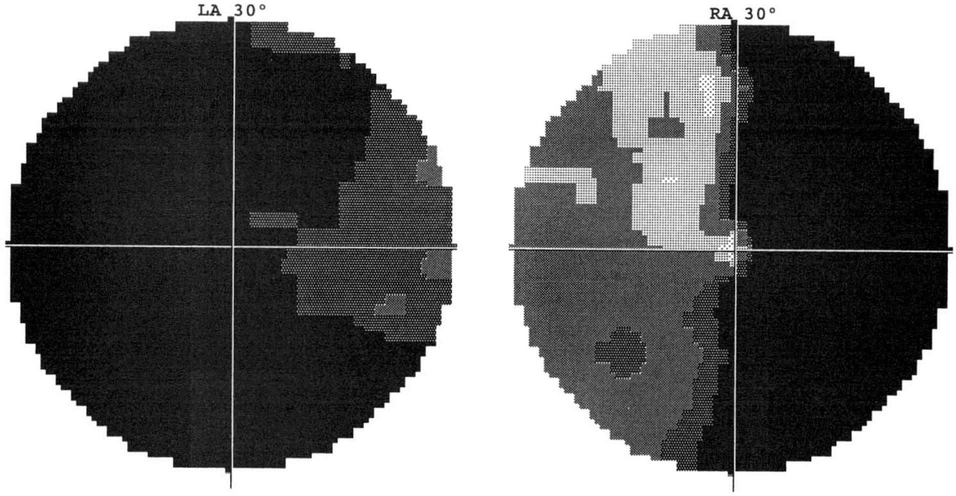

3.12S

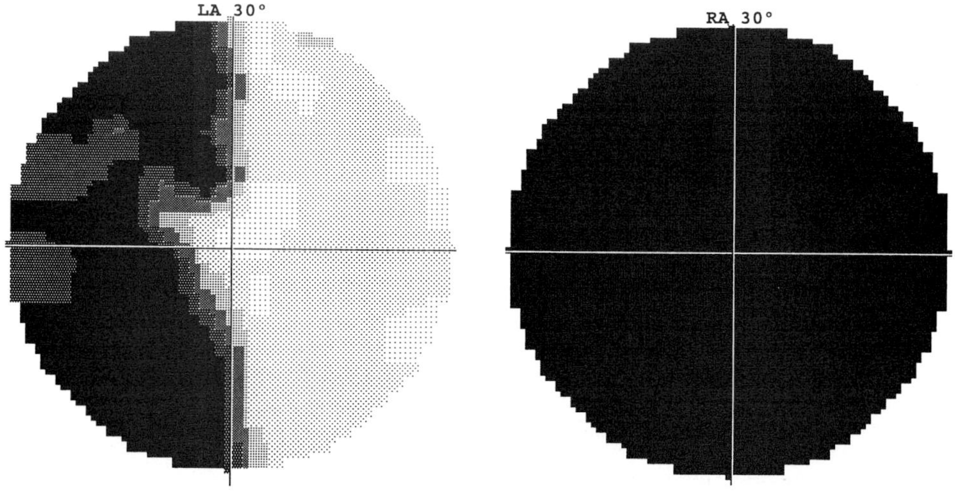

3.12T

3.13 OPTIC TRACT AND LATERAL GENICULATE BODY

Principle

The optic tract consists of fibers from the lateral retinal halves of both eyes. Posterior to the chiasm, their positions are rotated. The fibers of the lower retinal quadrant are lateral, and those of the upper retinal quadrant are medial (Fig. 3.13A). Because damage from the outside is more likely, partial damage affects the fibers of the lower retinal quadrants more frequently, producing an homonymous upper quadrantanopia. If quadrants are partially involved, the scotoma borders tend to radiate from fixation, and the scotoma itself appears as a circular sector.

Any irreversible interruption of the optic tract causes a descending optic atrophy, which can be observed ophthalmoscopically as a pale disk 4–6 weeks after the damage occurs. This phenomenon, called the *tract sign,* is an important criterion in differentiating a tract lesion from a suprageniculate lesion.

Congruent Defects in Lesions of the Optic Tract

Complete homonymous hemianopia from an interruption of the optic tract or the lateral geniculate body is always congruent. This condition can be distinguished from suprageniculate lesions by the presence of the tract sign.

Quadrantic defects, because of partial damage of fibers, tend to be congruent (Fig. 3.13B).

Figure 3.13A. Topographical principle of visual field defects in lesions of the optic tract. The more frequent compression from a lateral direction causes a homonymous upper quadrantanopia. In cases of complete damage, a homonymous hemianopia is found.

Figure 3.13B. Congruent lesion of the optic tract after pituitary surgery in a 52-year-old patient. Visual acuity was 1.0 in both eyes (program: HFA 30-2, representation: Peridata norm-related grayscale).

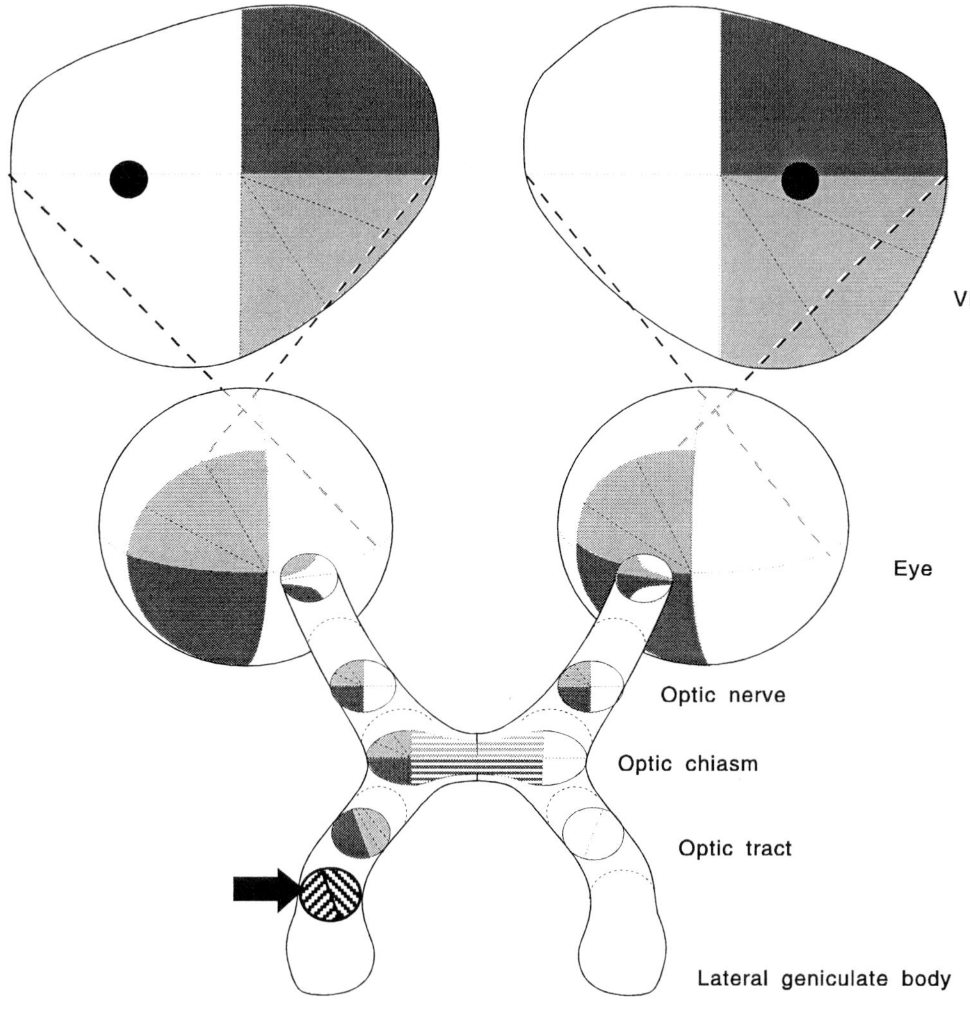
VF
Eye
Optic nerve
Optic chiasm
Optic tract
Lateral geniculate body

3.13A

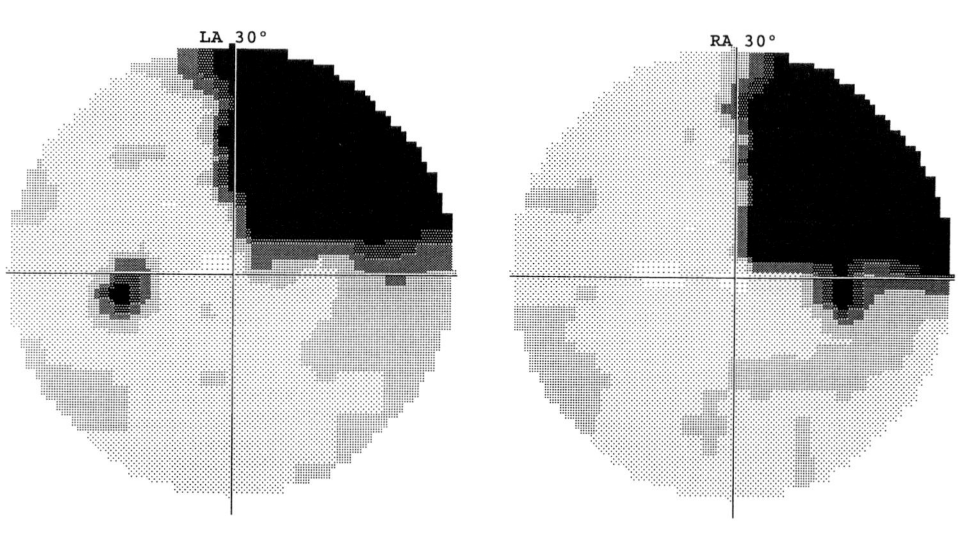
LA 30°
RA 30°

3.13B

Incongruent Defects in Lesions of the Optic Tract

If tract-related visual field defects are incongruent, the field on the side of the damage usually shows more damage. Figure 3.13C shows typical damage of the left optic tract. The ipsilateral left visual field has a nearly complete hemianopia; the right field has lost only an upper quadrant and a lower circular sector. The case in Figure 3.13D represents damage to the right optic tract. The homonymous hemianopia is complete in the right field; in the left field, an upper sector remains undamaged.

Figure 3.13C. Neoplasm in the left basal ganglia of a 15-year-old patient confirmed by computed tomography. Visual acuity was 1.0 in both eyes (program: HFA 30-2, representation: Peridata norm-related grayscale).

Figure 3.13D. Postsurgical status of an aneurysm of the right carotid artery in a 45-year-old patient. Visual acuity was 0.8 in both eyes (program: HFA 30-2, representation: Peridata norm-related grayscale).

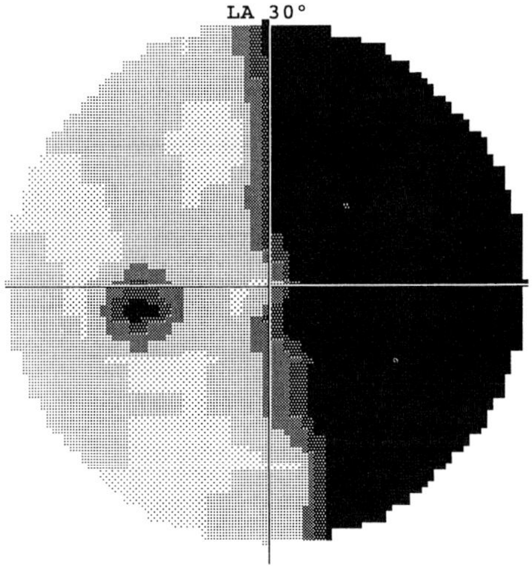

3.13C

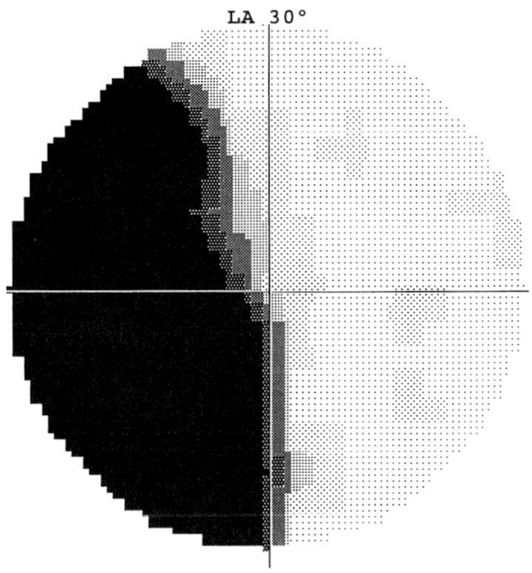

3.13D

3.14 OPTIC RADIATIONS

Principle

In the optic radiations, axons of the fourth order neurons spread out over a wide range. Damage is frequent but often only partial because of the large area over which the radiations spread. If the lower anterior horn is involved (temporal lobe), the contralateral upper quadrant of the visual field is defective (Fig. 3.14A). Other types of damage cause sector defects. Complete interruption of optic fibers causes a dense homonymous hemianopia.

In general, the defect pattern is very similar to that of tract lesions, with a tendency toward greater congruency the more posterior the lesion. In addition, the tract sign (optic nerve pallor) is absent.

Figure 3.14A. Topographical principle of a visual field alteration in lesions of the optic radiations. Lesions of the anterior lower horn cause a homonymous upper quadrantanopia. Other lesions cause sector defects. With complete damage, a homonymous hemianopia occurs.

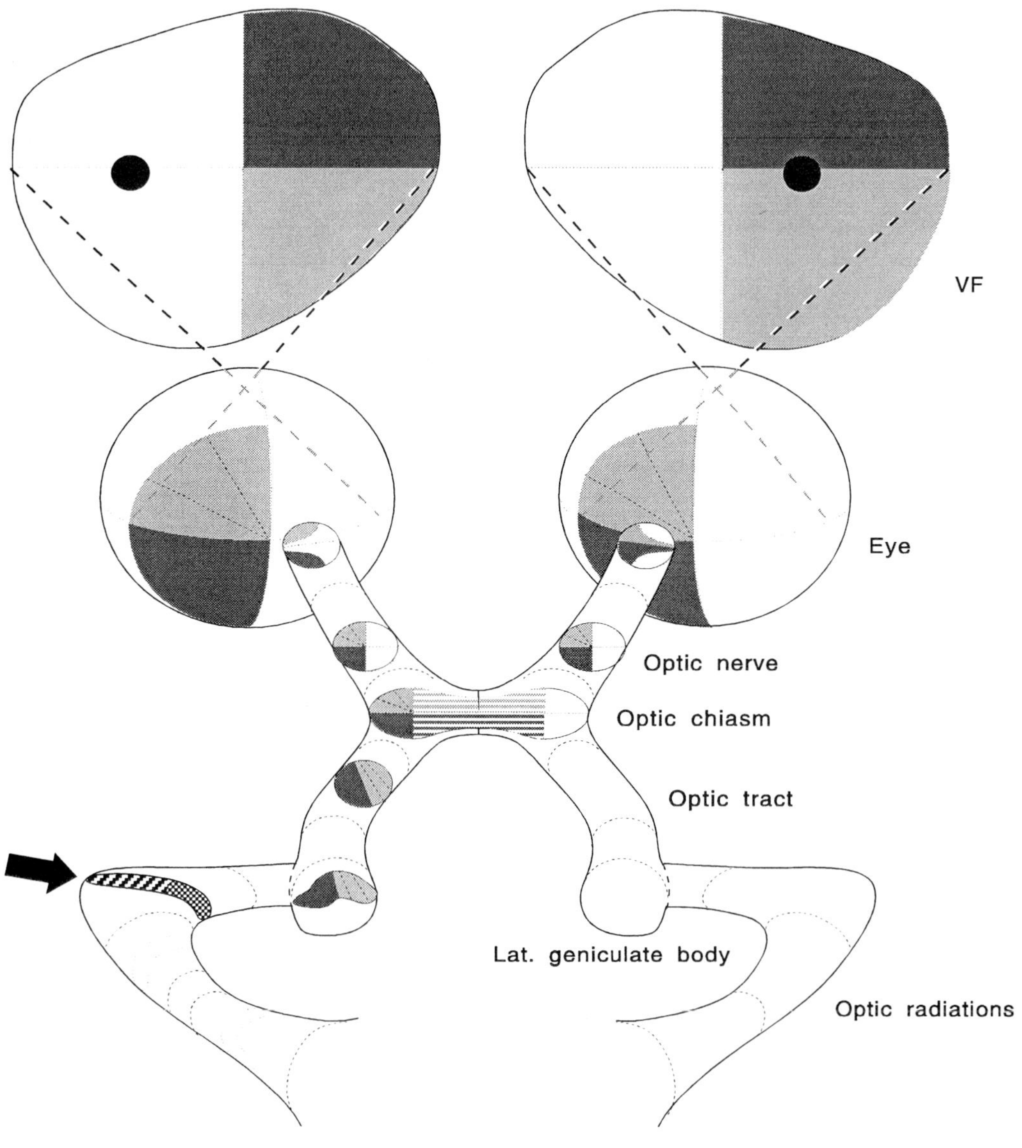
VF
Eye
Optic nerve
Optic chiasm
Optic tract
Lat. geniculate body
Optic radiations

3.14A

Homonymous Quadrant Defects

Upper quadrantic defects indicate a lesion of the anterior lower horn of the optic radiations which contain only fibers from lower retinal quadrants (Fig. 3.14B–C). Lower quadrantic defects can be caused by lesions that originate at the cerebral midline. They are very rare.

Congruent Partial Defects

Incomplete congruent defects often show radial borders, that is, they form circular sectors (Fig. 3.14D). The reason is the arrangement of fibers within the radiations, especially in the anterior part, where the fibers from sectors are close together. More posteriorly, approaching the cortex, they rearrange into groups of similar eccentricity.

Figure 3.14B. Astrocytoma of the left parietal lobe after surgery in a 36-year-old man. Visual acuity was 0.8 in the left eye and 0.1 in the right eye (program: HFA 30-2, representation: Peridata norm-related grayscale).

Figure 3.14C. Computed tomography of the patient shown in Figure 3.14B. In the left brain (right side in the image; the point of view of the tomogram is from caudal to cranial), large substance defects are visible.

Figure 3.14D. Occipital lobe infarct with an incomplete lesion of the optic radiation in a 76-year-old man. Visual acuity was 0.4 in the left eye and 0.5 in the right eye (program: HFA 30-2, representation: Peridata norm-related grayscale).

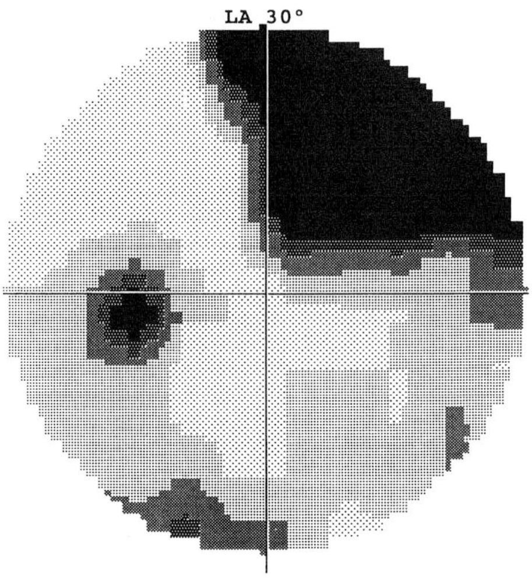

3.14B

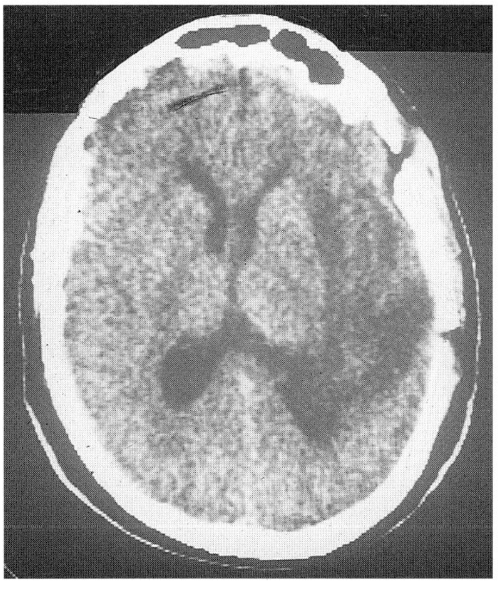

3.14C

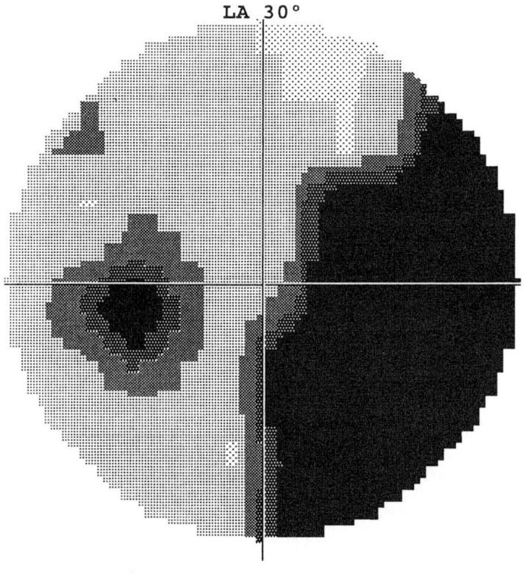

3.14D

Complete Hemianopia

If the radiations are completely interrupted, the visual fields show a homonymous hemianopia (Fig. 3.14E). In these cases, the lesion cannot be localized on the basis of visual fields.

Sparing of Fixation

Based on the topography of nerve fibers in the optic radiations, sparing of fixation is caused by partial, stratified damage of the radiations (Fig. 3.14F–G). It is important to distinguish this condition from a shift of fixation. Evidence of true sparing of the midline includes good central visual acuity and a normal position of the blind spot. Both conditions were found in the example.

Figure 3.14E. Lesion of the right temporal lobe and optic radiation in a 28-year-old man after an automobile accident, confirmed by computed tomography. Visual acuity was 0.2 in the left eye and 0.1 in the right eye (program: HFA 30-2, representation: Peridata norm-related grayscale).

Figure 3.14F. Astrocytoma in the medial cranial fossa of a 40-year-old man after surgery and radiation therapy. Visual acuity was 0.8 in the right eye and 0.1 in the left eye (program: HFA 30-2, representation: Peridata norm-related grayscale).

Figure 3.14G. Computed tomography scan of the patient in Figure 3.14F. In the left brain (see the label "LEFT" in the right part of the image; the point of view of tomography scans is from caudal to cranial), a cystic tissue defect and a bony defect after trephination can be seen.

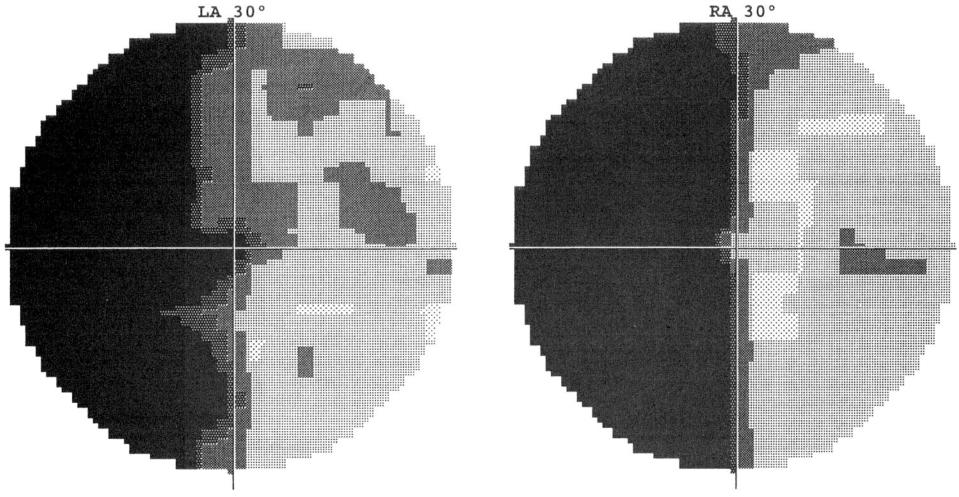

3.14E

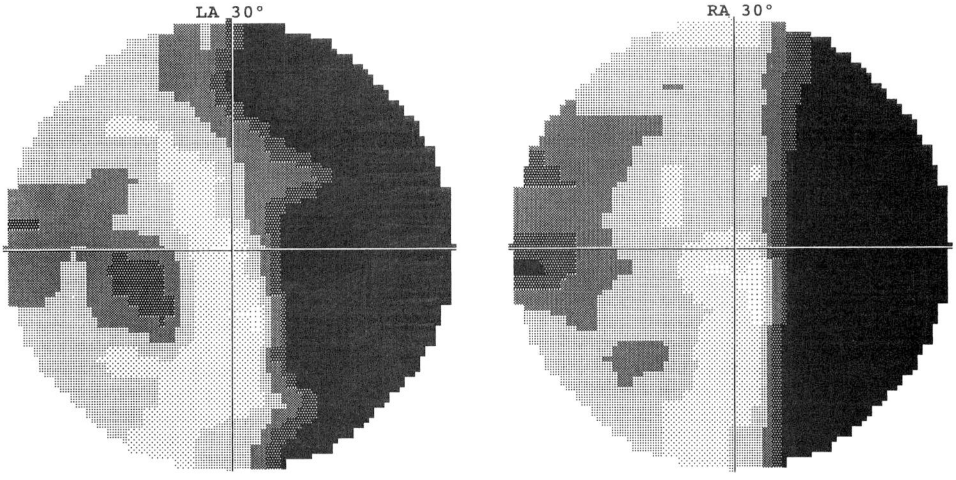

3.14F

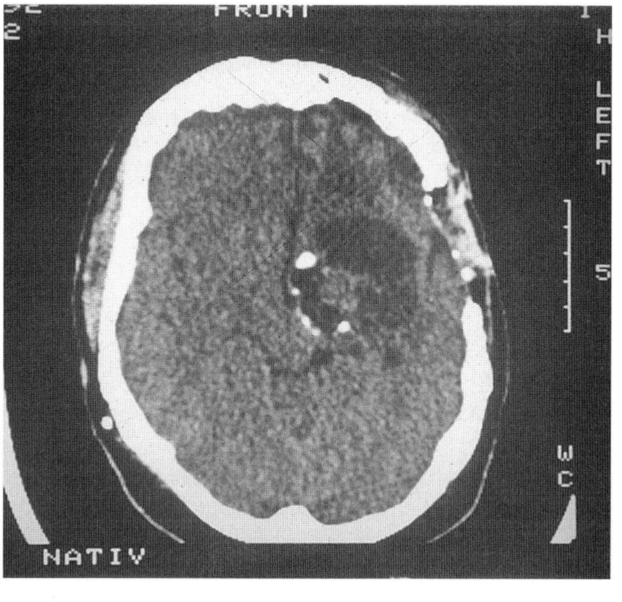

3.14G

Incongruent Partial Defects

Lesions of the optic radiation may show considerable incongruence of the fields (Fig. 3.14H). This characteristic may help to distinguish such lesions from cortical lesions, which are almost perfectly congruent. Smooth radial border lines also indicate damage of the radiation. Rarely, there are small, irregular defects that strongly resemble cortical lesions, but they are less congruent (Fig. 3.14J).

Figure 3.14H. Occipital lobe infarct affecting the optic radiations in a 64-year-old man. The cortex was normal in a computed tomography scan. Visual acuity was 0.8 in the right eye and 0.7 in the left eye (program: HFA 30-2, representation: Peridata norm-related grayscale).

Figure 3.14J. A 37-year-old patient with multiple sclerosis, full visual acuity in both eyes, and homonymous paracentral defects. The defects are best visualized in the 10° fields (bottom) and are more pronounced on the left side (program: HFA 30-2 and 10-2, representation: Peridata norm-related grayscale).

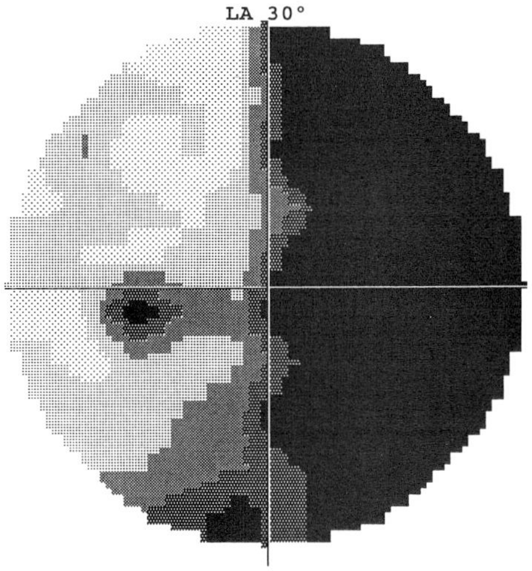

3.14H

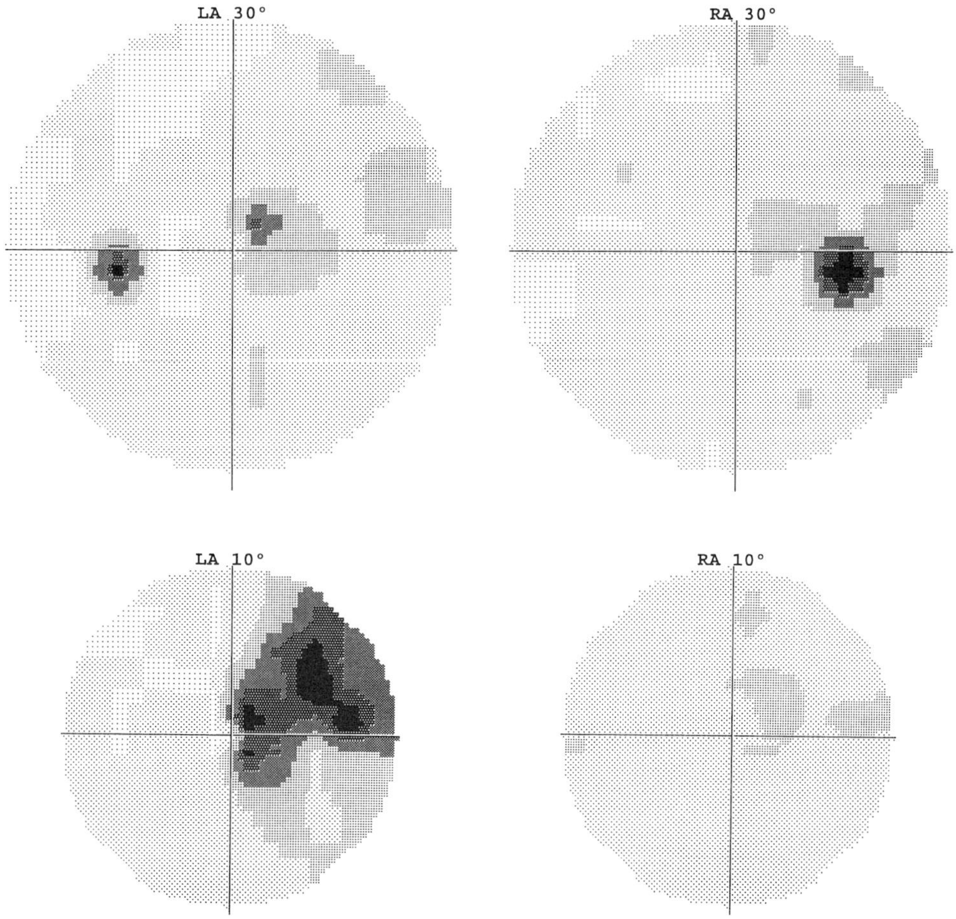

3.14J

3.15 VISUAL CORTEX

Principle

Like other suprachiasmal lesions, lesions of the visual cortex cause homonymous field defects, which are often limited to one-half of the fields. Congruence is considerably greater than with inferior lesions because corresponding fibers of the right and left eyes come together.

Due to the large extent of the visual cortex, partial lesions are frequent. The shape of the defect is often irregular because grouping of fibers—as it is found in inferior parts of the visual pathways—no longer exists (Fig. 3.15A). Because of topography and vascularization, the central field can be preserved (macular sparing) or damaged selectively (central hemianopia). In a few cases, these patterns may also occur with inferior lesions of the visual pathway. Therefore, the differential diagnostic weight of macular sparing or central hemianopia is limited. Increasingly, sophisticated imaging methods are providing precise localization of central lesions.

Figure 3.15A. Topographical principle of visual field alteration in lesions of the visual cortex. For a description, see the text.

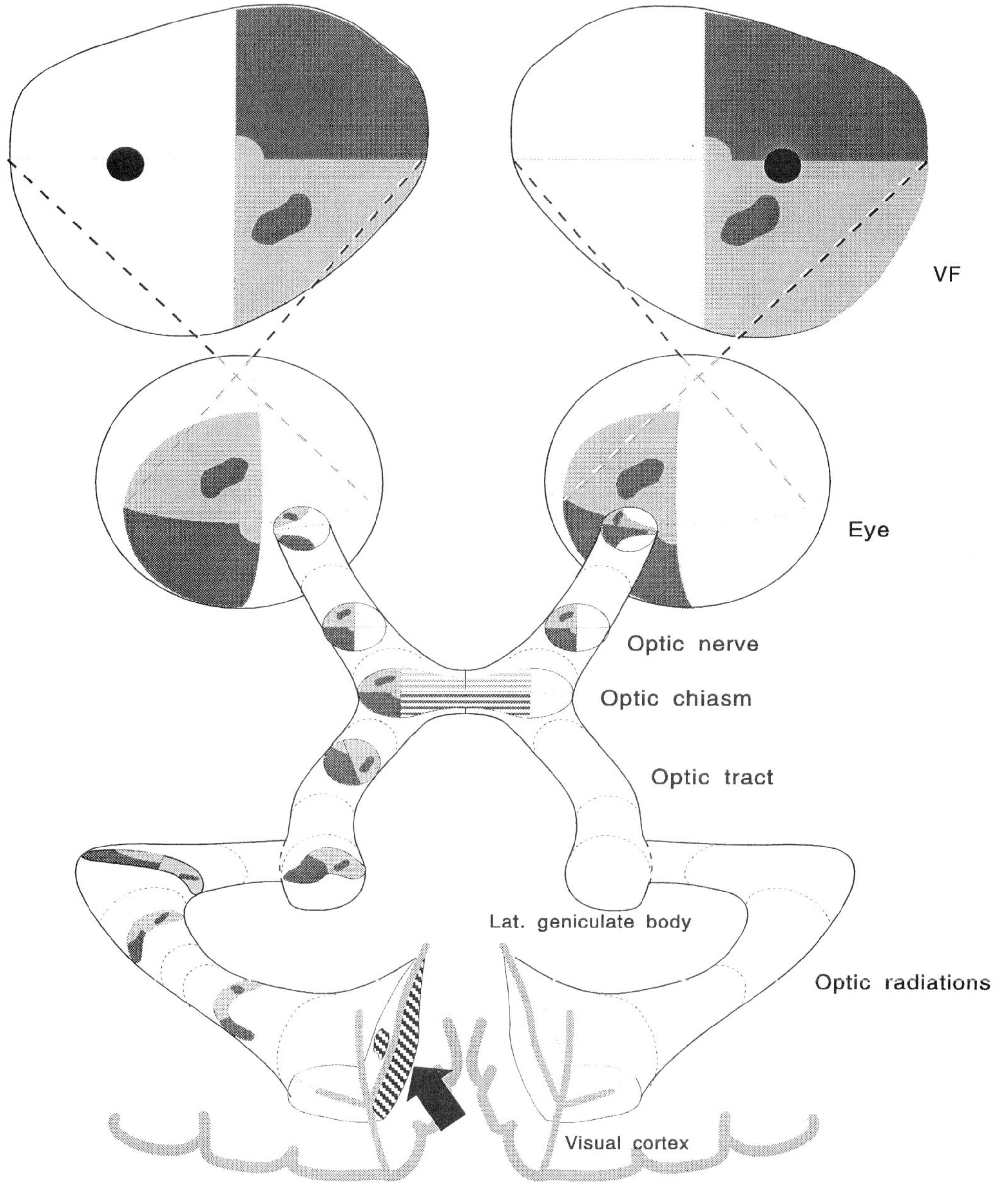
VF
Eye
Optic nerve
Optic chiasm
Optic tract
Lat. geniculate body
Optic radiations
Visual cortex

3.15A

Complete Homonymous Hemianopia

Hemianopic defects in lesions of the occipital cortex often have a small, semicircular field remnant in the center of the damaged half called *macular sparing*. The size of this remnant is not assessed properly with the usual perimetric programs, which have a resolution of 4°–6°. Also, Figures 3.15B and 3.15C are based on a paraxial 6° pattern. An additional measurement location is located in the center. Because this central point revealed normal sensitivity in both cases, interpolation led to a small apparent semicircle. Good visual acuity, good central sensitivity, and the subjective report of the patient are usually sufficient to diagnose macular sparing. For the purpose of follow-up or more precise diagnosis, a high-resolution program is preferable.

In the case of tumors, half of the visual field is usually normal (Fig. 3.15B). In occipital lobe infarcts, the most frequent cause of cortical lesions, there is often a generalized arteriosclerosis. The other cortical half also suffers from ischemia, showing microinfarctions and corresponding visual field alterations (Fig. 3.15C).

Incomplete Homonymous Defects

If incomplete cortical lesions do not cross over the calcarine fissure, quadrantic defects are found. They may be combined with limited damage to the other quadrant (Fig. 3.15D).

Figure 3.15B. Computed tomographically confirmed tumor in the right occipital cortex of a 50-year-old patient with visual acuity of 1.0 on both eyes (program: HFA 30-2, representation: Peridata norm-related grayscale).

Figure 3.15C. Occipital lobe infarct with a hypodense area in a left occipital computed tomography scan in a 54-year-old man with visual acuity of 1.0 in both eyes (program: HFA 30-2, representation: Peridata norm-related grayscale).

Figure 3.15D. Occipital lobe infarct caused by a hypoplastic vertebral artery in a 48-year-old man. Visual acuity was 0.8 in the right eye and 0.1 in the left eye (program: HFA 30-2, representation: Peridata norm-related grayscale).

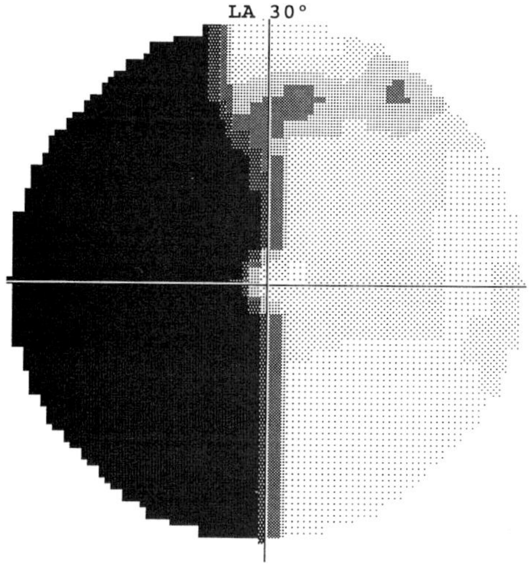

3.15B

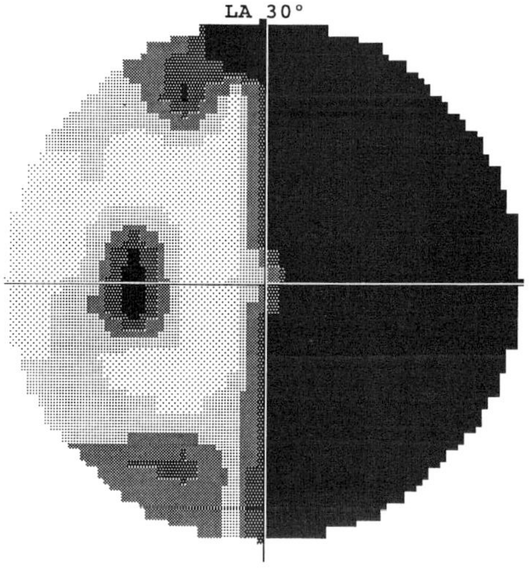

3.15C

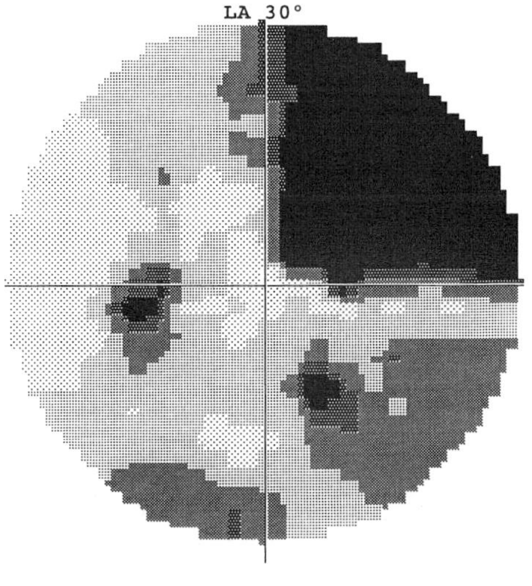

3.15D

Peripheral Homonymous Defects

Peripheral defects are either partially assessed or completely missed on computed perimetry, which is usually limited to the central 30° due to methodological time problems (Fig. 3.15E). The patient is seldom aware of these deficiencies. The patient in Figure 3.15E consulted a neurologist because of headache. Perimetry was ordered after the computed tomography scan revealed a hypodense area. Kinetic perimetry is clearly superior for assessing such defects. Suprathreshold peripheral tests are not reliable because of the high variation in normal values. Threshold measurements with fast algorithms are an interesting alternative, but they still take longer than kinetic perimetry.

Bilateral Homonymous Defects

Generalized extension of vascular processes often manifests as bilateral visual field defects. Each scotoma still demonstrates homonymity, that is, congruence between the eyes without mirror imaging. Figure 3.15F shows a combination of a homonymous upper left quadrantic defect, sector defects from 0 to 1 o'clock, and incomplete sector defects from 4 to 5 o'clock. In addition, there is a paracentral defect in the lower left quadrant. The left blind spot is merged with the defect and should be deleted before evaluation. This can be done by some sophisticated programs (Fig. 3.15F bottom).

Figure 3.15E. Occipital lobe infarct with a hypodense zone in a right occipital computed tomography scan in a 59-year-old woman with visual acuity of 1.3 in both eyes (program: HFA 30-2, representation: Peridata norm-related grayscale).

Figure 3.15F. Occipital lobe infarct with a right occipital malacia seen in this computed tomography scan in a 57-year-old woman. The visual field indicates that the left visual cortex is also involved. Visual acuity was 1.0 in the left eye and 0.8 in the right eye (program: HFA 30-2, representation: Peridata norm-related grayscale, top using standard mode, bottom with automated deletion of the blind spot area).

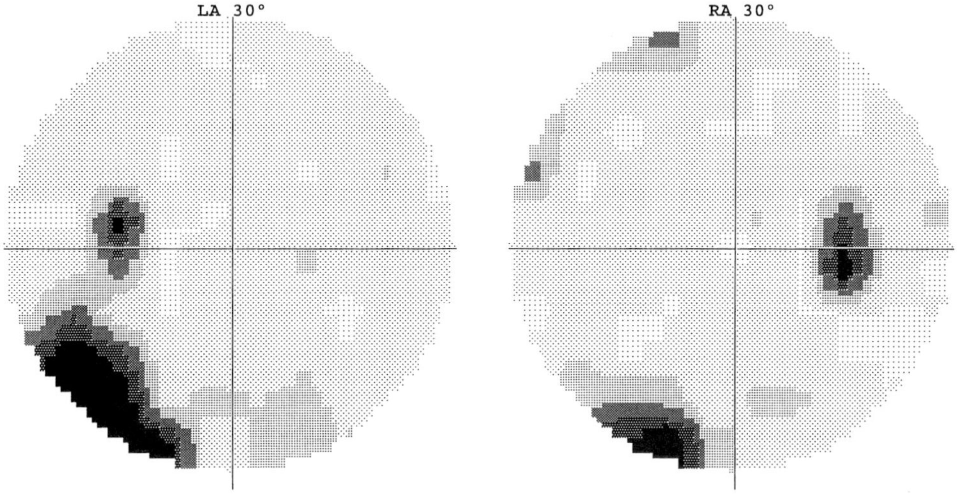

3.15E

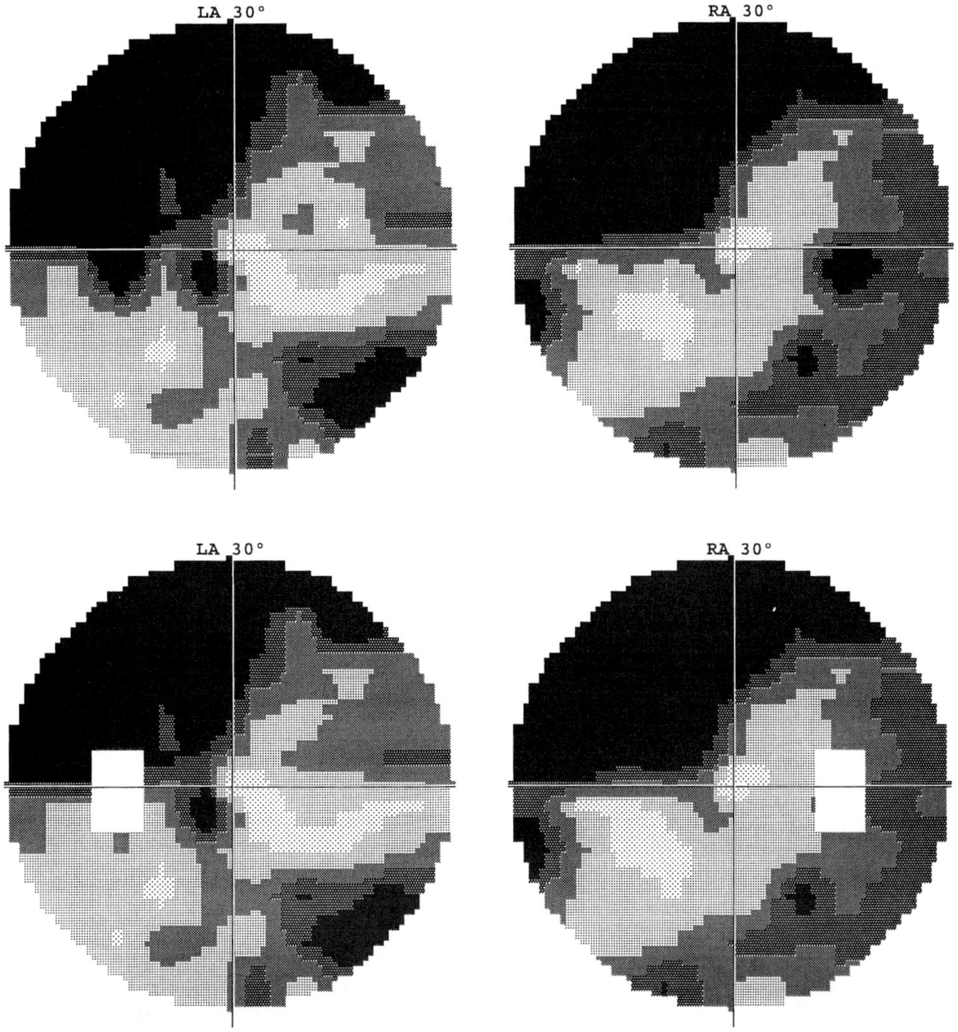

3.15F

Central Homonymous Defects

The most common symptom of homonymous defects is reading problems. Such defects are called *reading scotomas.* The impairment is larger if the scotoma is on the right side because the determination of the line and the recognition of the next letter for a saccade require paracentral vision to the right. The patient in Figure 3.15G had considerable problems; the patient in Figure 3.15H did not recognize her defects.

The shape of central defects is revealed as irregular by means of high-resolution static perimetry (Fig. 3.15G) and does not cover the entire inner semicircle. It can be argued that a central homonymous hemianopia with a purely semicircular shape probably does not exist.

Figure 3.15G. Postsurgical status of a 34-year-old man with an abscess of the left occipital lobe of the brain. Visual acuity was 0.8 in both eyes. In a standard 30° field, only one paracentral measurement point is involved. The 10° field with ninefold resolution discloses the bizarre shape, which does not follow any commonly recognized pattern (program: HFA 30-2 top, 10-2 bottom, representation: Peridata norm-related grayscale).

Figure 3.15H. Congenital arteriopathy (Moyamoya disease) in a 16-year-old patient. The computed tomography scan showed multiple focal necrosis in the occipital cortex. Visual acuity was 1.3 in both eyes (program: HFA 30-2, representation: Peridata norm-related grayscale).

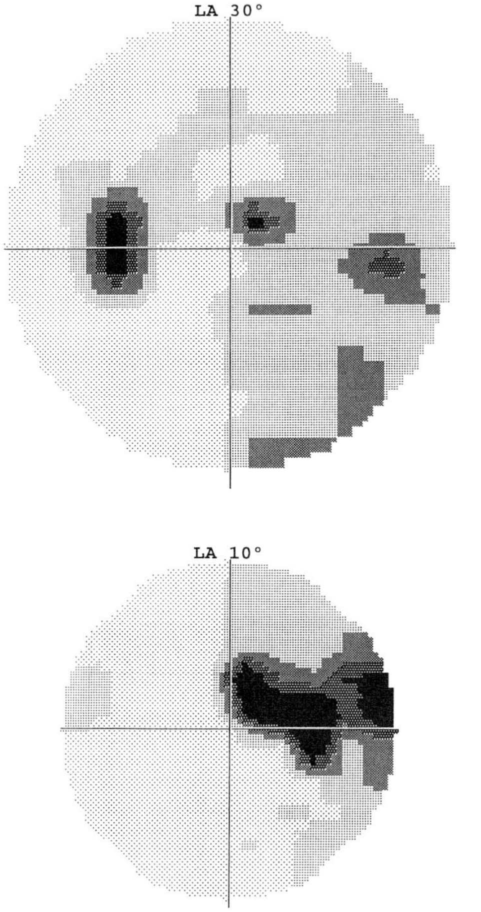

3.15G

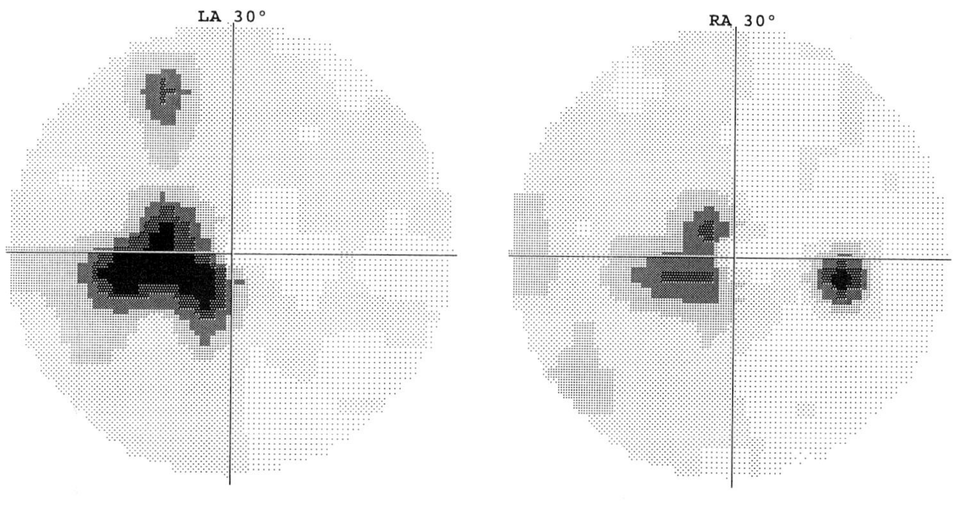

3.15H

3.16 PERMANENT FUNCTIONAL ALTERATIONS

Definition

Visual field alterations are termed *functional* if no organic cause can be detected and if the pattern of the field defect provides no indication of an organic cause. Functional alterations must be distinguished from erroneous measurements (*artifacts*) in which erroneous patient responses or instrument malfunction lead to anomalous results.

Simulation and Conversion Syndrome

Permanent functional disturbances may be conscious and intentional (simulation) or unconscious (psychic conversion syndrome). According to the definition above, simulation represents an artifact. Because the defect patterns of conscious and unconscious functional alterations are similar, they are discussed together.

Visual fields show severe concentric constriction. The sensitivity in the remaining field is usually reduced. The shape of the remaining field is nearly round (Fig. 3.16A, left eye), in contrast to the severe damage produced by glaucoma or central nervous system lesions. The rate of false-negative responses is elevated, but this should not be differential diagnostic criterion because this rate can also be elevated in organic visual field constrictions.

Simulation and conversion syndrome are distinguished from somatic alterations by means of simulation tests. One of these tests is objective pupil perimetry, which requires considerable experience. Automatic systems are now being developed. Another method is saccade perimetry. With this technique, the patient is informed that only the movements of the eye are tested. The patient is placed at a Goldmann perimeter with one eye patched, but with no answer button. He or she is then instructed to look at the fixation point. A stimulus which is likely to be visible, III/4 or I/4, is shown just inside the normal borders of the field, and the patent is told to look at this stimulus. A direct saccade toward the spot serves as proof of perception. An entire isopter is then mapped with a total of six to eight positions.

Patients with conversion syndrome (formerly called: *hysteric visual field constriction*) are often adolescents with vision of 0.1 to 0.3 in both eyes. They usually cooperate well during saccade perimetry. Other patients are older, often with other general diseases or after some sort of accident. Frequently, they have already applied for disability insurance without success. Their visual acuity is also usually between 0.1 and 0.3. During saccade perimetry they cooperate well at the beginning, but then they start to stare immovably at the fixation point after they realize the purpose of the test. If they are asked to search for the stimulus, they frequently look first in the opposite direction. Although the patient's behavior often provides clues, conscious and unconscious functional alterations cannot be distinguished with complete confidence.

Figure 3.16A. A 62-year-old man with nonspecific eye symptoms (pain, flickering vision) and visual acuity of 0.4 in both eyes. Concentric constriction is seen in static (top) and kinetic (bottom) perimetry. There is free orientation in the room, normal visual evoked cortical potentials, and no pathological findings on the computed tomography scan. The saccade field is normal (program: HFA 30-2, representation: Peridata norm-related grayscale).

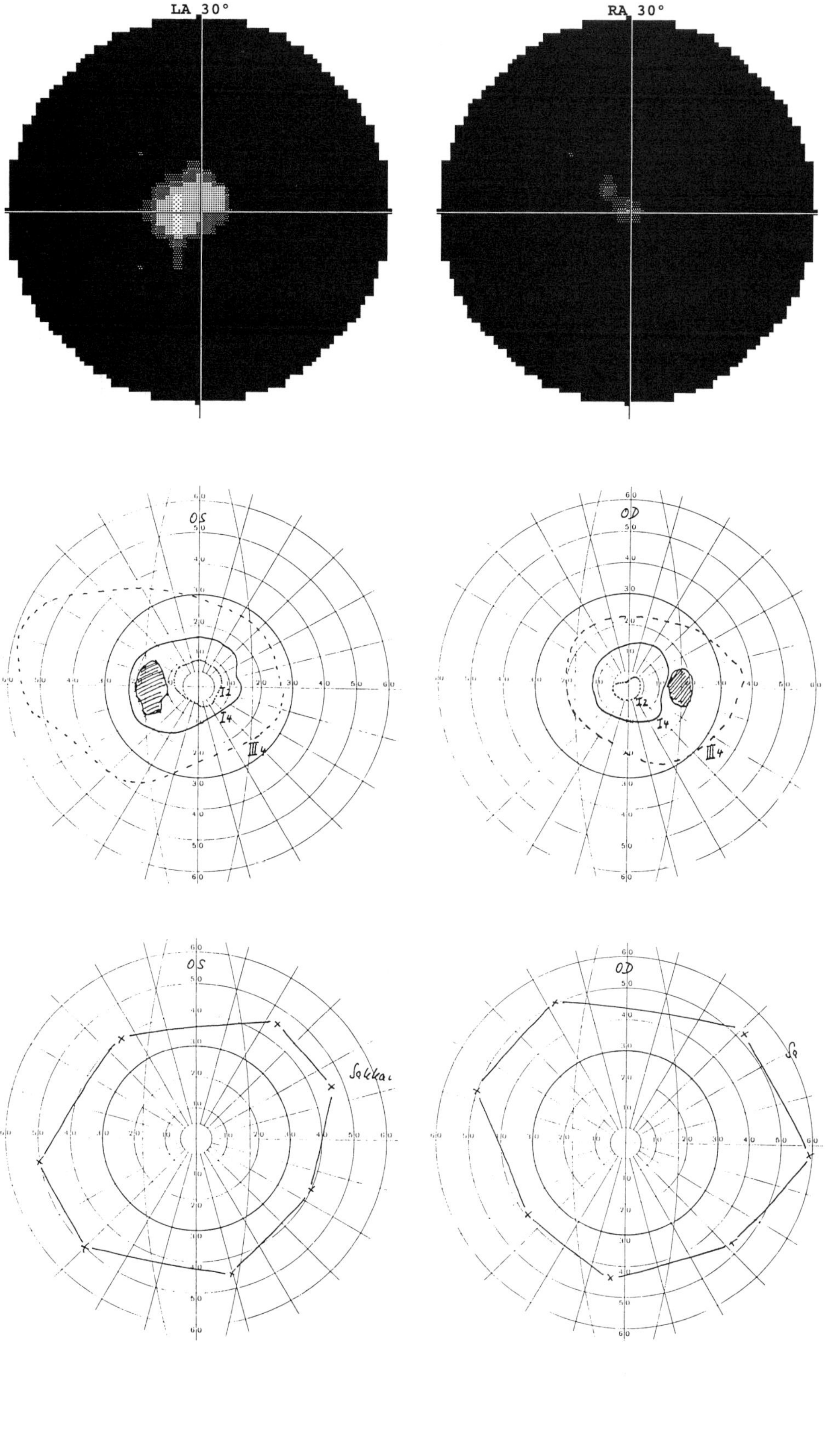

3.16A

Isolated Static Dysfunction

About 1% of all patients show loss of sensitivity in the static field, while the kinetic field is normal (Fig. 3.16B). In addition, patients do not complain of any visual impairment, in contrast to those with simulation and psychogenic dysfunction. Repeated examinations do not lead to any improvement, thus excluding lack of experience as a possible cause. The condition is an isolated static dysfunction. Further perimetric follow-up should be based on the kinetic fields.

Isolated static dysfunction must be distinguished from true defects, which are deeper and more extended in static perimetry than in kinetic perimetry. This phenomenon is called *stato-kinetic dissociation* and is discussed in Chapter 4.

Figure 3.16B. A 55-year-old man with a 2-year history of ocular hypertension, intraocular pressure of up to 28 mmHg, and disks with normal color and very small cups. Severe concentric constriction of the right visual field was found with automated perimetry in two examinations (top and center, program: HFA 30-2, representation: Peridata norm-related grayscale), but the kinetic field was normal (bottom, Goldmann perimeter).

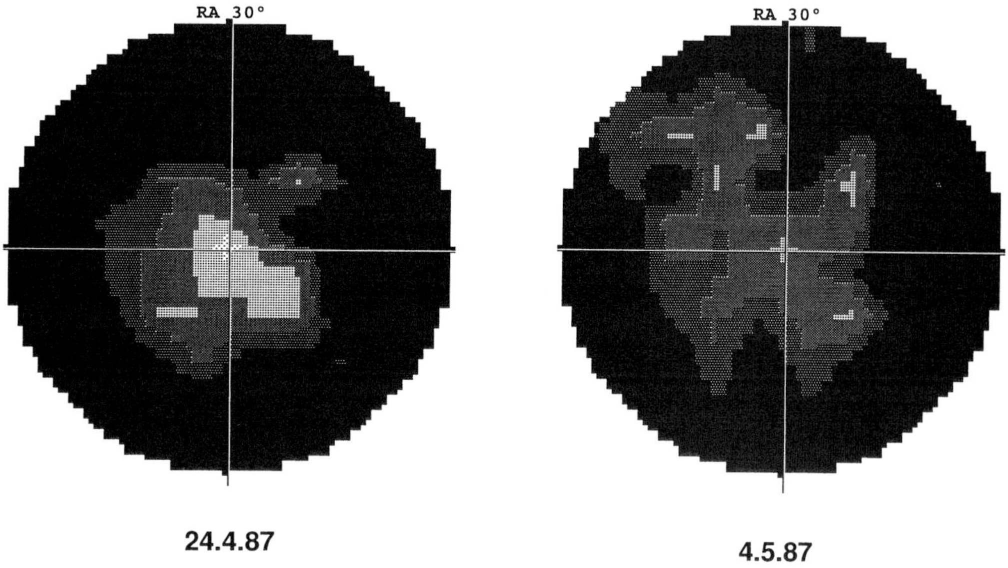
RA 30°
RA 30°
24.4.87
4.5.87

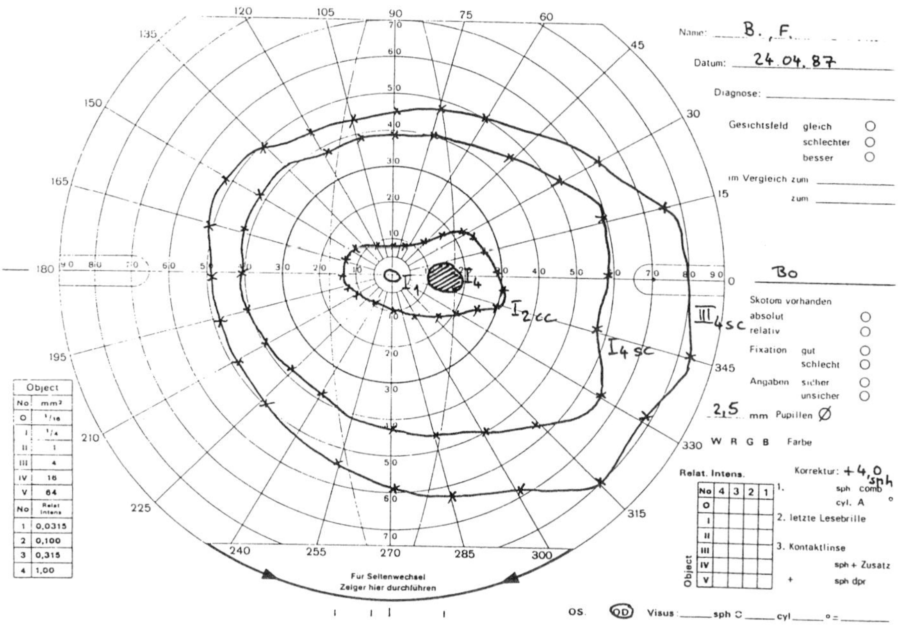
Name: B., F.
Datum: 24.04.87
Diagnose:
Gesichtsfeld gleich schlechter besser
im Vergleich zum
zum
Skotom vorhanden
absolut
relativ
Fixation gut schlecht
Angaben sicher unsicher
2,5 mm Pupillen Ø
W R G B Farbe
Relat. Intens.
Korrektur: +4,0 sph
sph comb
cyl. A
2. letzte Lesebrille
3. Kontaktlinse
sph + Zusatz
sph dpt
Object
OS OD Visus: sph cyl
Für Seitenwechsel Zeiger hier durchführen
Object No mm²
O 1/16
I 1/4
II 1
III 4
IV 16
V 64
No Relat. Intens.
1 0,0315
2 0,100
3 0,315
4 1,00
I1
I4
I2cc
III4sc
I4sc
Bo

3.16B

3.17 TRANSIENT FUNCTIONAL ALTERATIONS (LEARNING AND FATIGUE)

Learning

According to the definition of functional alterations, reduced sensitivity in untrained patients is also a functional alteration. This reduction can be conscious or unconscious. It is conscious if the untrained patient believes that he or she has to press the button only at the appearance of strong stimuli and that weak stimuli do not count. The reduction is unconscious if the patient does not perceive the stimuli knowingly. The learning experience varies from patient to patient. It may require one field or several fields; sometimes the performance is good from the very beginning (Fig. 3.17A).

The learning process is central and independent of the examined eye. Therefore, the visual field of the second eye on the first examination day is often better than the first eye.

The defect pattern in a learning deficit is usually spot-like and diffuse (Fig. 3.17A). Some fields resemble typical defect patterns, which may erroneously lead to extensive workup. Repeated field examinations usually turn out to be normal (Fig. 3.17B).

Fatigue

A decline in attention, and consequently reduced perception of weak stimuli, can occur during a standard examination of one eye. The perimetrist should provide breaks for the patient every 5 minutes or so. Many instruments allow an interruption on patient demand by removing the forehead from the headrest or keeping the button pressed down after a stimulus presentation. Fatigue is more frequent in the second eye or if a second examination on one eye is necessary for increased spatial resolution (Fig 3.17C). On the day of the first examination, learning effects and fatigue effects may overlap. Fatigue is reduced by the use of the newer fast algorithms.

Figure 3.17A. Learning effect in a 34-year-old woman with nonspecific ocular symptoms (photopsia) and no organic changes. Visual fields were measured with a 3-month interval (left eye, program: HFA 30-2, representation: Peridata norm-related grayscale).

Figure 3.17B. Learning effect in the right eye of the same patient. The measurement interval was 3 months (right eye, program: HFA 30-2, representation: Peridata norm-related grayscale).

Figure 3.17C. Fatigue in the left eye of a 63-year-old man with advanced glaucoma. Both examinations took about 15 minutes and were performed consecutively (program: HFA 30-2 [left] and 30-1 [right], representation: Peridata norm-related grayscale).

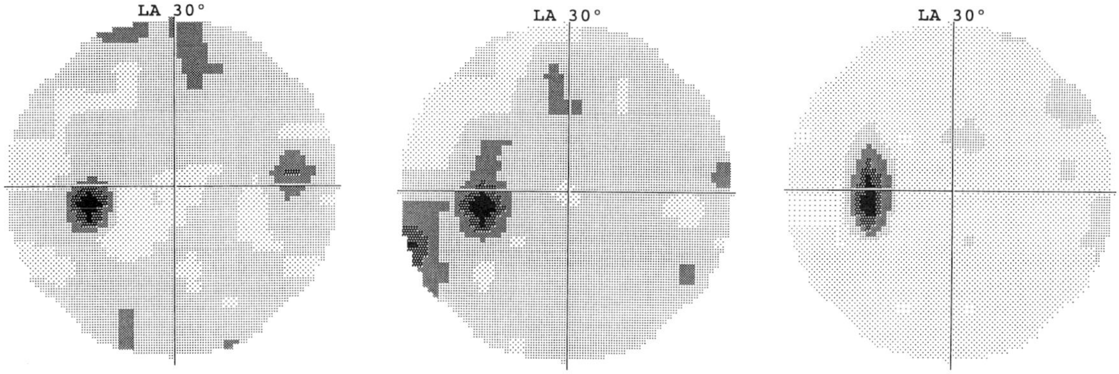

3.17A

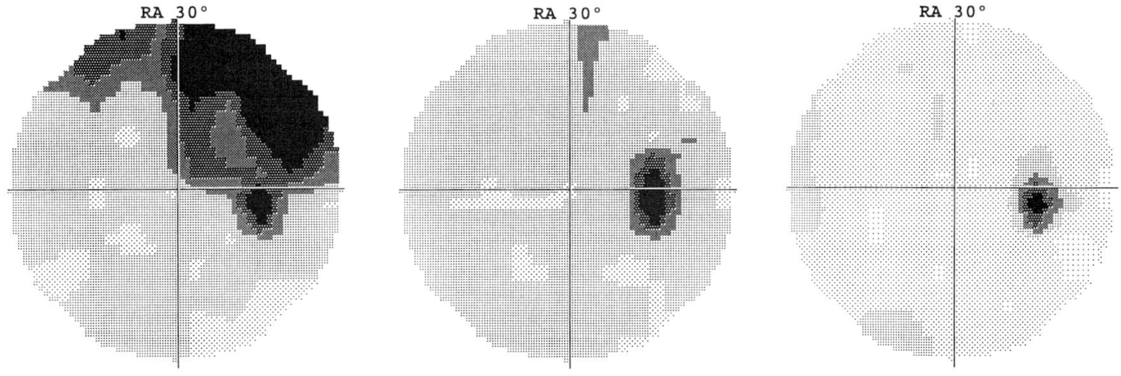

3.17B

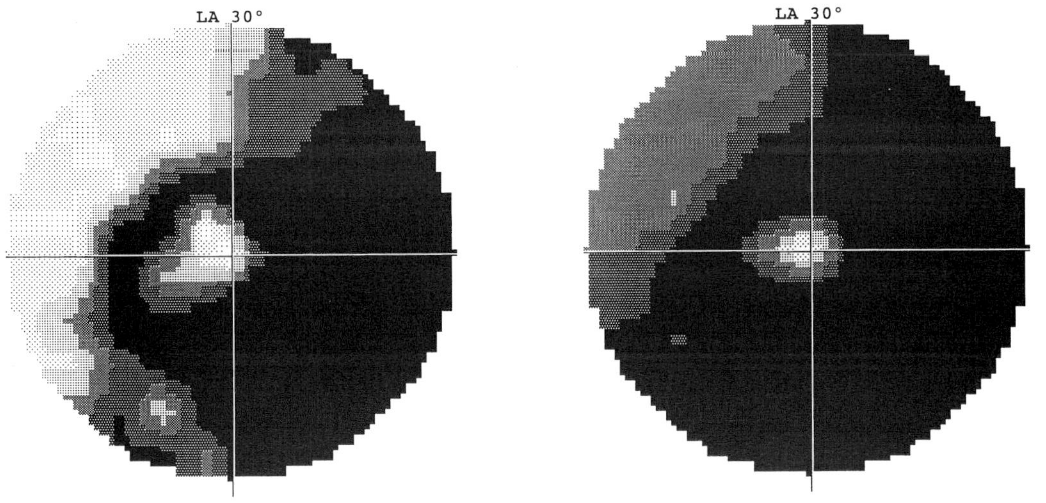

3.17C

3.18 ABNORMAL FINDINGS CAUSED BY ERRONEOUS PATIENT RESPONSES (PATIENT ARTIFACTS)

Dissimulation

Some patients press the button too often, even when the stimulus is not perceivable or no stimulus is shown. Possible causes are intentional influence on the examination result, especially in ability examinations (true dissimulation), ignorance of the examination rules (erroneous dissimulation), and extreme anxiety. The measured sensitivity becomes abnormally high, and the printout shows relative sensitivity values of more than 5 dB above normal. Absolute values are in the high 40s or 50s (Octopus and Humphrey scales). The grayscale shows *white scotomas,* or areas of abnormally high visual sensitivity (Swiss cheese syndrome; Fig. 3.18A). Dissimulation is recognized best in the cumulative defect curve that bends upward at the left end into the supranormal range (false-positive tail). Another fairly reliable criterion is the false-positive answer rate. The interpretation of this index will be discussed in detail in the following chapter.

Even with obvious dissimulation, the visual field findings are useful to some extent. If the true field is normal, the blind spot is present and the rest of the field is homogeneous (Fig. 3.18A). If the true field is pathological, defects are apparent, at least partially (Fig. 3.18B). The topography of the defects, however, can be altered considerably.

Figure 3.18A. Dissimulation in a 74-year-old patient with a normal true field. The rate of false-positive answers was 69%. Visual acuity was 1.0; ocular hypertension was present (program: HFA 30-2, representation: Peridata norm-related grayscale and cumulative curve).

Figure 3.18B. Dissimulation in a case of pathological true field in a 27-year-old patient with juvenile glaucoma. A series of a right field with 78% false-positive answers (top) and 30% false-positive answers (bottom) is shown. The bottom field can be considered the true field. Visual acuity was 0.7 (program: HFA 30-2, representation: Peridata "compressed" = grayscale, numerals, indices, and cumulative curve).

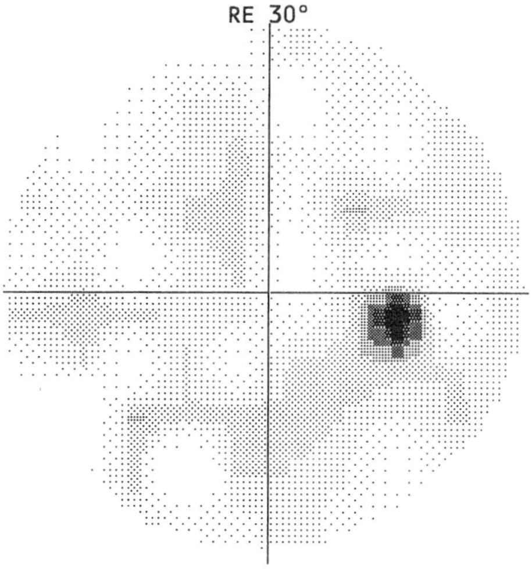
RE 30°

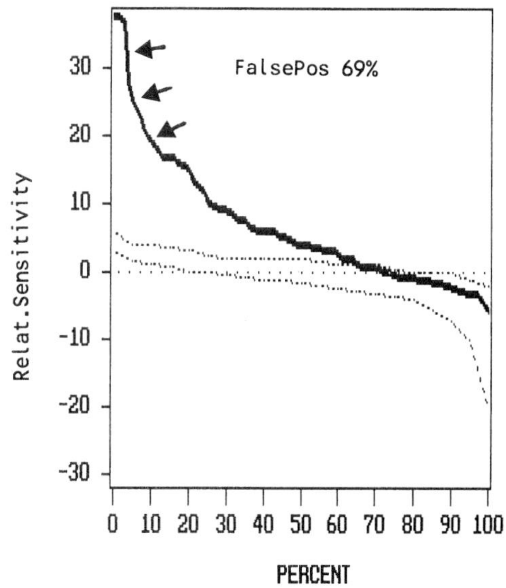
FalsePos 69%
Relat.Sensitivity
30
20
10
0
-10
-20
-30
0 10 20 30 40 50 60 70 80 90 100
PERCENT

3.18A

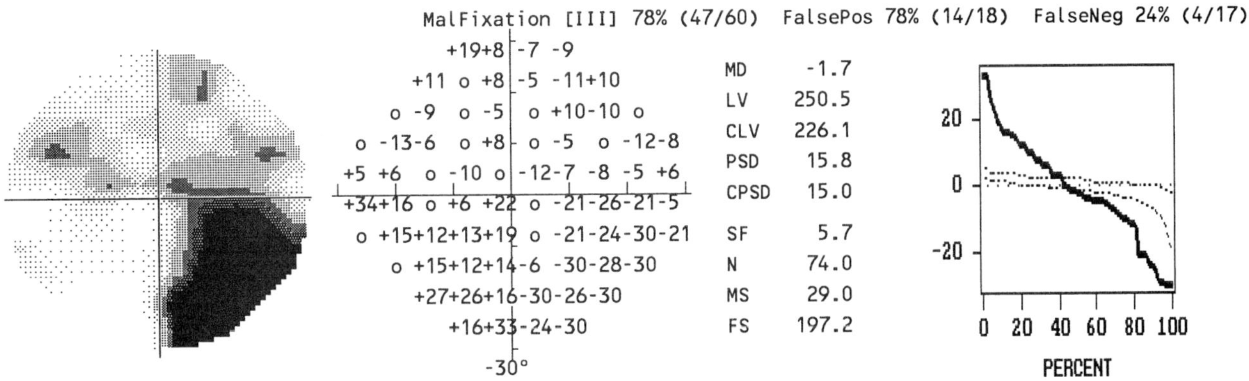
MalFixation [III] 78% (47/60) FalsePos 78% (14/18) FalseNeg 24% (4/17)
+19+8 -7 -9
+11 o +8 -5 -11+10
o -9 o -5 o +10-10 o
o -13-6 o +8 o -5 o -12-8
+5 +6 o -10 o -12-7 -8 -5 +6
+34+16 o +6 +22 o -21-26-21-5
o +15+12+13+19 o -21-24-30-21
o +15+12+14-6 -30-28-30
+27+26+16-30-26-30
+16+33-24-30
-30°
MD -1.7
LV 250.5
CLV 226.1
PSD 15.8
CPSD 15.0
SF 5.7
N 74.0
MS 29.0
FS 197.2
20
0
-20
0 20 40 60 80 100
PERCENT

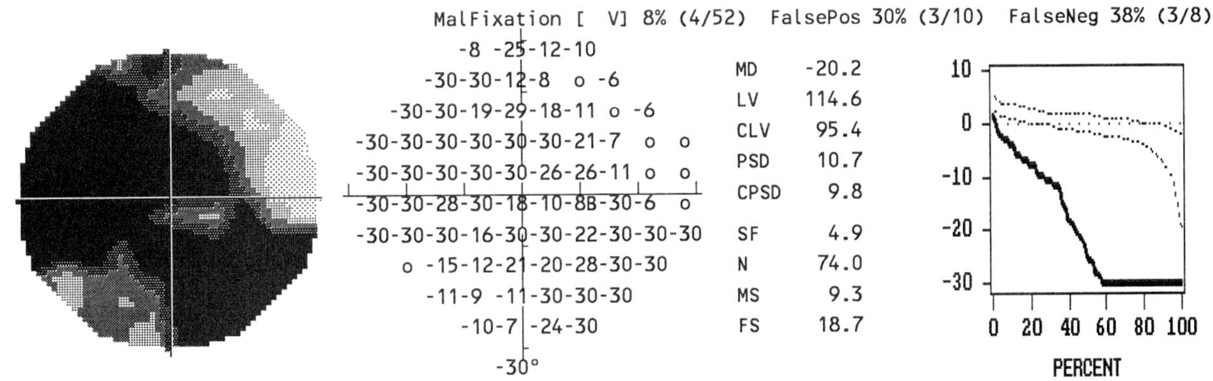
MalFixation [V] 8% (4/52) FalsePos 30% (3/10) FalseNeg 38% (3/8)
-8 -25-12-10
-30-30-12-8 o -6
-30-30-19-29-18-11 o -6
-30-30-30-30-30-30-21-7 o o
-30-30-30-30-30-26-26-11 o o
-30-30-28-30-18-10-8B-30-6 o
-30-30-30-16-30-30-22-30-30-30
o -15-12-21-20-28-30-30
-11-9 -11-30-30-30
-10-7 -24-30
-30°
MD -20.2
LV 114.6
CLV 95.4
PSD 10.7
CPSD 9.8
SF 4.9
N 74.0
MS 9.3
FS 18.7
10
0
-10
-20
-30
0 20 40 60 80 100
PERCENT

3.18B

Fixation Losses

Unsteady fixation (fixation losses) is a disturbance of the relationship between the perimeter bowl locations and the true visual field locations. As in a photograph that is out of focus, all contours (scotoma borders) are blurred, and small details (small scotomas) may vanish completely. In normal or mildly disturbed visual fields, the blind spot is shallow or missing (Fig. 3.18C). In pathological fields, the scotomas are smaller and shallower (Fig. 3.18D) or disappear. The assessment of large, absolute scotomas is only slightly influenced by poor fixation (Fig. 3.18E).

Fixation losses are measured by different types of fixation controls. The percentages used in this book are related to the Heijl-Krakau method, which uses bright stimuli at the location of the blind spot. The percentage of perceptions of these trial stimuli is the malfixation index. The evaluation of this indicator will be discussed in detail in the following chapter.

Figure 3.18C. Perimetric result with fixation losses (left) and the true visual field (right, examined later on the same day) of an eye with mild peripheral depressions. The blind spot is missing. This is the left eye of a 49-year-old patient with an orbital tumor without optic nerve compression. Visual acuity was 1.0 (program: HFA 30-2, representation: Peridata norm-related grayscale).

Figure 3.18D. Perimetric result with fixation losses (left) and true visual field (right) of an eye with deep but small scotomas. The blind spot is shallow, the paracentral scotoma is less deep and partly vanished, and the nasal wedge is displaced and shrunken. This is the right eye of a 77-year-old patient with an optic pit. Visual acuity was 0.7 (program: HFA 30-S custom program, representation: Peridata norm-related grayscale).

Figure 3.18E. Perimetric result with fixation losses (left) and the true visual field (right) of an eye with a deep, large defect in the lower temporal quadrant. The margins are shallower than in reality, and the area of absolute scotoma is narrowed, but the defect is well represented in general. This is the right eye of a 49-year-old patient with craniopharyngioma. Visual acuity was 0.6 (program: HFA 30-2, representation: Peridata norm-related grayscale).

Note: Fixation losses = fixation loss index; roman number in brackets = stimulus size (Goldmann's table) of the fixation loss test.

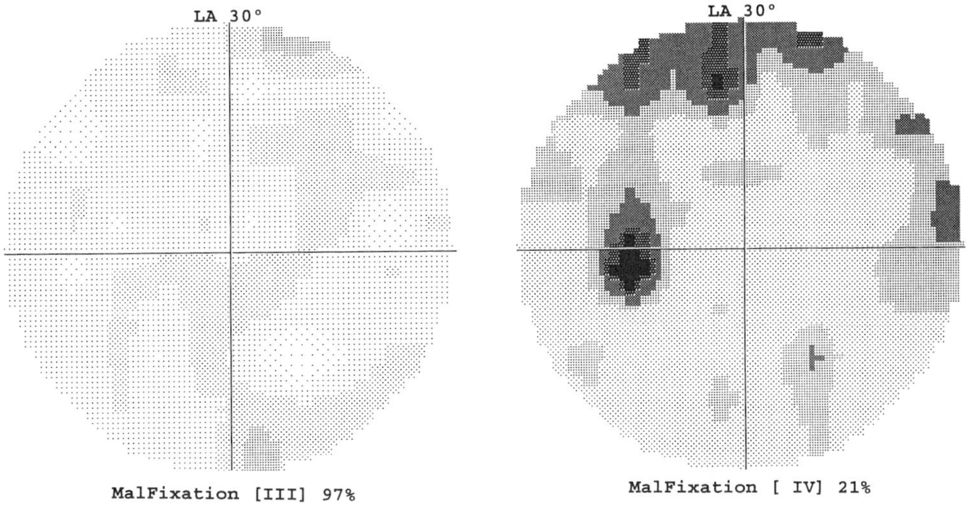

3.18C

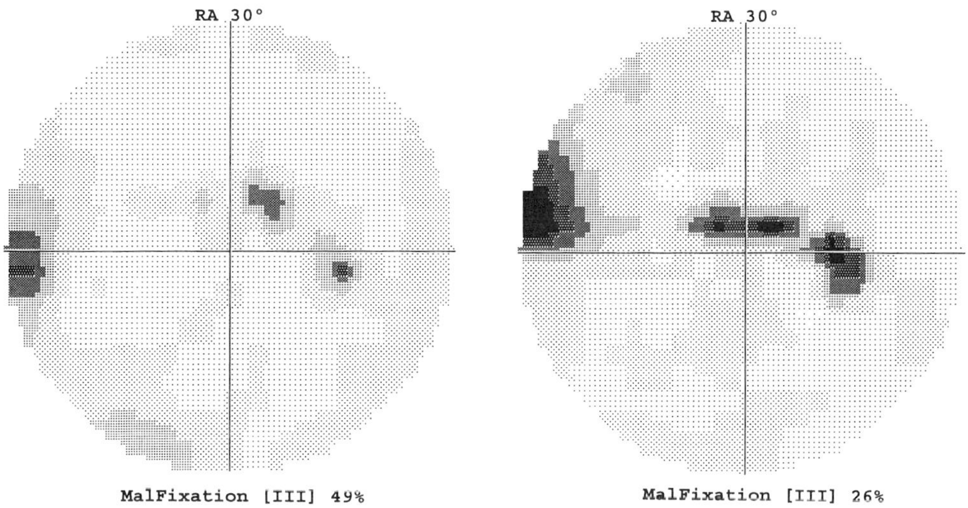

3.18D

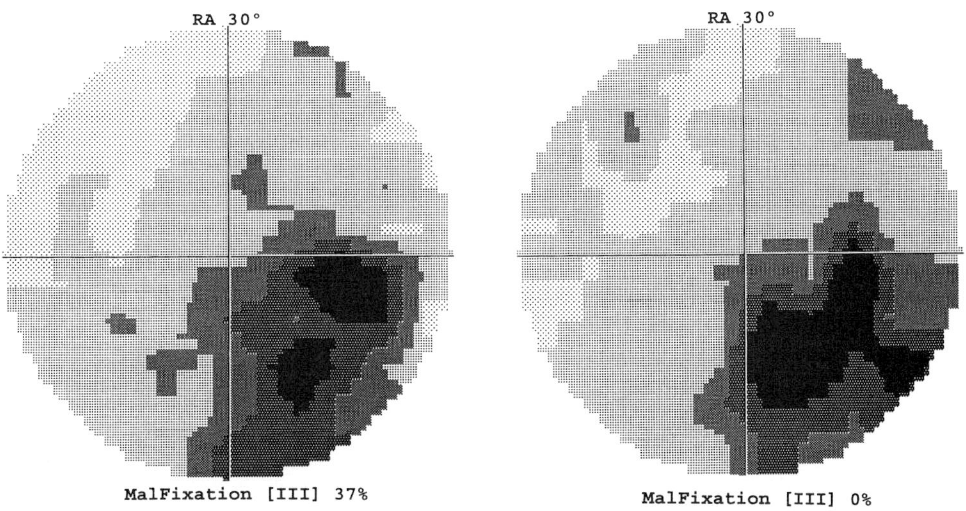

3.18E

Shift of Fixation

In contrast to patients with unsteady fixation, who move their eyes incessantly, other patients fixate steadily but aim at the wrong point. This erroneous shift in fixation may happen with the Humphrey Field Analyzer while using the fovea test option. In this case, the examination starts by presenting stimuli in the center of four eccentric fixation lights in the lower part of the bowl. Afterward, the patient is told to look at the usual single fixation point, which is located 7° above, and the other field locations are tested. If the examiner forgets to instruct the patient about the obligatory change in the fixation goal, he or she may continue to look 7° below the correct fixation point. The blind spot and all other parts of the visual field shift down by 7° (Fig. 3.18F). The blind spot is the best indicator of such a shift in fixation, provided that there is no optic disk ectopia. In addition, the applied normal values may not match, and the defect depth values may be wrong. The examiner should be aware of these potential problems.

There may also be a true shift in fixation in cases of central scotoma. It is reported by experts that fixation is most frequently shifted above and/or to the right. Figure 3.18G shows a typical example of a young patient with Stargardt's disease who dislocated her scotoma above and right (left eye) or above alone (right eye). In the right eye, the blind spot confirms the shift. In the left eye, the blind spot is not apparent. It is located between test locations because of its abnormal position.

Figure 3.18F. Erroneous shift of fixation by 7° below (left) and correct fixation (right). This is the right eye in a 65-year-old man with chronic angle-closure glaucoma and depression of the superior field. Visual acuity was 1.0 (program: HFA 30-2, representation: Peridata norm-related grayscale).

Figure 3.18G. True shift of fixation superiorly. Both eyes of a 24-year-old patient with Stargardt's disease were tested. Visual acuity was 0.1 in both eyes (program: HFA 30-S custom program with 3° resolution in the center, representation: Peridata norm-related grayscale).

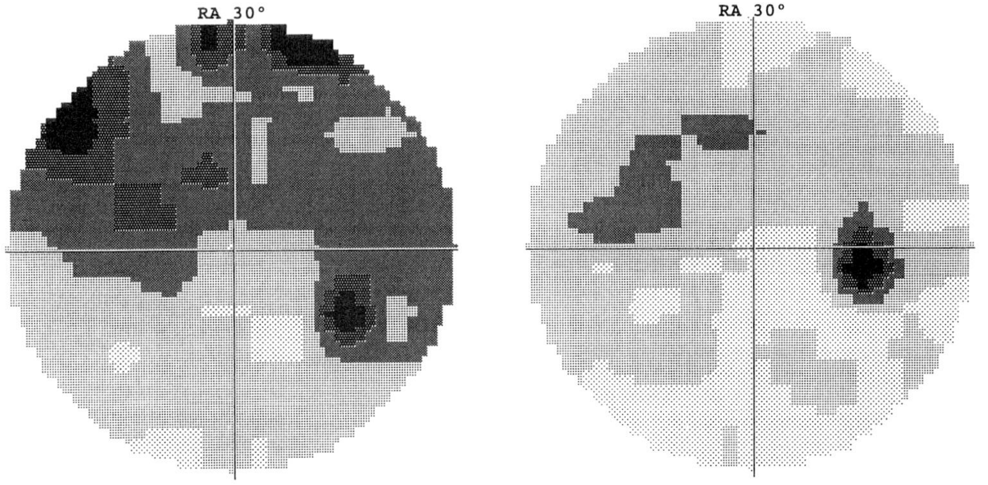

3.18F

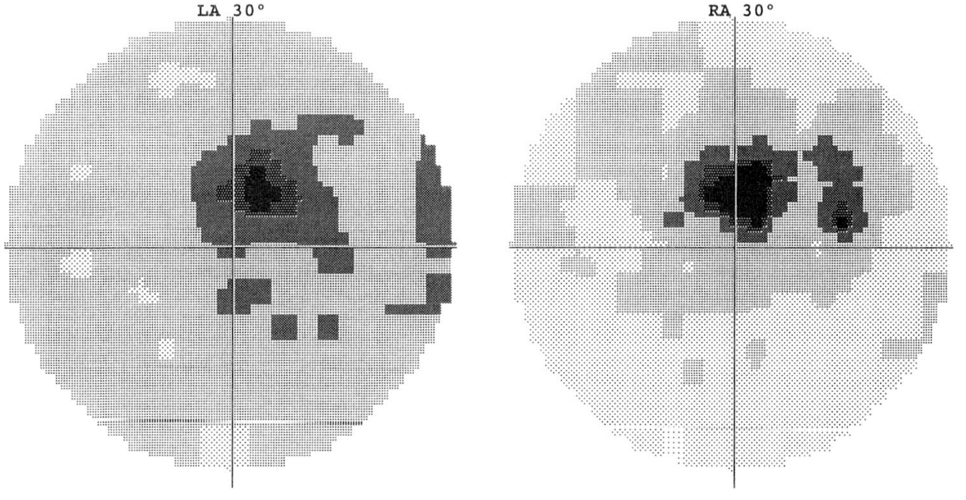

3.18G

3.19 ABNORMAL RESULTS CAUSED BY METHODICAL PECULIARITIES (INSTRUMENT ARTIFACTS)

Starting Point Effect

Starting points are the locations where a perimetric program begins its measurements. They usually are in the center of the four quadrants. Threshold measurements start with a medium luminance. In badly affected fields, up to eight stimulus presentations may be required until the low threshold or the lower end of the measurement range has been reached. This means up to 32 stimulus presentations which cannot be perceived by the patient. The chance that the patient will press the response button accidentally during these presentations is relatively high. A single wrong answer may raise the sensitivity result considerably. Neighboring points are started at a lower level, and the chance of an erroneous elevation in sensitivity is much lower. These wrong values appear as four bright spots in the grayscale or as four high values in the numerical display (Fig. 3.19A).

Missing the Blind Spot Caused by Gaps in the Point Pattern

The pattern of measured points varies considerably among examination programs. The assessment of the blind spot, which has a fairly constant position of 15° temporally and 2° below the horizontal axis, depends greatly on the pattern used. The common paraxial 6° pattern of Fankhauser (Octopus program 32 or Humphrey program 30-2 or 24-2) provides a measurement point (coordinates: $x = 15°$, $y = -3°$) which is very close to that position and nearly always assesses the blind spot. The complementary axial 6° pattern (Octopus program 31 or Humphrey program 30-1) has measurement points at the border of the normal blind spot. In about 10% to 20% of cases, it is not assessed (Fig. 3.19B).

The Octopus program G1 omits the blind spot region intentionally because it is of little use for quantitative analysis of visual damage (Fig. 3.19C). As a side effect, important information is lost about false-positive behavior and fixation losses provided by the blind spot as a "test scotoma."

Figure 3.19A. Starting point effect on a severely damaged field in the left eye of a 78-year-old patient with pigmentary glaucoma. Visual acuity was 0.5. There was loss of orientation, presumably due to a miniature central island (program: HFA 30-2, representation: Peridata grayscale and numerals/absolute sensitivity).

Figure 3.19B. Missing blind spot caused by a gap in an axial measurement point pattern. The blind spot (BS) lies between the measurement points. In this printout, BS indicates the location where the trial stimuli for the fixation test are shown. It is determined by a cross-axis search algorithm (right eye, program: HFA 30-2, representation: Peridata grayscale and numerals/relative sensitivity).

Figure 3.19C. Missing blind spot caused by a measurement point gap in the Octopus program G1. The blind spot is excluded intentionally (left eye, program: Octopus 1-2-3/G1x, representation: Peridata grayscale and numerals/relative sensitivity).

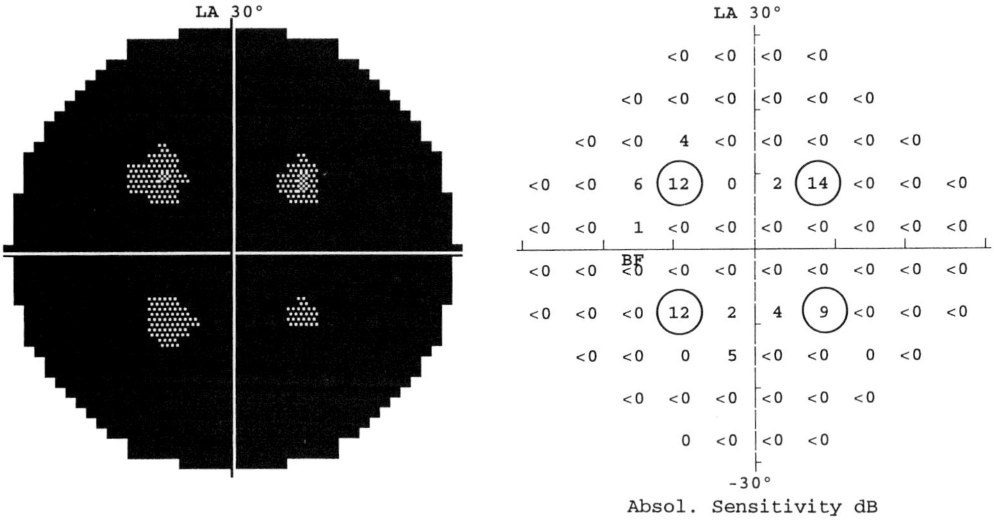

3.19A

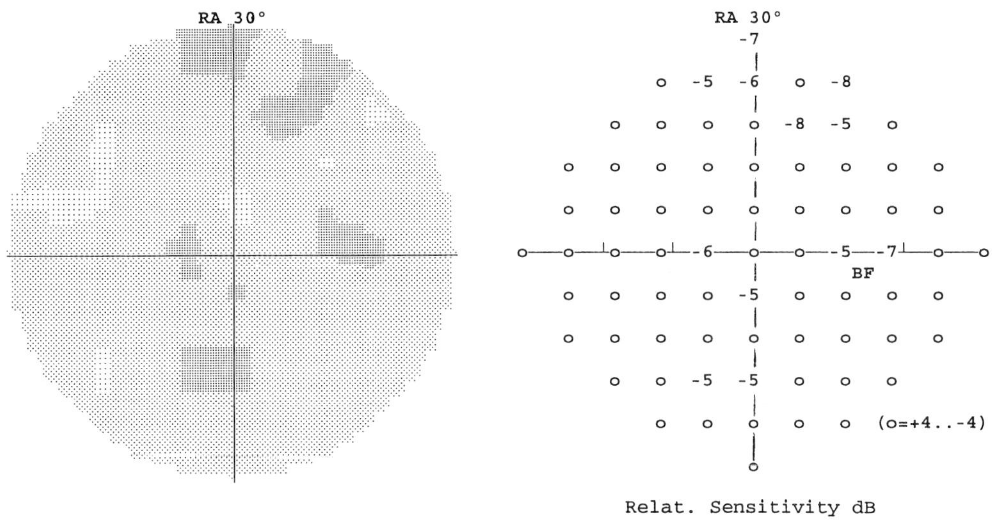

3.19B

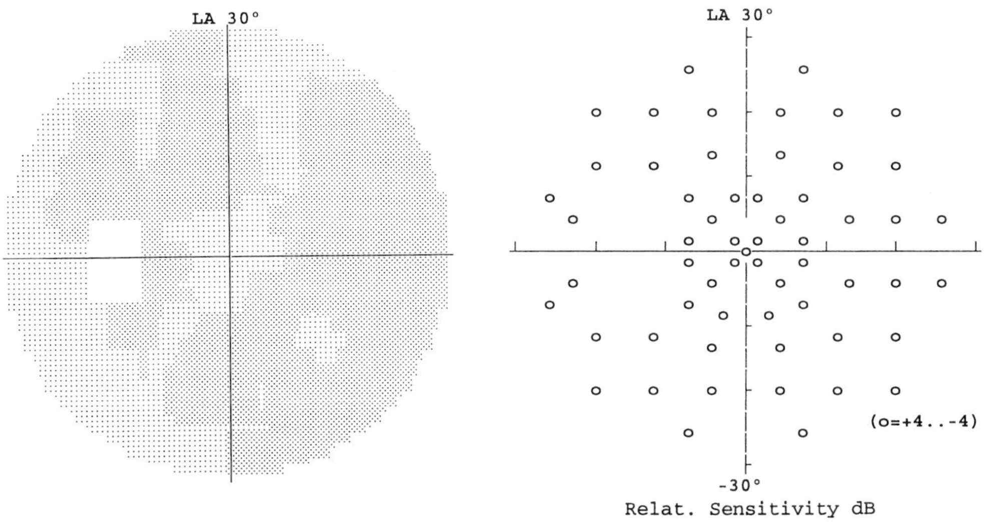

3.19C

4 Interpretation and Differential Diagnosis

4.1 THE DIAGNOSTIC PATHWAY

Analysis of the automated visual field examination results can be divided into several steps.

First, the quality of the result is determined. Loss of fixation index, false-positive and false-negative answer rates, and representation of the blind spot indicate the reliability of the patient's performance. However, unreliable fields provide at least a limited impression of the true field and should not be entirely disregarded. A repeat test, preferably performed on a different day, is always recommended for unreliable fields.

Next, the normality of a field is checked by inspecting its quantitative and topographical properties. If the field is normal in all respects, the examiner concludes that there are no functional disturbances in the examined visual field area.

If the visual field is abnormal a differential diagnosis follows, based on the topographical pattern of the defects. A list of all known typical defect patterns that resemble the current pattern is developed. If there is a diagnosis in the list that harmonizes with other findings (fundus, computed tomography scan, etc.) or is in accordance with the suspected diagnosis, a diagnostic decision can be made. Otherwise, the information from the field may be improved by repetition and refinement (resolution). Alternatively, other examinations may be completed or repeated.

In addition, the amount of damage should be compared with other findings (e.g., the appearance of the optic nerve). If discrepancies occur, additional diseases should be considered. Further examination may be indicated. Alternatively, the visual field result may be unreliable. This problem can often be handled by repeating the test. If the amount of damage is in accordance with the clinical picture and this was the first visual field, therapy should be discussed if appropriate. In a follow-up field exam, the series is inspected for significant trends. If deterioration is found, the therapeutic plan may need revision. Otherwise, continuation of the current therapy seems justified (Fig. 4.1).

In this chapter, the steps of visual field evaluation are described. The special problems of follow-up evaluation are discussed in Chapter 5.

Figure 4.1. Flow chart of visual field evaluation.

Diagnostic algorithm

reliable

yes / no → *repeat VF*

↓

normal

no / yes → *no functional damage*

↓

topography of defects
in accordance with the other findings

yes / no → *e.g. repetition of VF, other examinations*

↓

degree of damage
correlates with other findings

yes / no → *e.g. repetition of VF, other examinations*

↓

first field

no / yes → *start therapy*

↓

deterioration

no / yes → *reconsider therapy*

↓

continue therapy

4.1

4.2 QUALITY OF THE RESULT

Measurement Error (Short-Term Fluctuation)

Accidental measurement error at a single visual field location depends on the instrument and the program. This error is about 1.5 to 2 dB using the traditional double-bracketing staircase method. A number of perimetric programs determine the measurement error by repetitive measurements and display it as a short-term fluctuation (SF) index. The perimetric measurement error depends mainly on the variability with which the patient responds. This variability rises in cases of inattention or hypersensitive behavior. It is greater in peripheral field regions and especially at locations with depressed sensitivities. It increases with age.

A normal visual field with increased SF will present more supranormal points and more defect points. The SF index helps to avoid misinterpretation. In an abnormal field with increased SF, defect depths are less accurate but interpretation is not significantly altered. Whether isolated elevation of the SF index in fields with normal sensitivity is a precursor to deterioration has not been proven.

Hypersensitive Behavior

The patient's tendency to push the button frequently causes a systematic measurement error with an upward shift in sensitivity values. This behavior is assessed by false-positive catch trials (see Chapter 1). The rate of false-positive answers is given in the report. Rates above 20% usually cause considerable bias of measurement results.

A normal visual field with hypersensitive behavior is characterized by single or grouped sensitivity values more than 5 dB above normal (see Section 3.18). In a pathological field, defects are abnormally flat and interrupted. In suprathreshold tests, hypersensitive behavior is even more serious: several defect points are not assessed, and the field appears falsely normal. A 10% false-positive answer rate in a suprathreshold test is a clear indication for repetition of the test, preferably with a full threshold strategy (Fig. 4.2A).

Hyposensitive Behavior

The patient's tendency to not push the button even when a stimulus is perceived causes a downshift in sensitivity values. Normal visual fields with hyposensitive behavior show single or spot-like adjacent locations with reduced sensitivity. In abnormal visual fields, defects appear deeper than they really are.

Hyposensitive behavior is assessed by trial questions with very bright stimuli (false-negative catch trials). The false-negative answer rate is provided in the report. In damaged fields, the brightness of these trial stimuli is often well within the threshold zone. Therefore, the false-negative rate may be elevated even with correct behavior. The value of this index is limited in markedly abnormal fields (Fig. 4.2A).

Figure 4.2A. Types of errors in sensitivity measurement.

ERRORS OF SENSITIVITY MEASUREMENT

TYPE	HIGH FLUCTUATION	HYPERSENSITIVE	HYPOSENSITIVE	NORMAL
DISTRIBUTION of results at a single test location	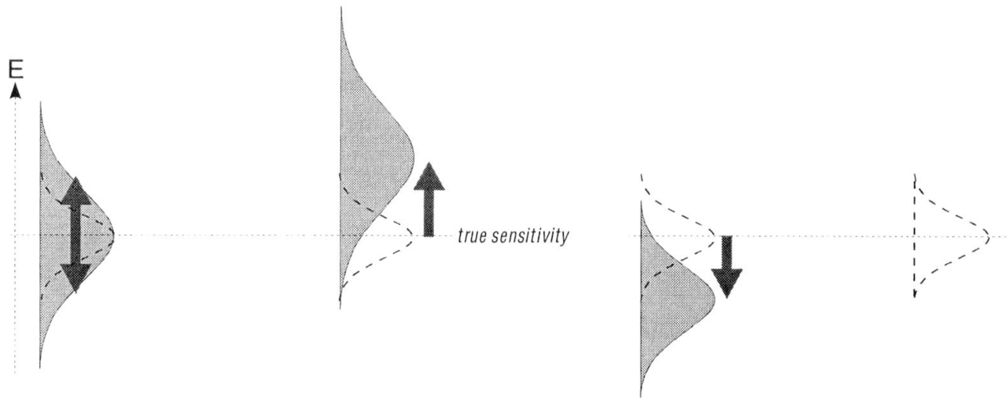			
INDEX	SF	FALSE POSITIVE	FALSE NEGATIVE	
NORMAL LIMIT	< 2 dB	< 20%	< 33%	
EFFECTS on normal VF	single defects single supranormals	spotty supranormal thresholds	spotty defects	
EFFECTS on patholog. VF	not considerable	defects too shallow spotty supranormal thresholds	defects too deep	
EFFECTS on global MD	none	better than true value	worse than true value	
EFFECTS on suprathreshold tests	sometimes single defects	many defects missed	too many defects	

4.2A

Fixation

Poor fixation blurs all contours in the visual field. In normal fields, the blind spot becomes shallow or vanishes. In abnormal fields, scotomas become smaller and the borders become softer. Small scotomas may vanish completely (see Chapter 3).

Different methods are used to monitor fixation behavior, which is described by a fixation loss index (see Chapter 1). The meaning of this index depends on the method used and on the perimeter.

Sensory fixation monitoring uses trial stimuli projected into the blind spot (Heijl-Krakau method). The fixation loss index is the percentage of positive answers related to all trial stimuli presented in the blind spot. The higher the index, the worse the fixation. "Normal" limits are defined somewhat arbitrarily. The manufacturer of the Humphrey Field Analyzer suggests a limit of 33%. Our own examinations suggest reliable results with a rate as high as 40%.

The sensory fixation loss index may be erroneously low if the range for undetected fixation loss is enlarged by scotomas near the blind spot. The index may be erroneously high if the test location for the trial stimulus is in the wrong position. This happens often because localization of the supposed blind spot uses a crossed-axis search algorithm in which a single wrong response may shift its position. In Figure 4.2B, the location of the trial stimuli for the blind spot is dislocated superiorly and centrally. The fixation loss index was high. In a visual field measured independently, the blind spot was accurately assessed. Fixation was therefore fairly good. The index may be erroneously high if the patient has a high false-positive index (Fig. 4.2C). Because the patient likes to push the button without a stimulus, the patient also pushes it if he or she does not see the trial stimulus in the blind spot. A third reason for a high index despite good fixation is cataract. Optical divergence of the stimulus may fall on the peripapillary retina and allow perception even in cases of good fixation (Fig. 4.2D).

Electronic-optical fixation monitoring is independent of the topography of the visual field and the patient's behavior. In some Octopus models, it is based on the position of the pupil. The correct position of the eye and a suitable size of the monitor window inside the pupil must be set in advance and tested. Every stimulus which occurs at the same time as a fixation loss is canceled and repeated. The fixation loss index is the number of repeated stimuli relative to all stimuli. In the new Humphrey Field Analyzer, monitoring is based on Purkinje's reflexes. It is centered automatically and is independent of the pupil size. There is no fixation loss index, but the decentration angle is plotted versus time on a graph.

An additional clue to fixation quality is the presence or absence of the blind spot, especially with the borderline fixation loss index. This can be determined only if there are measured locations in the area of the blind spot. They are missing in Octopus program G1, and they are not very suitable in programs 31 (Octopus) or 30-1 (Humphrey-Perimeter).

Figure 4.2B. Erroneously high fixation loss index caused by a wrong position of the trial location (BS = blind spot; program: HFA 30-2).

Figure 4.2C. Erroneously high fixation loss index caused by hypersensitive behavior (program: HFA 30-2).

Figure 4.2D. Erroneously high fixation loss index caused by cataract (program: HFA 30-2).

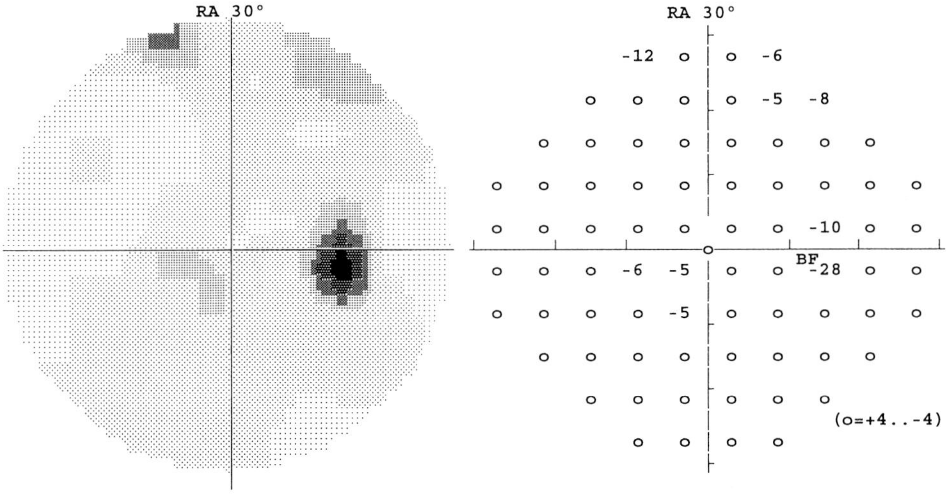

Malfixation	64%
False Pos	0%
False Neg	6%

4.2B

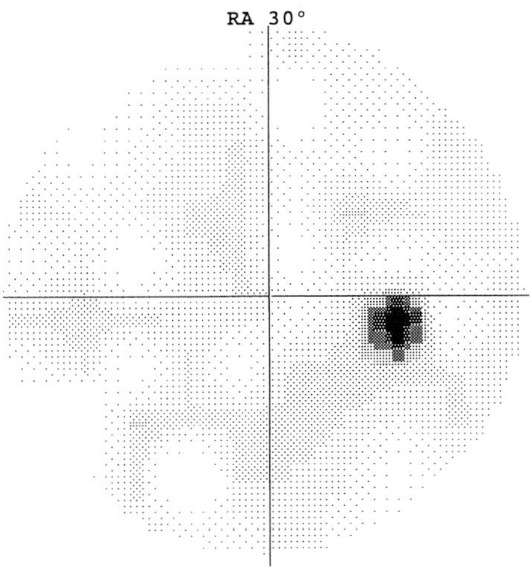

Malfixation	59%
False Pos	69%
False Neg	6%

4.2C

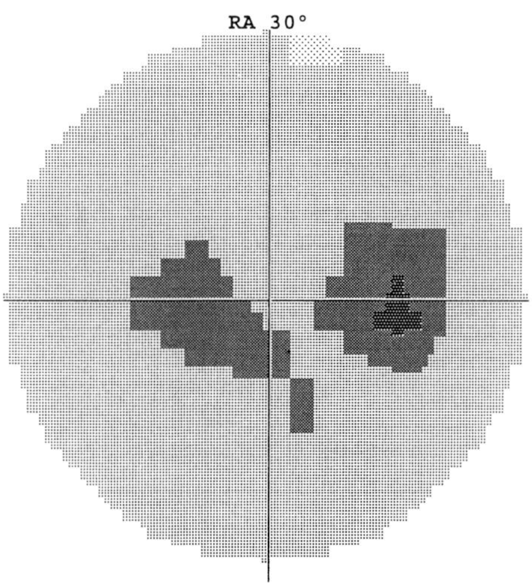

Malfixation	32%
False Pos	0%
False Neg	0%

4.2D

Fatigue and Examination Time

During the course of a perimetric examination, patients may become fatigued and their sensitivity decreases. Fatigue depends on the patient and the examination time. After more than 10 minutes, fatigue effects become increasingly likely. Nearly all perimeters report and store the duration of the examination (Fig. 4.2E). If the examiner suspects fatigue based on direct observation or the result of the test, perimetry should be repeated with sufficient breaks, comfortable clothing, a proper sitting position, and fresh air in the room to avoid fatigue.

Pupil Diameter

An abnormally large or small pupil may significantly affect the interpretation of visual field results. Thus, documentation of pupil diameter is very important (Fig. 4.2E) and should be recorded in every case. If the pupil size is abnormal, the examination may need to be repeated. In glaucoma patients with small pupils, pilocarpine therapy should be discontinued at least 24 hours before perimetry. The use of irreversible cholinesterase inhibitors should be discontinued several weeks before perimetry, but they may be replaced by pilocarpine during that period. If the pupil diameter is still less than 3 mm, sphincter sclerosis or synechia is probably present. Short-acting mydriatics may be given, with some effect.

Learning Effect

Lack of experience during the first examination with an automated perimeter will result in reduced sensitivity, often with increased measurement error (SF index) and sometimes unexplained defects (see Section 3.18 in Chapter 3). The quality of the result is better when the examiner has had prior experience with manual perimeters, and it is better in the second eye tested on the first day.
The order in which the eyes were examined can be deduced from the stored examination times (Fig. 4.2E). If a learning deficit is suspected, the examination has to be repeated on another day. If a longer follow-up interval is planned (as in glaucoma patients), repetition is always recommended because the first examination should be discarded routinely.

Unreliable Results

If the results are unreliable the test should be repeated, preferably on a different day. Examination results, however, should never be deleted. They always contain some—though perhaps limited—information. The first result in Figure 4.2F is sufficient for diagnosis because, despite a false-positive index of 43%, the arcuate scotoma is easily recognized. However, this result cannot be used for follow-up comparisons, because all values are shifted. This is very well illustrated by the index mean defect MD in Fig. 4.2F, which was about 3 dB better in the first, unreliable field exam than in the second exam representing the true visual field.

Figure 4.2E. Header in the Peridata Standard Printout. Important quality data are the reliability indices, time of the test (order of eyes tested), pupil diameter, and test duration (fatigue).

Figure 4.2F. Series of a patient with a glaucomatous arcuate scotoma in his left eye and a high false-positive index for the first examination (HFA program 30-2, Peridata "compressed").

PERIDATA Professional 7.0 PRIVATDOZ. DR. MED. JOERG WEBER, COLOGNE
1 TEST * SINGLE RESULT (08-10-98 D:\PROJEKTE\ETLAS\GF\ETLAS.PHF)

4.02E NAME, FIRSTNAME *09-08-35 ID: +51875 (LE: Glaucoma chronicum simplex)

LE 04-03-89 10.04 HFA1 30-2 ZENTRALFELD SCHWELLENTEST Stim III (200ms) Full threshold
Pupil 3.5 mm VA 0.50 Fixation Target Central RX Used 3.00 DS -2.00 DC 90° axis
Test Duration 19:42 min Questions 571 MalFixation [III] 0% (0/28) FalsePos 0% (0/17) FalseNeg 0% (0/14)

4.2E

LE 04-27-87 7.09 HFA1 30-2 ZENTRALFELD SCHWELLENTEST Stim III (200ms) Full threshold
Pupil 4.0 mm VA 1.30 Fixation Target Central RX Used 5.00 DS 0.00 DC 0° axis
Test Duration 26:51 min Questions 730 MalFixation [IV] 51% (18/35) FalsePos 43% (9/21) FalseNeg 16% (3/19)

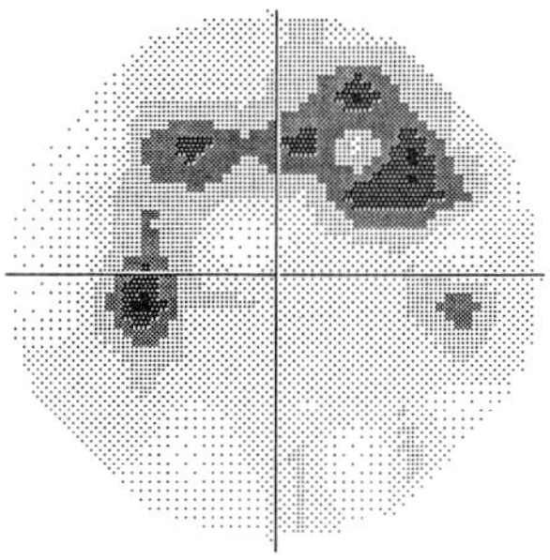

```
                o  o -6  o
             o  o  o -7 -21-5
        +13-11-18-12-20  o -23  o
      +12  o -8 -9 -5  o -18-20-12  o
      +7   o -12-6 +10  o  o -6 +6  o
      +14  o BS-25-5 -5  o  o -5 -14  o
       o   o -7  o  o  o  o  o -5  o
           o -5  o  o  o  o -5 +10
              o +9  o -6 +11-8
                 o  o -5  o
                   -30°
```

MD	-3.4
LV	57.3
CLV	37.1
PSD	7.6
CPSD	6.1
SF	5.3
N	75.0
MS	26.3
FS	89.1

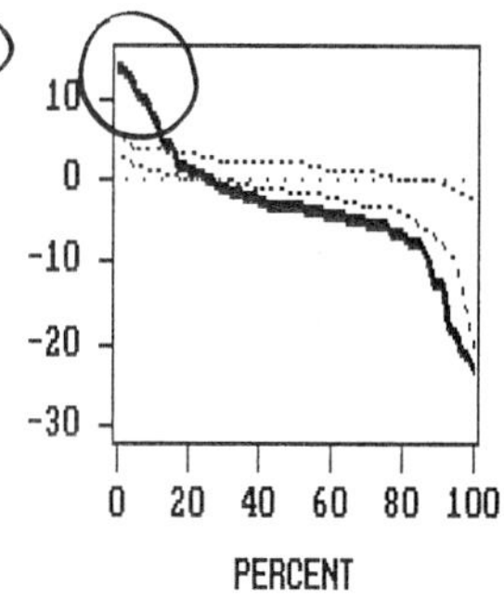

LE 04-29-87 14.22 HFA1 30-2 ZENTRALFELD SCHWELLENTEST Stim III (200ms) Full threshold
Pupil 4.0 mm VA 1.30 Fixation Target Central RX Used 5.00 DS 0.00 DC 0° axis
Test Duration 17:46 min Questions 517 MalFixation [IV] 7% (2/27) FalsePos 0% (0/18) FalseNeg 0% (0/10)

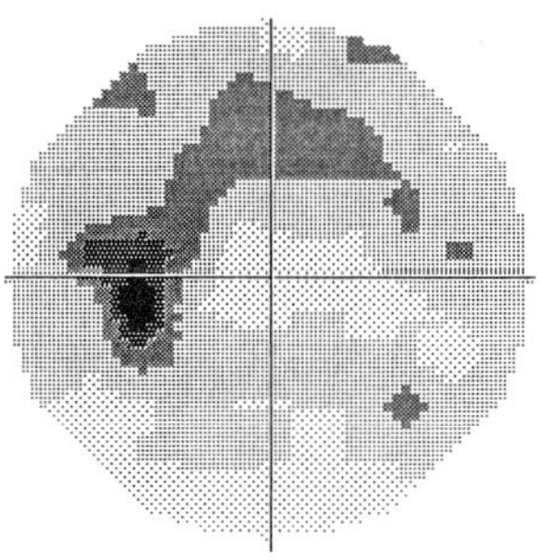

```
               -5 -6  o -11
            -11-7 -13-9 -7 -9
         -9 -7 -10-13-12-15-5  o
      -5 -5 -7 -12-7 -8 -6 -12-6 -7
       o -17-19-12  o  o  o -8 -10-8
      -8 -6 BS-29-5  o  o  o  o -6 -8
      -8 -6 -12-7 -8 -5 -5 -7  o -7
            o  o -6  o -5 -5 -12-7
              -5 -6 -6  o -5 -6
                 o  o  o  o
                   -30°
```

MD	-6.7
LV	12.7
CLV	4.1
PSD	3.6
CPSD	2.0
SF	3.2
N	75.0
MS	22.9
FS	51.0

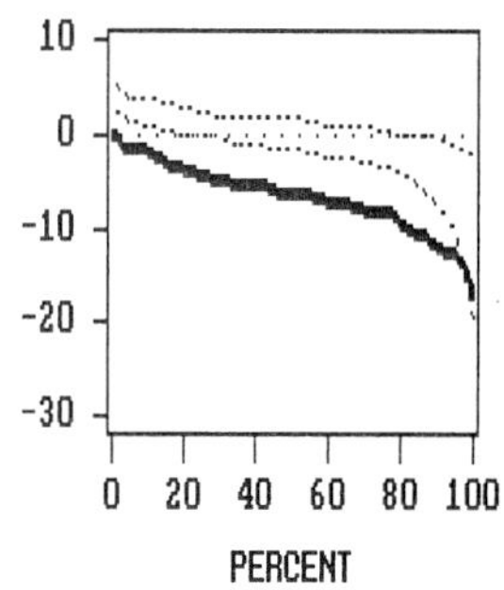

4.2F

4.3 NORMALITY

Prerequisites

The determination of whether a visual field test result is normal or pathological is based on a comparison with normal data from a group of healthy subjects. The normal value in its true sense is the mean value for a given field location or an index. The normal range depends on the scatter of the values. Depending on the definition, it may include 80% (10th to 90th percentile) or 90% (5th to 95th percentile) of the values from the group of normal subjects.

It is good practice to define normal data according to age. Additional factors are stimulus size, stimulus duration, stimulus color, and background luminance. In general, normal values are known only for the standard configuration of stimulus and background.

Normal data are different for each type of instrument even when stimulus and background values are similar. Therefore, universal analytical programs use different normal data sets for each instrument.

Pointwise Evaluation

Pointwise normality is checked by looking at the numerical display. With norm-related sensitivity values (synonyms: *relative sensitivity, defect values, difference values, deviation*), a value of 0 dB is normal. The normal range (5th to 95th percentile) is usually from +4 dB to −4 dB. Some perimeters and printouts suppress values within the normal range and show a "symbol of normality" (e.g., a cross or a small circle) instead of a number (Fig. 4.3A).

A caveat should be mentioned here: not all numerical representations with the label "defect" are really norm related. "Defects" in the three-in-one printout of the Humphrey Field Analyzer are related to individually adjusted reference values based on a simple, age-independent, normal hill of vision. With predominantly homonymous (diffuse) depression (e.g., cataract or early glaucomatous damage), no defects are indicated. Such representations are often useless and misleading.

With the Humphrey Field Analyzer, the normal range increases considerably toward the periphery. Therefore, an alternative normal evaluation is carried out pointwise and indicated in a *probability plot.* Defect depth is replaced by symbols which indicate how far the result is from the normal range (Fig. 4.3B, Section 2).

An overall evaluation of the normality of a visual field based on pointwise data is difficult. Even in a normal field, every 20th value may exceed the 5th percentile or 4 dB defect depth. Abnormality requires a larger number of defect points or deeper defects. Also, neighboring depressed points (defect cluster, Fig. 4.3C) are more likely to be abnormal. There are some rules of thumb which take these probabilities into account. For example, typical early glaucomatous visual field defects can be defined as two or more contiguous points with $p < 0.01$ (or 10 dB loss) or greater in the superior or inferior arcuate areas, compared with perimeter-defined, age-matched controls; or three or contiguous points with $p < 0.05$ (or 5 dB loss) or greater in the superior or inferior arcuate areas; or a 10 dB difference across the nasal horizontal midline in two or more adjacent locations.

Figure 4.3A. Numerical display of relative sensitivity (defects) with the analysis Peridata program (left: Octopus program 32; right: HFA program 30-2).

Figure 4.3B. Total deviation and probability plot of the Humphrey Field Analyzer (Statpac Analysis).

Figure 4.3C. Defect cluster (Peridata: numerals and grayscale).

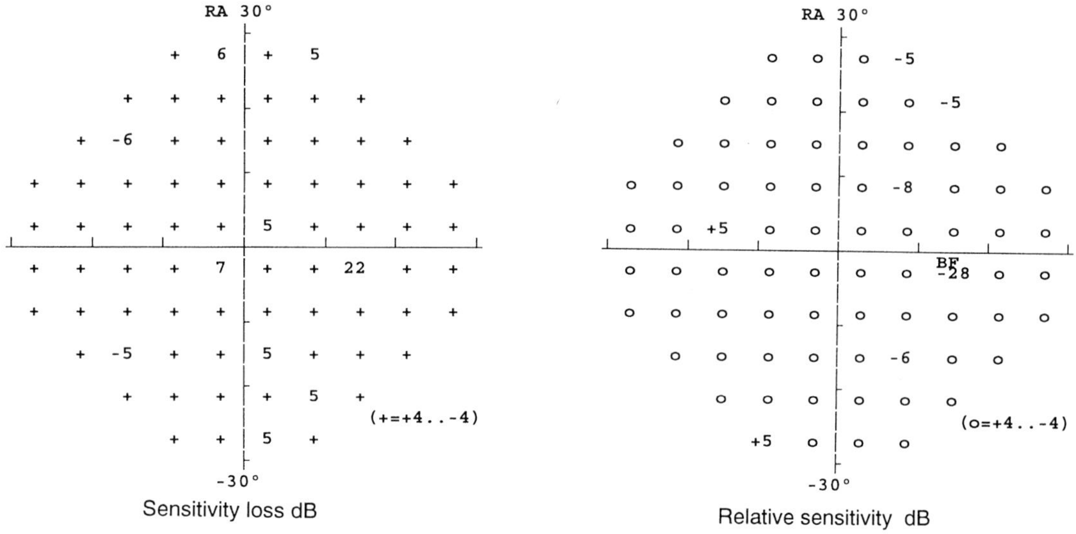
RA 30°
-30°
(+=+4..-4)
Sensitivity loss dB
RA 30°
BF -28
(o=+4..-4)
-30°
Relative sensitivity dB

4.3A

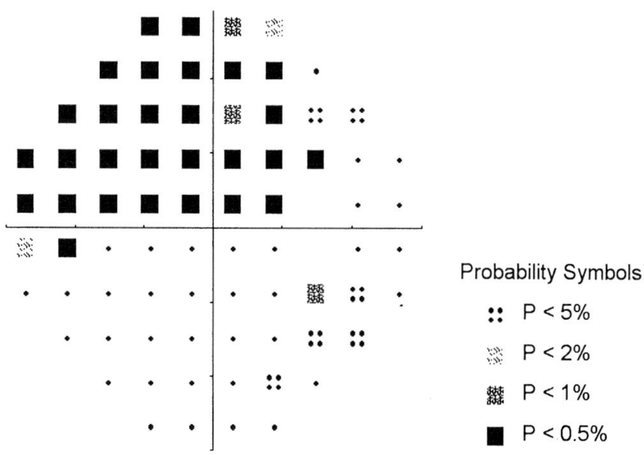
Probability Symbols
P < 5%
P < 2%
P < 1%
P < 0.5%

4.3B

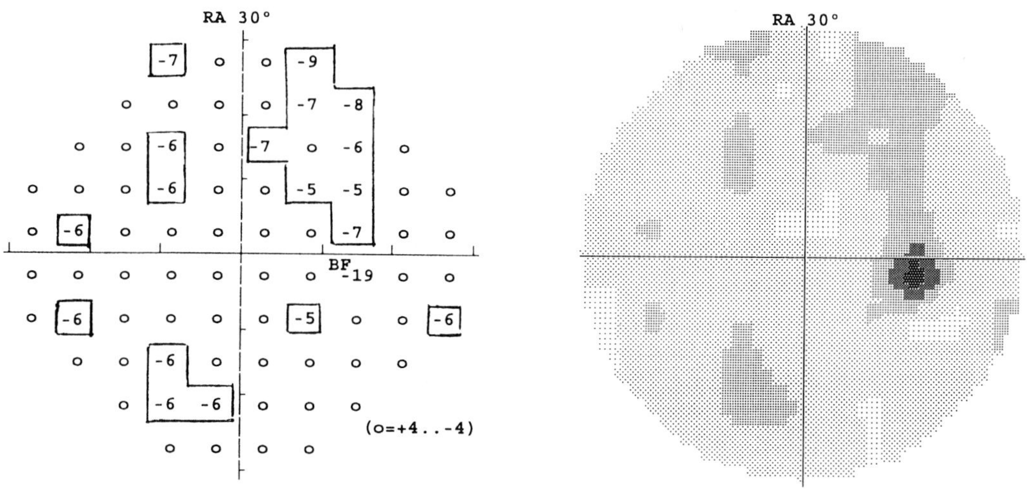
RA 30°
BF -19
(o=+4..-4)
RA 30°

4.3C

Pointwise deviation from normality is also shown in a norm-related grayscale display. Defect clusters are also easily identified because interpolation increases the "dark" area disproportionately, whereas a single defect point is represented by a very small dark spot (Fig. 4.3C). Interpolation is therefore a type of graphical cluster analysis.

Global Normality

The global MD index is the mean value of all measured data. Using this index, the influence of accidental variation (pointwise measurement error and spatial variation) is reduced considerably. Consequently, the normal MD range is smaller (from about +2dB to −2dB) than the pointwise normal range (+4 to −4 dB or, for the periphery of the Humphrey Field Analyzer, from +6 to −10 dB). The other global indices are also stabilized by the use of many data points. Figure 4.3D shows normal ranges as they are supplied for the Octopus program G1.

The cumulative defect curve represents single values, but due to the sort process, the single values at a given rank depend on their global distribution. By that distribution, the values are stabilized similarly to the global indices, and the cumulative defect curve has a small normal range of about 2 dB. The normal range (5th to 95th percentile) is drawn on the graph (Fig. 4.3E).

Topographical Normality

In addition to global field indices, there are topographical indices (Glaucoma Hemifield Index, Clusterindex, Conformity indices) which quantify the clustering of defects with a given topography. They will be discussed below. These indices have normal ranges.

Summary Evaluation

A visual field is abnormal if the normal range is exceeded in any of the data representations (pointwise, global indices, cumulative curve, topographical indices, lateral difference).

The relative significance of these data representations depends on the type of visual field damage. In cases of homogeneous damage, the MD index and the cumulative defect curve become abnormal at a relatively early stage (Fig. 4.3F). In cases of heterogeneous damage, pointwise values, the indices of variation (pattern standard deviation/loss variance [PSD/LV]), and the cumulative defect curve (right half) become abnormal at a relatively early stage (Fig. 4.3G). In our experience, the cumulative curve is the most significant tool for the overall identification of abnormalities.

Figure 4.3D. Table of visual field indices with normal ranges for program G1 (Octopus).

Figure 4.3E. Cumulative defect curve with normal range (5th and 95th percentiles).

Figure 4.3F. Homogeneous sensitivity loss in the right eye of a 52-year-old patient with primary open-angle glaucoma and visual acuity of 1.3 (program: HFA 30-2, representation: Peridata "compressed").

Figure 4.3G. Heterogeneous, clearly localized sensitivity loss in the left eye of a 49-year-old patient with primary open-angle glaucoma and visual acuity of 1.3 (program: HFA 30-2, representation: Peridata "compressed").

		Normal	Phase 1	Phase 2	Mean
			59	0	0
MS	[dB]		8.0		
MD	[dB]	-2..2	21.2		
LV	[dB²]	0..6	58.6		
CLV	[dB²]	0..4			
SF	[dB]	0..2			
RF	[%]				18.2

4.3D

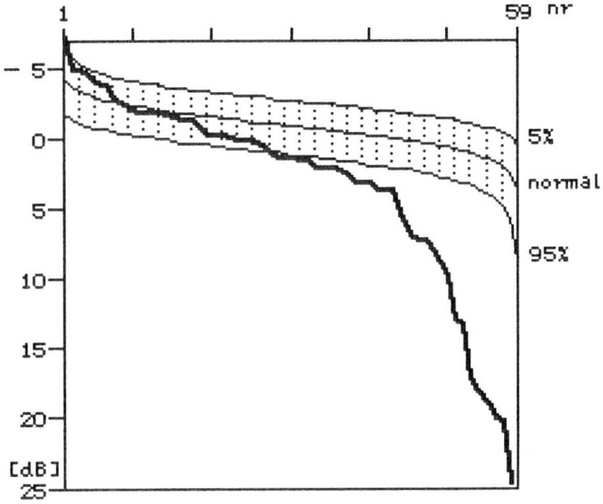

4.3E

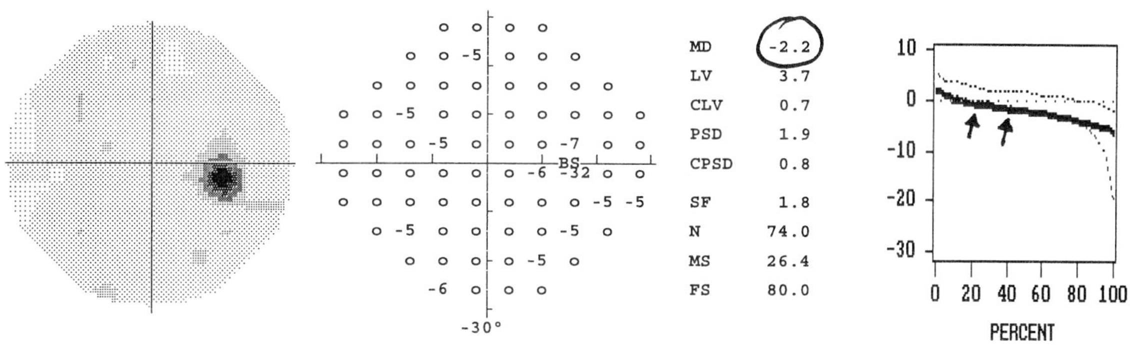

4.3F

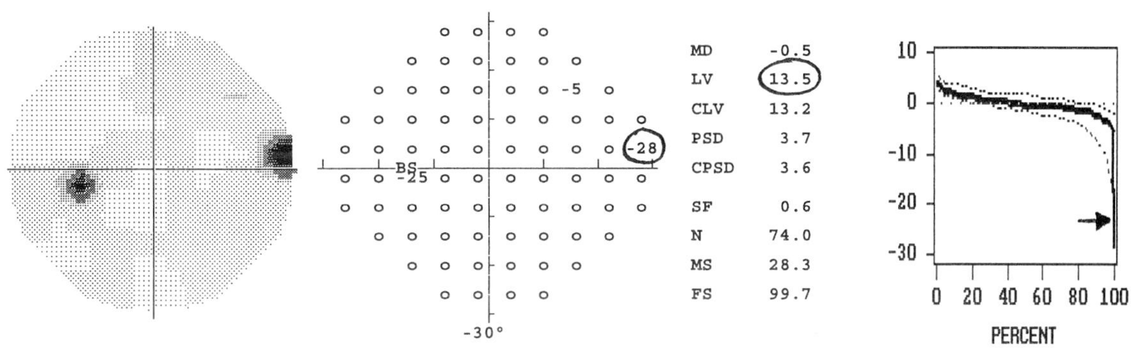

4.3G

However, the decision to declare a field abnormal is individual and also depends on the purpose of the examination. Normal ranges are based on normal percentiles and thus on a given specificity. If we choose a high specificity, we get wider ranges and, of course, lose sensitivity, and vice versa. The art of interpretation lies in choosing a test with adequate specificity. For example, in deciding whether to see a patient again, low specificity but high sensitivity is adequate. If we choose the wide range of the 90th percentile, we obtain high sensitivity, but we also classify 10% of all true normal patients as abnormal. This is acceptable since the only drawback is an additional visit. A decision on whether to start treatment, however, requires higher specificity. If we choose the 95th percentile, 5% of all true normals would be treated. Depending on the severity of the treatment (e.g. surgery), even higher specificity (98th or 99th percentile)—meaning deeper defects in the visual field—might be required. These examples show that one should never interpret a visual field in a vacuum without evaluating all the clinical circumstances.

Pseudonormal Results

Normal results can be falsely produced by inadequate printouts (e.g., defects in the Humphrey Field Analyzer three-in-one printout). Misinterpretation is also possible if the analysis is correct but the examination program is not problem oriented. The most frequent problem is the use of inadequate measurement strategies which miss shallow and diffuse damage, although such a defect may be found in high-tension glaucoma, for example (see Section 3.9 in Chapter 3).

Another cause of pseudonormal results is inappropriate test patterns. In low-tension glaucoma, for example, small and short arcuate scotomas are frequent. The 6° Humphrey Field Analyzer programs 31 and 30-1 assess them incompletely. Programs 32 and 30-2 assess them, but only a combination (with a subsequent point density of 4.2°) shows the arcuate topography accurately and thus allows a differential diagnosis (Fig. 4.3H).

Figure 4.3H. Short paracentral arcuate scotoma in the right eye of a 49-year-old patient with low-tension glaucoma and visual acuity of 1.0. Program HFA 30-1 (top) does not assess the defect sufficiently; the field is pseudonormal. Program HFA 30-2 (center) discovers a deep scotoma. Only the combination of both programs (bottom) shows the topography and thus the diagnosis accurately (representation: Peridata grayscale and numerals, both norm-related).

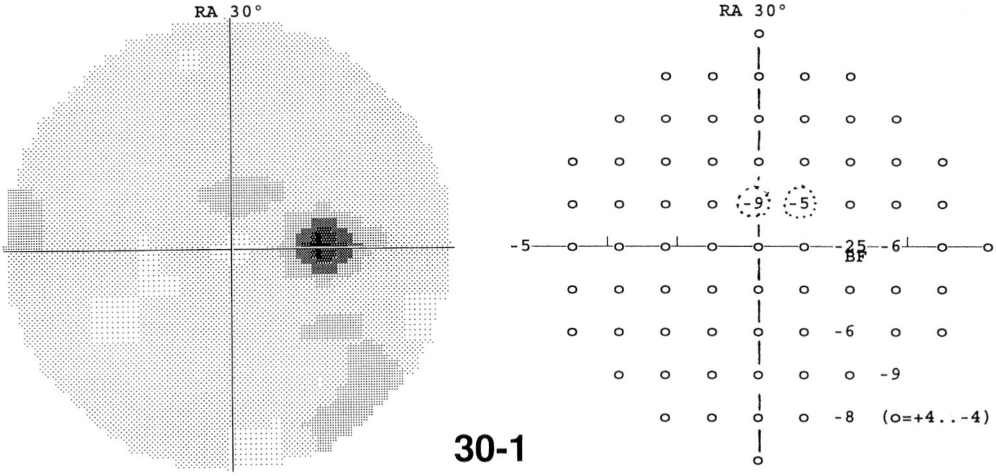

30-1

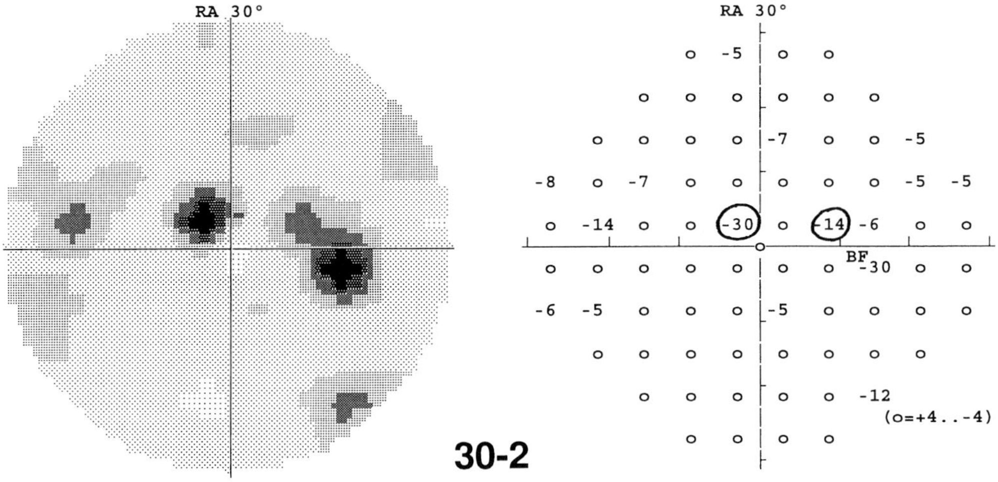

30-2

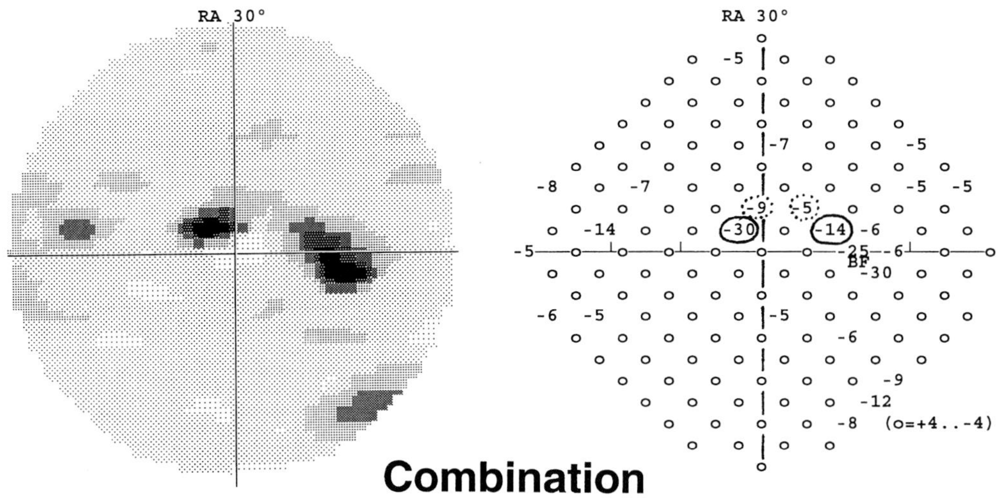

Combination

4.3H

4.4 DIFFERENTIAL DIAGNOSIS

General Considerations

There are different ways to determine the origin of damage from visual field defects. All of these methods depend on topography, that is, the spatial pattern of defects. However, although the site of the damage may be pinpointed, the nature of the damage cannot be determined in most cases. It is mainly the topography of visual projection which determines the topography of the field defects. The following subsection describes two ways to approach diagnosis, or at least localization of the damage, to answer the question "Where is the lesion located?" For further analysis, see Chapter 3. No schemes or rules are absolute; there are many exceptions.

Differential Diagnosis Using Laterality, Congruence, and Ophthalmoscopy

Unilateral visual field defects are caused by changes anterior to the chiasm. Two exceptions are unilateral learning deficit and unilateral fatigue. Another exception is a temporal crescent scotoma in cortical processes at the apex of the calcarine sulcus, which is called a homonymous hemianopia *minus*. However, these scotomas are often missed with computerized perimetry. Lesions that cause bilateral visual field defects can be located anywhere. If they are homonymous, they are likely to be postchiasmal. An exception is asymmetric retinal disease. If bilateral field defects are heteronymous or irregular, the lesion is in the chiasm or anterior to it. If prechiasmal or chiasmal lesions (unilateral, bilateral heteronymous/irregular) are associated with a poor view of the fundus, a media opacity or irregularity may be present (in the cornea, lens, or vitreous). If the fundus image is clear, the lesion is more posterior. If ophthalmoscopy reveals changes in the choroid, retina, or retinal vessels, the lesion is anterior to the optic nerve. If the fundus is normal, the lesion is in the optic nerve or, in the case of bilateral field defects, in either the nerve or the chiasm (Fig. 4.4A).

Postchiasmal lesions (bilateral, homonymous field defects) can be classified based on the appearance of the optic disc if the lesion is more than 4–6 weeks old. If the disc shows pallor, the optic tract or the lateral geniculate body is involved (tract sign). Otherwise, a suprageniculate lesion is present. If the congruence of field defects is high, the lesion is more likely to be in the cortex; if congruence is low, it is more likely to be in the optic radiation.

Mathematical Tools: Congruence Index

The combined congruence index determines, by its sign, which type of congruence is present. Homonymous defects have a positive sign, heteronymous defects a negative sign (Fig. 4.4B–C). The size of the value determines the significance of this decision. Values above 0.1 are considered good proof of congruence. Homonymous and heteronymous congruence indices indicate the degree of congruence.

Figure 4.4A. Decision tree for differential diagnosis using laterality, congruence, and ophthalmoscopy.

Figure 4.4B–C. Examples of the congruence index (see text).

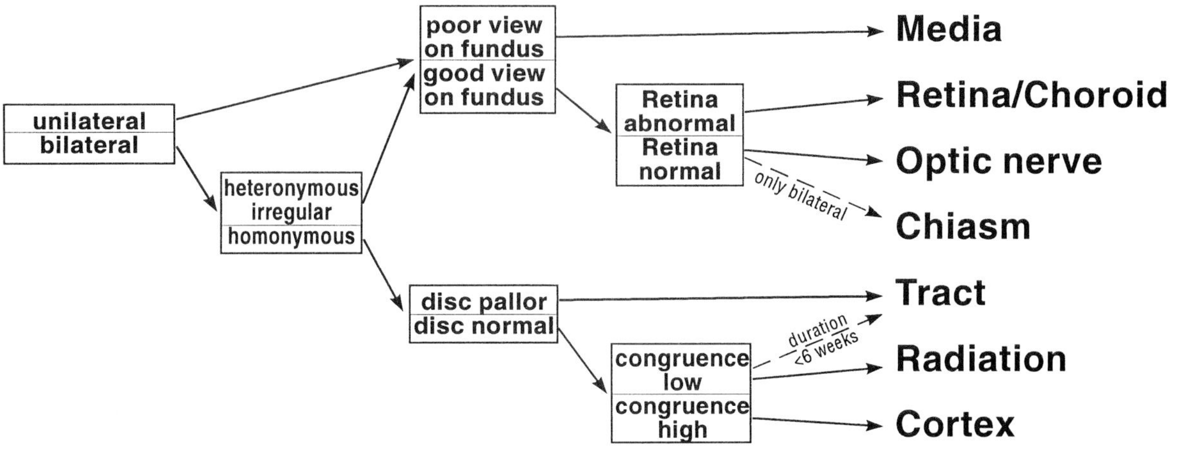

unilateral
bilateral
heteronymous
irregular
homonymous
poor view on fundus
good view on fundus
disc pallor
disc normal
Retina abnormal
Retina normal
congruence low
congruence high
only bilateral
duration <6 weeks
Media
Retina/Choroid
Optic nerve
Chiasm
Tract
Radiation
Cortex

4.4A

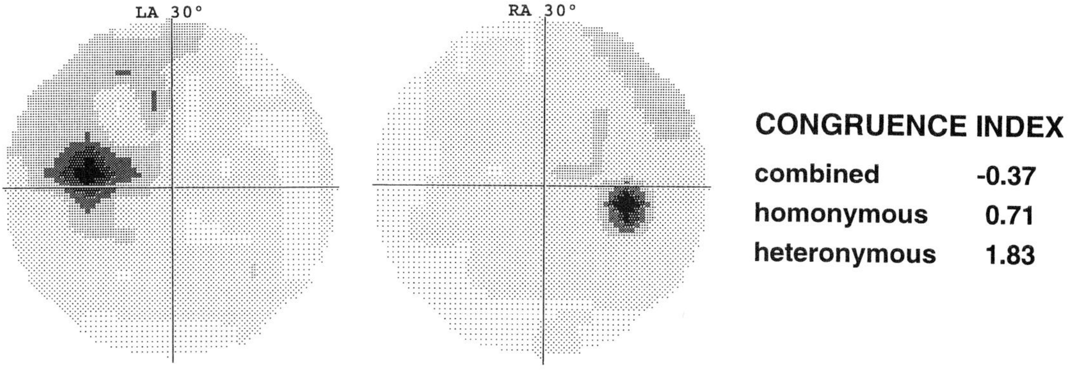

LA 30°
RA 30°
CONGRUENCE INDEX
combined -0.37
homonymous 0.71
heteronymous 1.83

4.4B

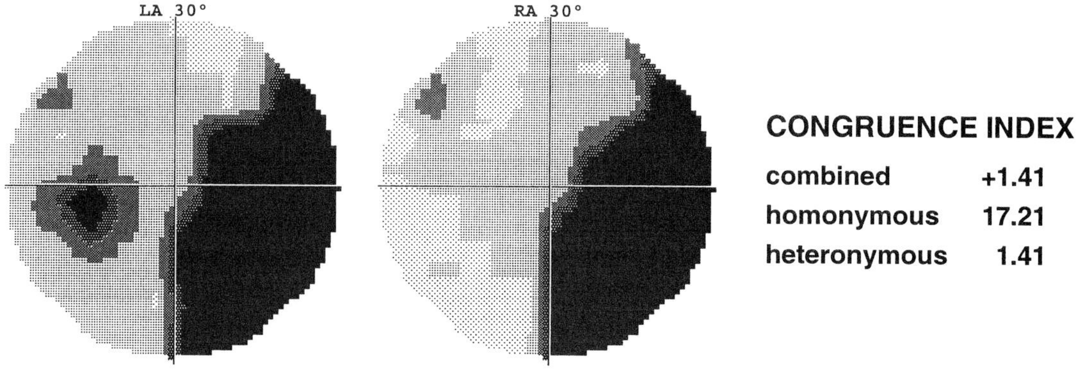

LA 30°
RA 30°
CONGRUENCE INDEX
combined +1.41
homonymous 17.21
heteronymous 1.41

4.4C

Differential Diagnosis Using Defect Shape

Another method for reaching a differential diagnosis is based on the shape of the visual field defect. Shape has two aspects: form (e.g., quadrant, ring, sector) and location (e.g., quadrant: upper nasal, ring: between 20° and 30°). Shape has more variants than laterality and congruence. Both decision pathways are complementary and should be combined. The following lists of shapes also contain hints about laterality (MO = monolateral, BI = bilateral) and congruence (HO = homonymous, HE = heteronymous).

The shape of the defect is determined by the anatomy of the visual pathway and the topography of the damage. True damage, however, may deviate from idealized patterns. For example, nerve fiber bundle defects, which may be peripheral, may appear as sector defects, quadrant defects, or half-ring-shaped peripheral defects. The following lists denote the true appearance of the defect. Because the number of possible combinations is almost unlimited, those listed are the ones which are most frequent in our experience. Exceptions are always possible, of course.

Hemianopia

Nasal (similar: long (NFB)-related arcuate scotomas): optic disc/glaucoma (MO/HE), neuritis (MO), chiasm from lateral (HE, very rare), tract/radiation/ cortex (HO)

Temporal: myopic staphyloma (MO/HE), neuritis (MO), center of chiasm (HE), tract/radiation/cortex (HO)

Altitudinal Hemianopia (Upper/Lower Half)

Lower (similar: long + short NFB-related arcuate scotoma): (NH): retinal detachment/retinoschisis upper (MO), retinal vessel occlusion (MO), optic disc/ glaucoma (MO/BI), orbita (MO/BI), cortex (BI, excessive blood loss, very rare)

Upper (similar: long + short NFB-related arcuate scotoma): NH: retinal detachment/retinoschisis lower (MO), retinal vessel occlusion (MO), optic disc/glaucoma (MO/BI), orbita (MO/BI)

One Quadrant

Upper/lower nasal (similar: long NFB-related arcuate scotoma): retinal vessel occlusion (MO), optic disc/glaucoma (MO/HE/rare HO), orbita (MO/HE), chiasm from lateral (MO/HE, rare), tract/radiation/cortex (HO)

Upper temporal (similar: upper NFB defect/arcuate scotoma nach upper): myopic staphyloma (MO/HE), optic disc/glaucoma (MO/HE), orbital papilledema (MO/HE), center of chiasm from below (HE), tract/radiation/cortex (HO)

Lower temporal (similar: lower NFB-related arcuate scotoma): optic disc/glaucoma (MO/HE), orbital papilledema (MO/HE), center of chiasm from above (HE), tract/radiation/cortex (HO)

Two Quadrants

Optic disc/glaucoma (MO/HE), cortex (HO)

Three Quadrants

Optic disc/glaucoma (MO/HE), center of chiasm (HE), tract/radiation/cortex (HO)

Figure 4.4D. Shapes (patterns) of visual field defects.

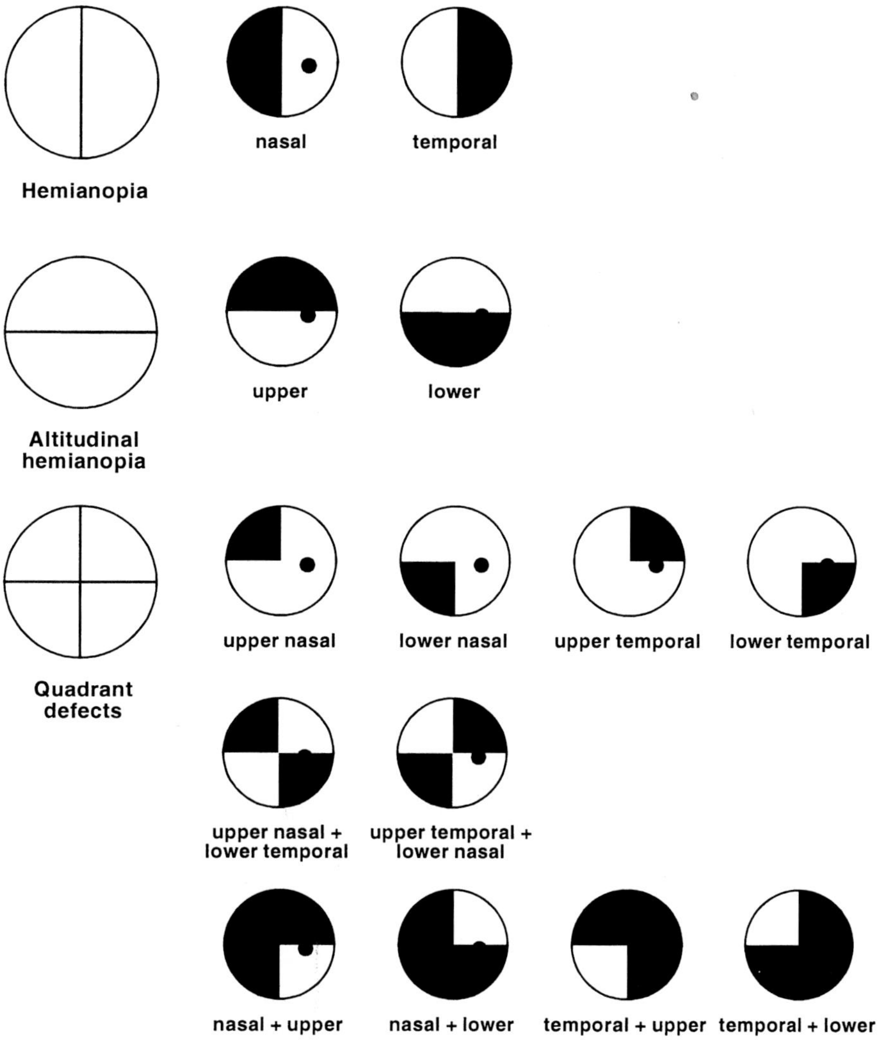
nasal
temporal
Hemianopia
upper
lower
Altitudinal hemianopia
upper nasal
lower nasal
upper temporal
lower temporal
Quadrant defects
upper nasal + lower temporal
upper temporal + lower nasal
nasal + upper
nasal + lower
temporal + upper
temporal + lower

4.4D

Small Sector

Upper/lower temporal (similar: NFB-related arcuate scotoma): optic disc/glaucoma (MO/HE), chiasm (HE), tract/radiation/cortex (HO)

Upper/lower nasal: tract/radiation/cortex (HO)

Nasal horizontally (similar: long NFB-related arcuate scotoma): optic disc/glaucoma (MO/HE), cortex (HO)

Temporal horizontally (similar: temporal NFB sector): optic disc/glaucoma (MO/HE), cortex (HO)

Large Sector

Temporal (similar: quadrant, hemianopia, large temporal NFB sector): myopic staphyloma (MO/HE), orbital disc edema (MO/HE), chiasm (HE), tract/radiation/cortex (HO)

Nasal (similar: quadrant and hemianopia, long NFB-related arcuate scotomata): optic disc/glaucoma (MO/HE), orbital (MO/HE), chiasm from lateral (MO/HE, rare), tract/radiation/cortex (HO)

Two Sectors

Nasal + temporal: theoretical, never seen

Upper + lower: optic disc/glaucoma (MO/HE)

Nerve Fiber Bundle Shape

Temporal NFB sector (originating at the blind spot; similar: temporal sector): myopic staphyloma (MO/HE), optic disc/glaucoma (MO/HE), neuritis (MO), orbital (MO/HE)

Long arcuate scotoma (similar: nasal quadrant, nasal hemianopia, temporal sector, nasal sector): retinal vessel occlusion, retinochoroiditis juxtapapillaris (MO), optic disc/glaucoma (MO/HE), neuritis (MO), orbital/anterior chiasm (MO/HE)

Short arcuate scotoma: like long arcuate scotoma

Cecocentral scotoma (similar: central scotoma, partial central scotoma): eccentric macular degeneration (MO/HE), optic disc/glaucoma (MO/HE), optic nerve degeneration/congenital + acquired (HE), neuritis (MO/rare HE)

Ring/Circle

Outer (10°/20° to outer border of the measured area/30°): lens rim, plus lens effect, retinitis pigmentosa, central venous occlusion, diabetic retinopathy, orbital, functional

Inner (2° to 5°): toxic macular degeneration (HE)

Central scotoma (similar: cecocentral scotoma, partial central scotoma): hereditary and acquired macular degeneration/macular edema (MO/HE), central retinitis/choroiditis (MO), neuritis

Pericecal Scotoma (Enlarged Blind Spot)

Conus circularis papillae (MO/BI), fibrae medullaris (MO/BI), papilledema (MO/BI)

Figure 4.4E. Shapes (patterns) of visual field defects.

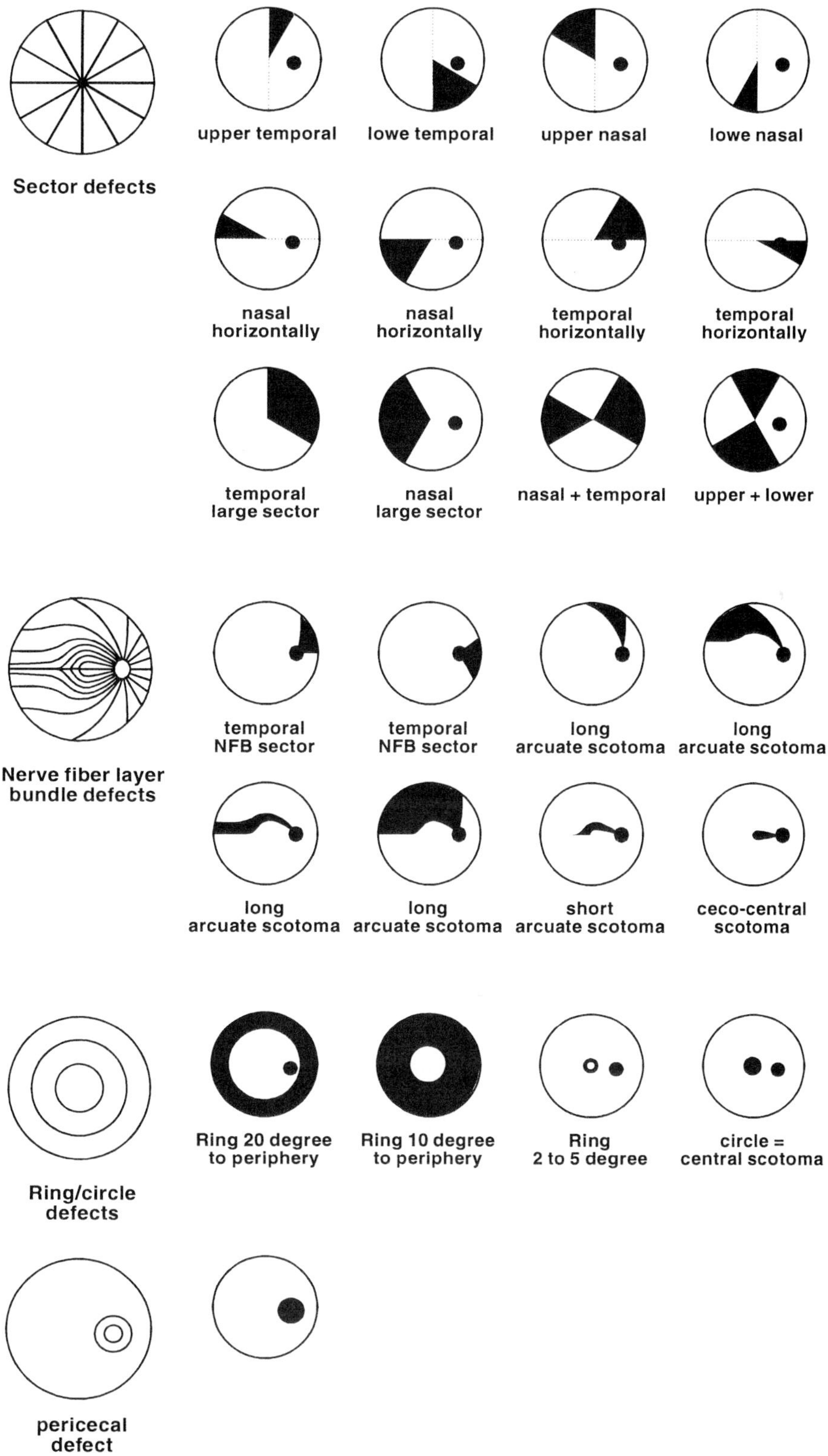
Sector defects
upper temporal
lowe temporal
upper nasal
lowe nasal
nasal horizontally
nasal horizontally
temporal horizontally
temporal horizontally
temporal large sector
nasal large sector
nasal + temporal
upper + lower
Nerve fiber layer bundle defects
temporal NFB sector
temporal NFB sector
long arcuate scotoma
long arcuate scotoma
long arcuate scotoma
long arcuate scotoma
short arcuate scotoma
ceco-central scotoma
Ring/circle defects
Ring 20 degree to periphery
Ring 10 degree to periphery
Ring 2 to 5 degree
circle = central scotoma
pericecal defect

4.4E

Peripheral Constriction

Upper: lens rim/brow/upper lid (MO/BI), retinal vessel occlusion (MO), optic disc/glaucoma (MO/BI), orbital (MO/HE)

Lower: lens rim (MO/BI), retinal vessel occlusion (MO), optic disc/glaucoma (MO/HE), orbital (MO/HE)

Nasal: lens rim (MO/HO/HE), optic disc/glaucoma (MO), tract/radiation/cortex (HO)

Temporal: lens rim (MO/HO/HE), myopic staphyloma (MO/HE), chiasm (HE), tract/radiation/cortex (HO)

Partial Central Scotoma

One half (similar: central scotoma, cecocentral scotoma): hereditary and acquired macular degeneration (MO/HE), central retinitis/choroiditis (MO), radiation/cortex (HO)

Both halves (similar: central scotoma, cecocentral scotoma): hereditary and acquired macular degeneration (MO/HE), central retinitis/choroiditis (MO)

Diffuse

False correction (MO), ptosis (MO/BI), corneal opacification/cataract/vitreal opacification (MO/BI), small pupil (MO/BI), glaucoma (MO/BI), neuritis (MO), orbital/anterior chiasm (MO)

Mathematical Tools to Assess Shape

Several mathematical methods are used to assess the topographical properties of a visual field numerically. Such indices are called *topographical indices*. The cluster index (Peridata program) tests, by calculation, whether an extraordinarily high clustering of defects is present. It is normal in cases of diffuse damage and large, homogeneous defects (e.g., hemianopia). The conformity index (Peridata program) tests the accordance of the defect pattern with several standard patterns. Location is not considered. The index is calculated for every standard shape and presented in a list which is sorted by the degree of conformity. The first pattern in the list fits best (Fig. 4.4G–H).

The glaucoma hemifield test (program Statpac, Humphrey Field Analyzer) depends on sensitivity differences between the upper and lower hemifields. The sum of these differences represents an index. The program does not show the index, but it does show whether this index is normal, borderline, or abnormal compared to its normal range. This test is positive for all defects located predominantly in one hemifield. Because spatial variance is not considered (in contrast to the conformity index), it may be positive in irregular fields with no significant hemifield predominance.

Figure 4.4F. Shapes (patterns) of visual field defects.

Figure 4.4G. Conformity indices in a glaucoma field with an absolute quadrant defect and an arcuate scotoma.

Figure 4.4H. Conformity indices in a glaucoma field with an absolute sector defect and a relative quadrant defect which is not limited by the vertical axis.

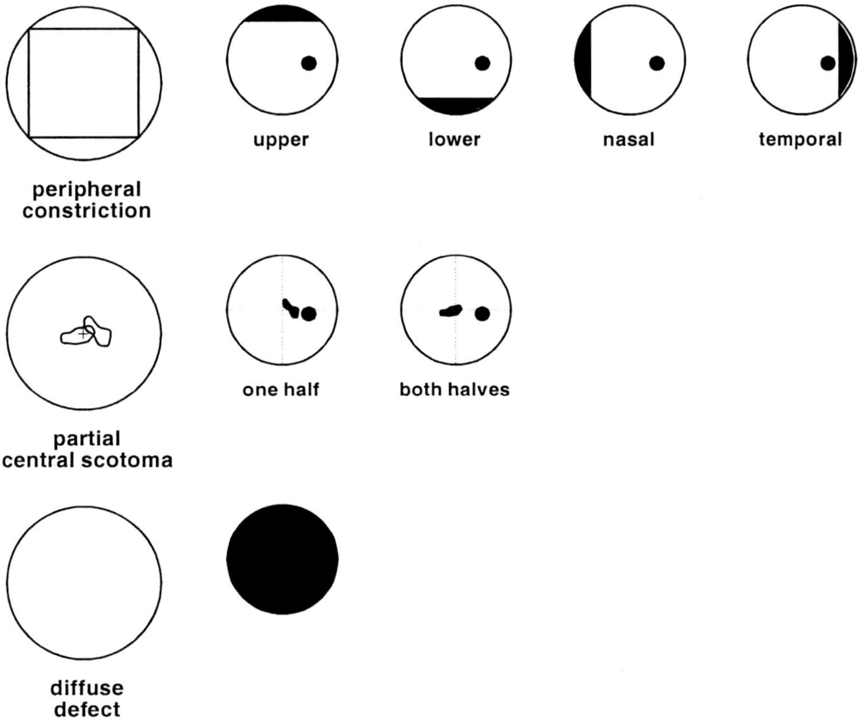

4.4F

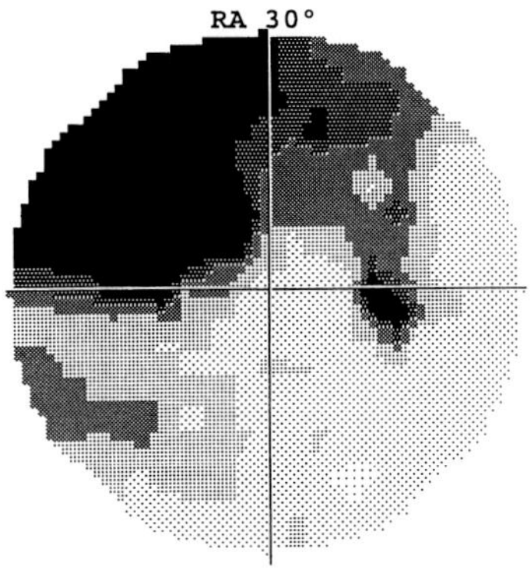

CONFORMITY INDEX	
Quadrants	2.11xx
NerveFibreBundles	1.80xx
Sectors	1.74xx
21 NerveFibreBundles	1.69xx
UpperLower-Hemifield	1.54xx
RightLeft-Hemifield	1.37xx
Rings	1.03
Center	1.02

4.4G

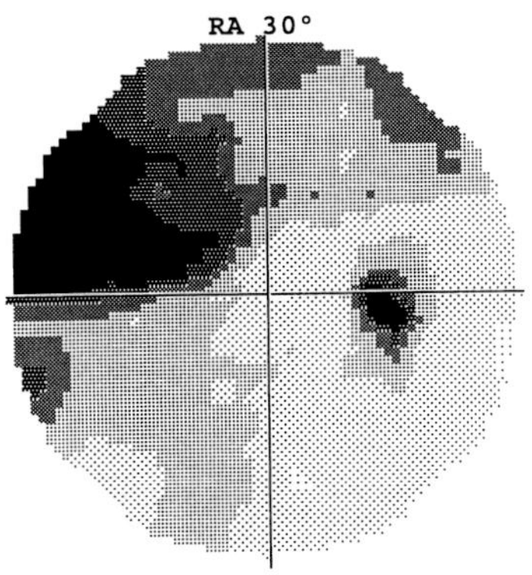

CONFORMITY INDEX	
Sectors	1.69xx
Quadrants	1.66xx
RightLeft-Hemifield	1.50xx
NerveFibreBundles	1.45xx
21 NerveFibreBundles	1.36xx
UpperLower-Hemifield	1.25xx
Center	1.03
Rings	1.02

4.4H

Shape and Pattern Density

Insufficient density of the test point pattern may lead to inaccurate or false assessment of a defect's shape. Differential diagnostic difficulties and errors may follow. Especially in the center, assessment of the alignment of defect borders and axis, of nerve fiber bundle shape, or of congruence is important and requires a resolution higher than the traditional 6° (Fig. 4.4J).

Shape and Pattern Geometry

The geometry of a test point pattern influences the shape of visual field defects. Rectangular patterns create rectangular and rhomboid defects in interpolated representations. Scotoma borders on the axis become more linear than they really are. Diagonal patterns may show zigzag borders (Fig. 4.4K). Circular patterns may look like arcuate scotomas. These pseudoshapes have to be considered in visual field interpretation.

Figure 4.4J. Long NFB-related arcuate scotoma in a case of low-tension glaucoma. Insufficient assessment with a 6° pattern (upper, program HFA 30-2) and clear representation using a 4.2° pattern (lower, program HFA 30-1 and 30-2 combined) representation with Peridata grayscale and a numeral plot.

Figure 4.4K. Hemianopia with macular sparing in a case of sphenoidal meningioma. Unnatural linearity is produced with a rectangular pattern (upper, program HFA 30-2). The indented line has a pseudoshape with a diagonal pattern (lower, programs HFA 30-1 and 30-2 combined). The representation uses the Peridata grayscale and a numeral map.

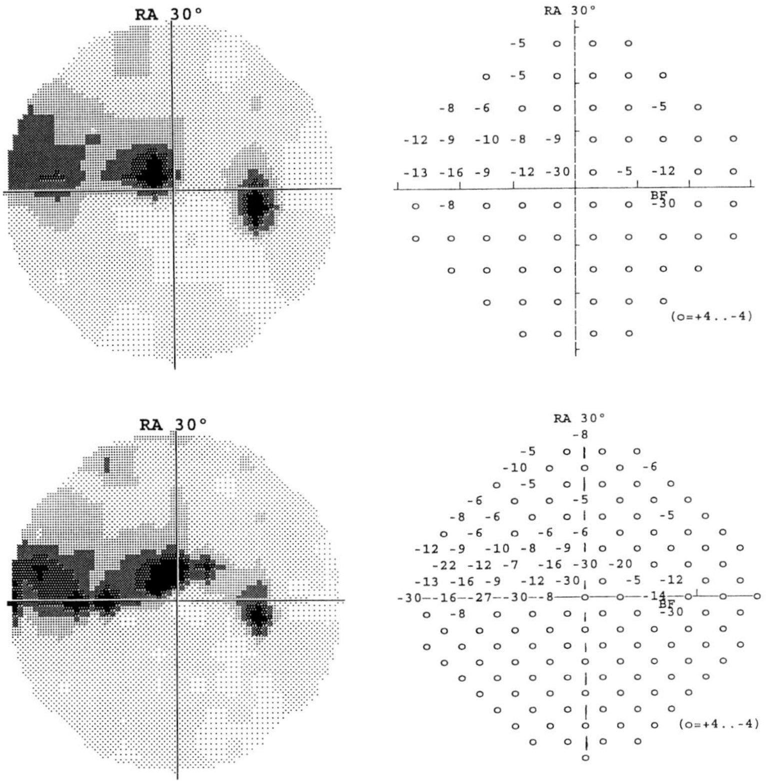

4.4J

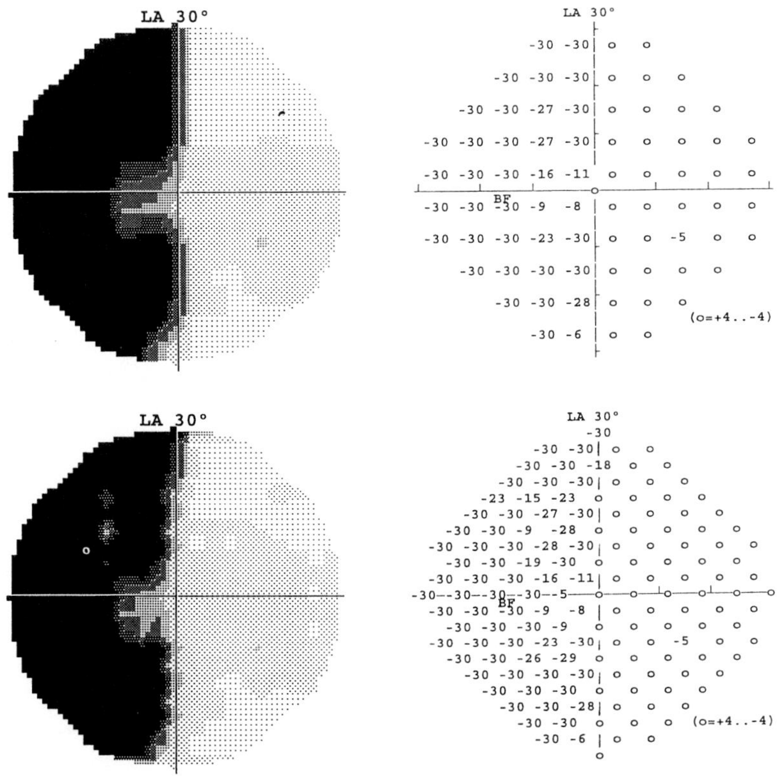

4.4K

4.5 EVALUATION OF THE DEGREE OF DAMAGE

Correlation Between Static and Kinetic Visual Fields

To evaluate the degree of functional damage, the results of computerized perimetry must be related to other findings. First, the familiar kinetic field is considered. Frequently, defects are deeper in static perimetry. This phenomenon, called *stato-kinetic dissociation,* has partly methodological and partly psychophysical origins (Fig. 4.5A). Often, the worse results of static perimetry are in closer agreement with other findings, suggesting that static perimetry is more sensitive.

Correlation of the Static Visual Field, Spatial Resolution, and Ganglion Cell Count in Diseases of the Optic Nerve

In diseases involving only retinal ganglion cells, one can assume that the spatial resolution of the eye diminishes in proportion to the number of intact axons. The spatial resolution (square of visual acuity) serves as an absolute value of function. With acuity perimetry (Frisen) it can be shown that there is a strong relationship between the spatial resolution and intensity thresholds of conventional perimetry, allowing conversion of decibel values to functional values given in percentages (Fig. 4.5B left). This relationship is an exponential function in which every 6 dB of loss is equivalent to a halving of function (Fig. 4.5B, thick line). The first decibel of sensitivity loss is equivalent to 10% of functional loss. This relation is in good agreement with histological findings regarding ganglion cell counts in glaucomatous eyes (Fig. 4.5B right). Discrepancies between decibel values in the visual field and visible morphological changes may be a scaling problem which is overcome by using the true exponential relationship.

Figure 4.5A. Stato-kinetic dissociation: static computerized perimetry (upper, program: HFA 30-2, representation: Peridata norm-related grayscale) shows much deeper defects than the constriction of the isopters of kinetic perimetry (lower) suggests. The patient suffered from a neurofibroma in the chiasmal region.

Figure 4.5B. Spatial resolution (left) is an exponential function of sensitivity loss. A similar relationship is found for ganglion cell loss (right) (after Bartz-Schmidt KU, Weber J: Comparison of spatial thresholds and intensity thresholds in glaucoma. Int Ophthalmol 17:171–178, 1993).

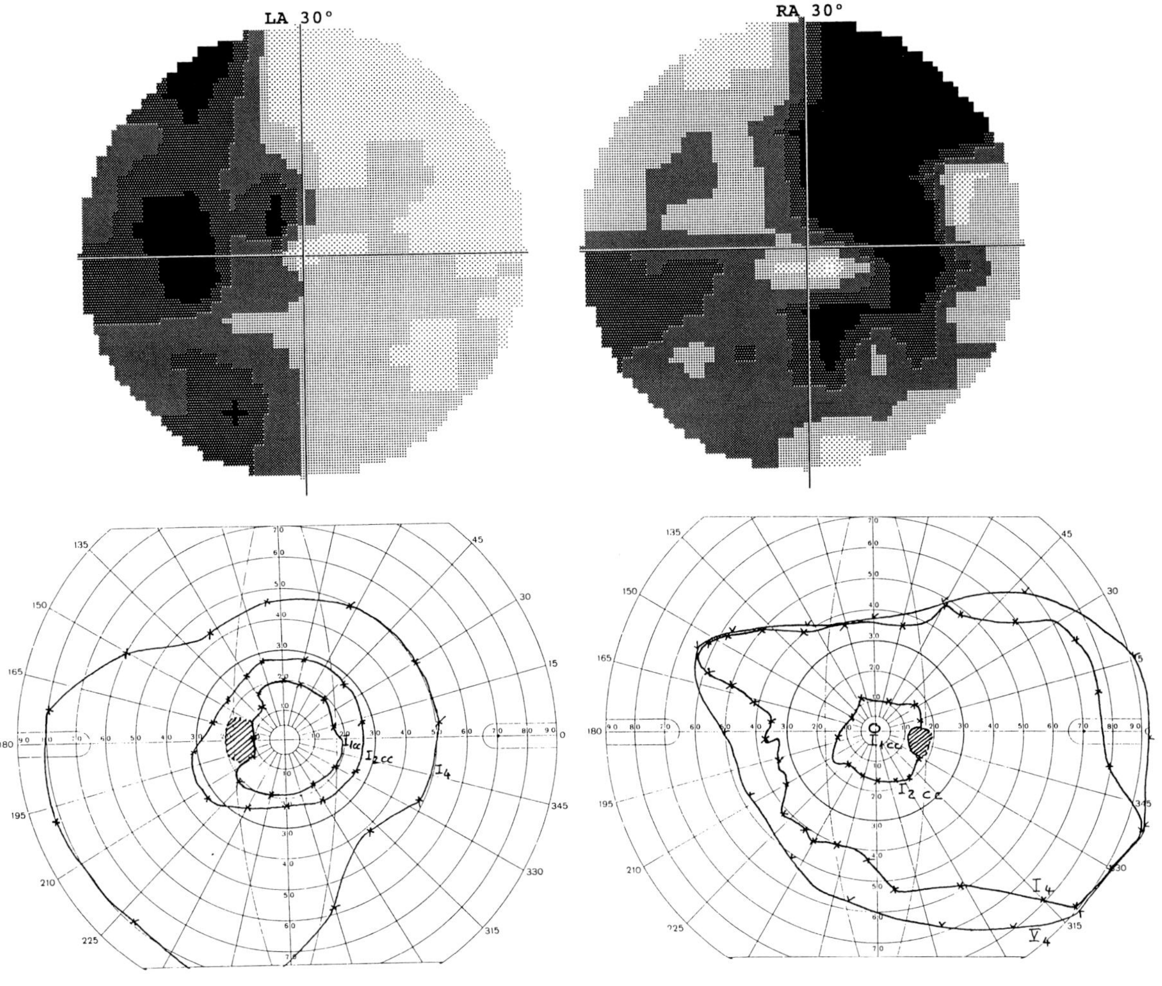
LA 30°
RA 30°

4.5A

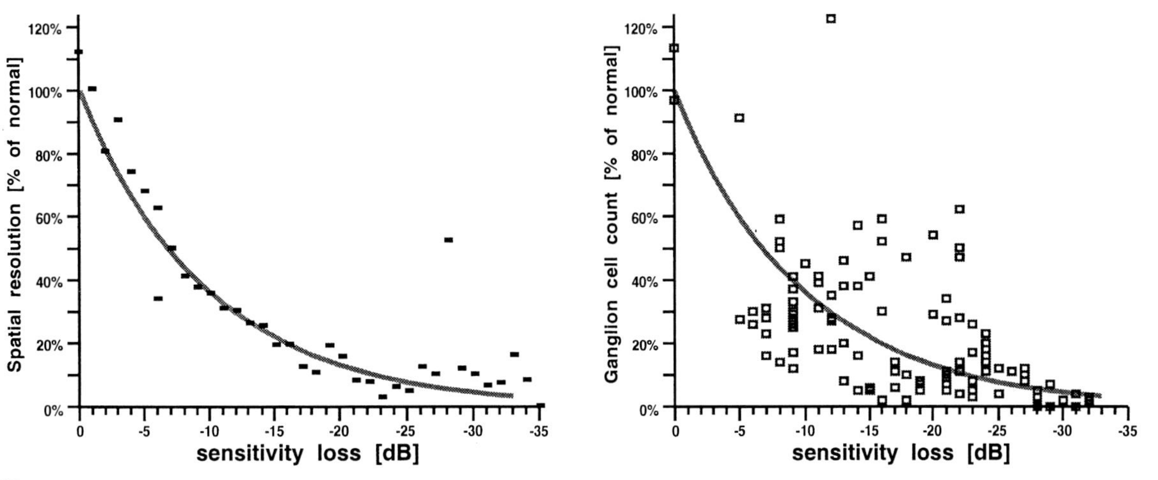
Spatial resolution [% of normal]
120%
100%
80%
60%
40%
20%
0%
0
-5
-10
-15
-20
-25
-30
-35
sensitivity loss [dB]
Ganglion cell count [% of normal]
120%
100%
80%
60%
40%
20%
0%
0
-5
-10
-15
-20
-25
-30
-35
sensitivity loss [dB]

4.5B

5 Follow-Up

5.1 SYNOPSIS

Principle

The time-honored method of visual field follow-up is the simultaneous review of several visual fields in a series *(synopsis)*. The printouts are often skimmed through or spread out on a table. Problems with this method of interpretation are the changing intensity of the ink (with respect to the grayscale), changes in normal values with age (with respect to defect depth and indices), and changes in print modes of newer software versions. These problems may be overcome if the data are stored electronically. A series of visual fields can then be printed at the same time with the same software or analysis package, or they can be viewed on a display screen (Figs. 5.1A, 5.1B).

Numerical Series

Numerical series displays consist of hundreds of numbers. It is practically impossible to get an accurate impression of the behavior of a visual field by simply looking at these figures. However, they may be useful in following up a particular suspicious test location or area in the field numerically.

Grayscale Series

Serial displays of grayscales or color scales are suitable for identifying substantial changes in the degree of damage. The number of fields that can be viewed simultaneously is two to four on a printout and three to six on a computer screen. Some programs allow the user to scroll through the fields or display them dynamically like a movie. In this mode, up to 25 fields can be displayed. For series as well as for single fields, it is generally better to use grayscales based on relative, norm-related sensitivity instead of raw data.

Series of Cumulative Defect Curves

Changes in the degree of damage can be recognized by looking at a series of cumulative defect curves. The Peridata program, for example, prints four curves on a sheet or displays six curves simultaneously on a computer screen.

Series of Indices Tables

Most perimetric analysis programs contain statistically derived indices in their series printouts or displays. As with all numerical representations, their meaning is not intuitive or graphical. One or two preferred indices, such as MD and PSD, can be followed well using the numbers alone. Alternatively, there are graphical representations of the time course of indices (see below).

Figure 5.1A. Serial printout ("compressed" format, Peridata program): norm-related grayscale, norm-related numerals (defects), standard indices, and a cumulative defect curve are printed in a smaller size. With high printer resolution, all details are visible. Four fields fit on a sheet.

PERIDATA Professional 7.0 PRIVATDOZENT DR. MED. JOERG WEBER, COLOGNE

TREND (REGRESSION) * SINGLE RESULT (08-14-98 D:\PROJEKTE\ETLAS\GF\ETLAS.PHF)

PATIENT 5., E. *11-02-18 ID: 75599

RE 07-05-85 11.43 hours HFA1 30-2 ZENTRALFELD SCHWELLENTEST Stim III (200ms) Full threshold
Pupil 4.0 mm VA 1.00 Fixation Target Central RX Used 6.00 DS -1.50 DC 100° axis
Test Duration 15:18 min Questions 520 MalFixation [III] 2% (1/49) FalsePos 25% (3/12) FalseNeg 13% (2/15)

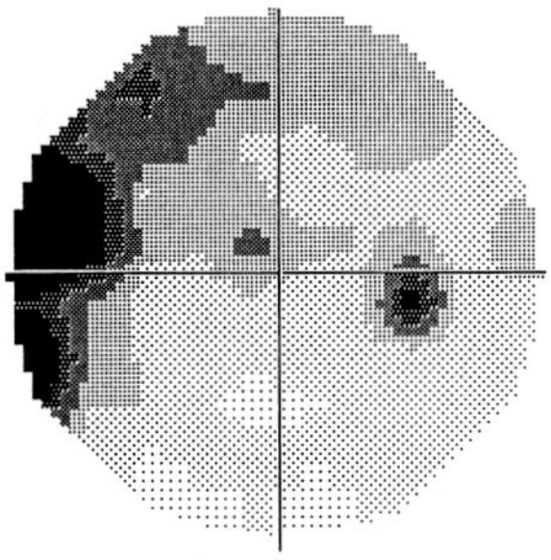

```
           -9 -5|-5 -7
        -16-12-10|-8 -7 -5
     -12-13-10 o| o -7 -9 o
  -30-23 o -8 -6| o  o  o  o  o
  -30-25-5 -5 -11-7  o -9  o -8
  -18-9  o  o  o| o  oB-27 o  o
  -30-7  o  o  o| o  o  o  o  o
     -5  o  o  o| o  o  o  o
         o  o  o| o  o  o
            o  o| o  o
              -30°
```

MD	-5.8
LV	52.3
CLV	45.1
PSD	7.2
CPSD	6.7
SF	2.9
N	74.0
MS	21.7
FS	68.6

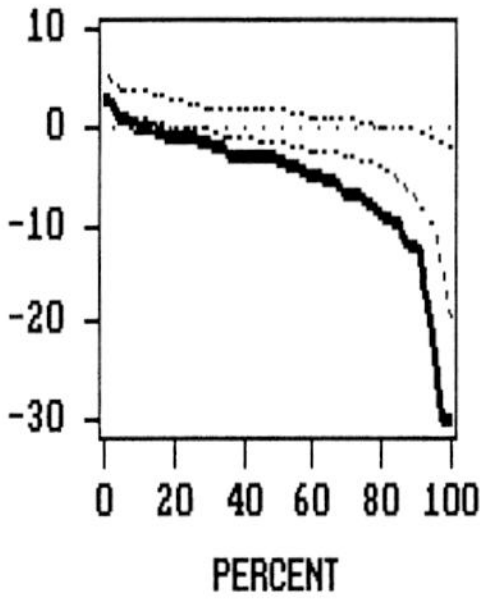

RE 02-28-91 13.53 hours HFA1 30-2 ZENTRALFELD SCHWELLENTEST Stim III (200ms) Full threshold
Pupil 4.0 mm VA 0.00 Fixation Target Central RX Used 4.00 DS 0.00 DC 0° axis
Test Duration 17:35 min Questions 497 MalFixation [I] 12% (3/26) FalsePos 8% (1/12) FalseNeg 25% (3/12)

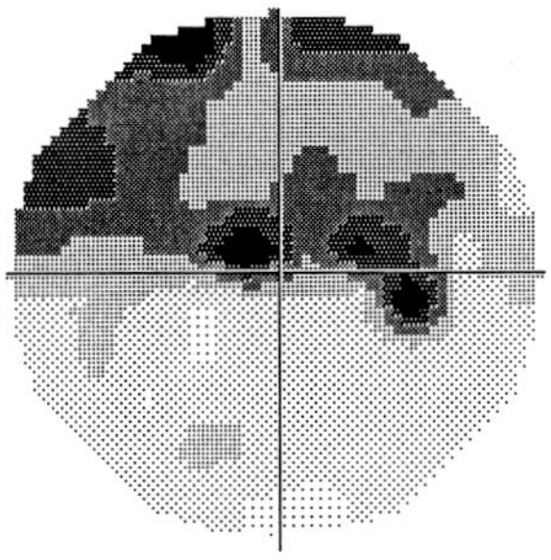

```
           -30-7|-17-17
        -11-11-8|-8 -7 -12
     -15-12-10-5|-9 -7 -6 -6
  -16-16-12-8 -8|-13-9 -11-10 o
  -11-7 -10-12-30-10-22-13 o -7
   o -5  o  o  o| o  o BS-30 o -5
   o -6  o  o  o| o  o  o  o  o
      o  o  o  o| o  o  o  o
         o -6  o| o  o  o
            o  o| o  o
              -30°
```

MD	-6.8
LV	41.9
CLV	34.4
PSD	6.5
CPSD	5.9
SF	2.9
N	74.0
MS	20.2
FS	61.1

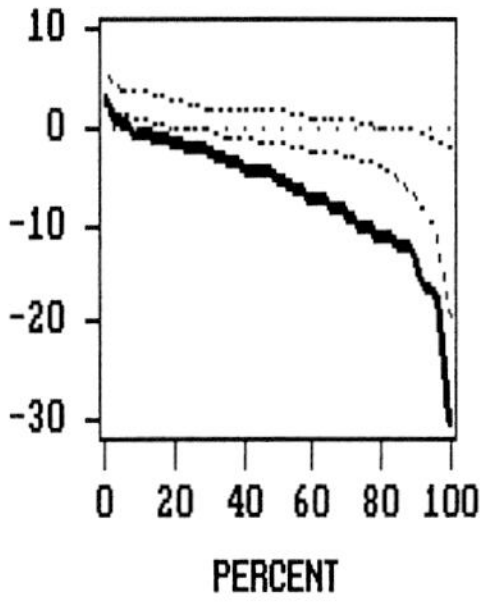

RE 08-29-91 11.49 hours HFA1 30-2 ZENTRALFELD SCHWELLENTEST Stim III (200ms) Full threshold
Pupil 2.0 mm VA 0.00 Fixation Target Central RX Used 3.00 DS 0.00 DC 0° axis
Test Duration 16:33 min Questions 531 MalFixation [III] 7% (2/27) FalsePos 0% (0/16) FalseNeg 7% (1/15)

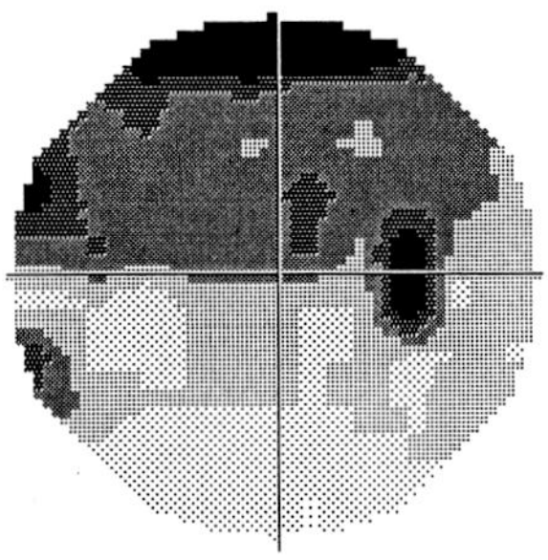

```
           -30-30-30-30
        -18-12-16-10-11-12
     -11-14-12-8|-11-8 -12-10
  -22-12-12-11-12-17-12-11-12-8
  -13-15-12-14-12-16-9 -28-6 -5
   o -5  o -6 -8|-5 -5 BS-30 o -7
  -17 o  o -5 -5| o -5  o -5  o
     -8 -5 -5 -5| o -6  o -7
         o  o  o| o  o -5
            o  o| o  o
              -30°
```

MD	-9.3
LV	48.1
CLV	39.4
PSD	6.9
CPSD	6.3
SF	3.2
N	74.0
MS	18.0
FS	47.2

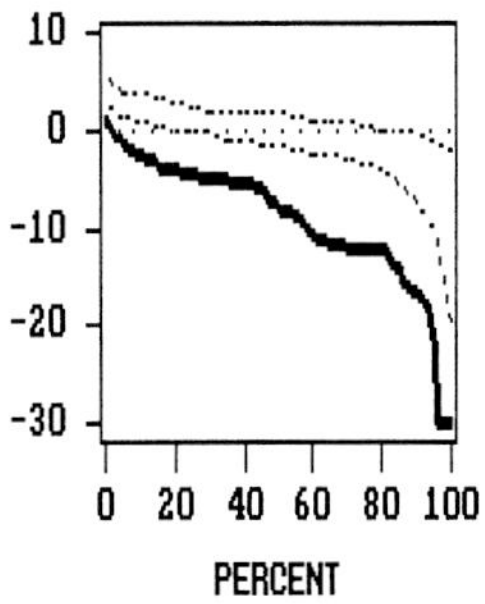

RE 03-09-92 9.59 hours HFA1 30-2 ZENTRALFELD SCHWELLENTEST Stim III (200ms) Full threshold
Pupil 3.0 mm VA 0.00 Fixation Target Central RX Used 0.00 DS 0.00 DC 0° axis
Test Duration 15:59 min Questions 518 MalFixation [III] 8% (2/26) FalsePos 18% (2/11) FalseNeg 7% (1/15)

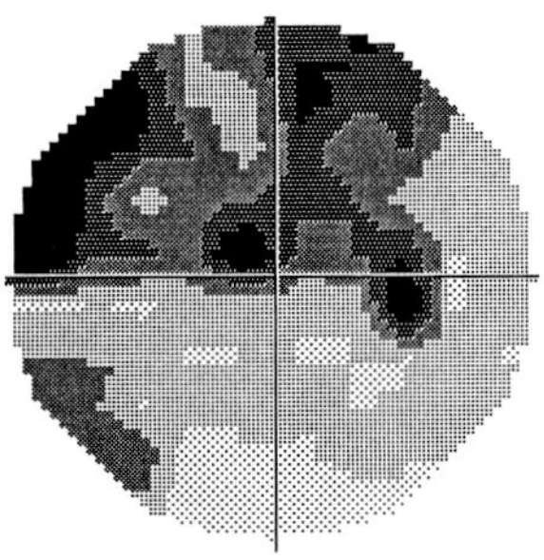

```
           -8 -14-18-20
        -23-9 -6|-22-17-16
     -22-19-16-6|-17-9 -16-6
  -30-18-6 -12-14-17-14-6 -6 -6
  -30-16-16-12-28-12-15-20-5 -6
   o -5  o -8 -6|-6 -7 BS-30 o -7
  -10-9 -9  o -5| o -5  o -7  o
     -10 o -7 -7|-6  o -6 -5
        -14 o  o| o -8 -5
            o  o| o  o
              -30°
```

MD	-9.9
LV	48.4
CLV	35.6
PSD	7.0
CPSD	6.0
SF	3.9
N	74.0
MS	17.0
FS	44.3

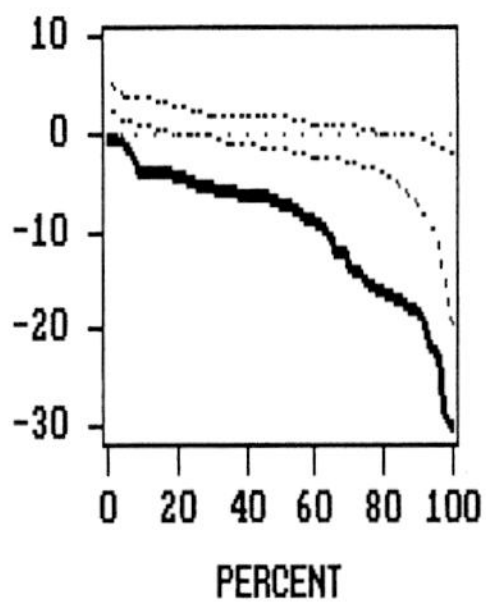

5.1A

Series of Probability Maps

Probability maps consist of noninterpolated grayscale symbols where defect depth is converted to a probability value (see Chapter 2). Because they are norm-related, their usefulness is comparable to that of interpolated, norm-related grayscale maps. Because there are always black squares in deeper defects and points in normal values, changes within these ranges are not represented.

Series of Other Representation Modes

All other representations of the visual field can be displayed in a series. For example, the Peridata program offers series of the three-dimensional hill of vision, the profile, regional and global statistics, a noninterpolated grayscale, and histograms. This information may be of additional help in visualizing and interpreting the results.

Figure 5.1B. Serial printout overview (Statpac program, Humphrey Field Analyzer), same patient as Figure 5.1A. grayscale and numerical map (absolute values), probability map, and pattern deviation probability map. The indices and the Glaucoma Hemifield Test are printed in the interspaces. Any number of fields can be printed out at a density of three fields per sheet.

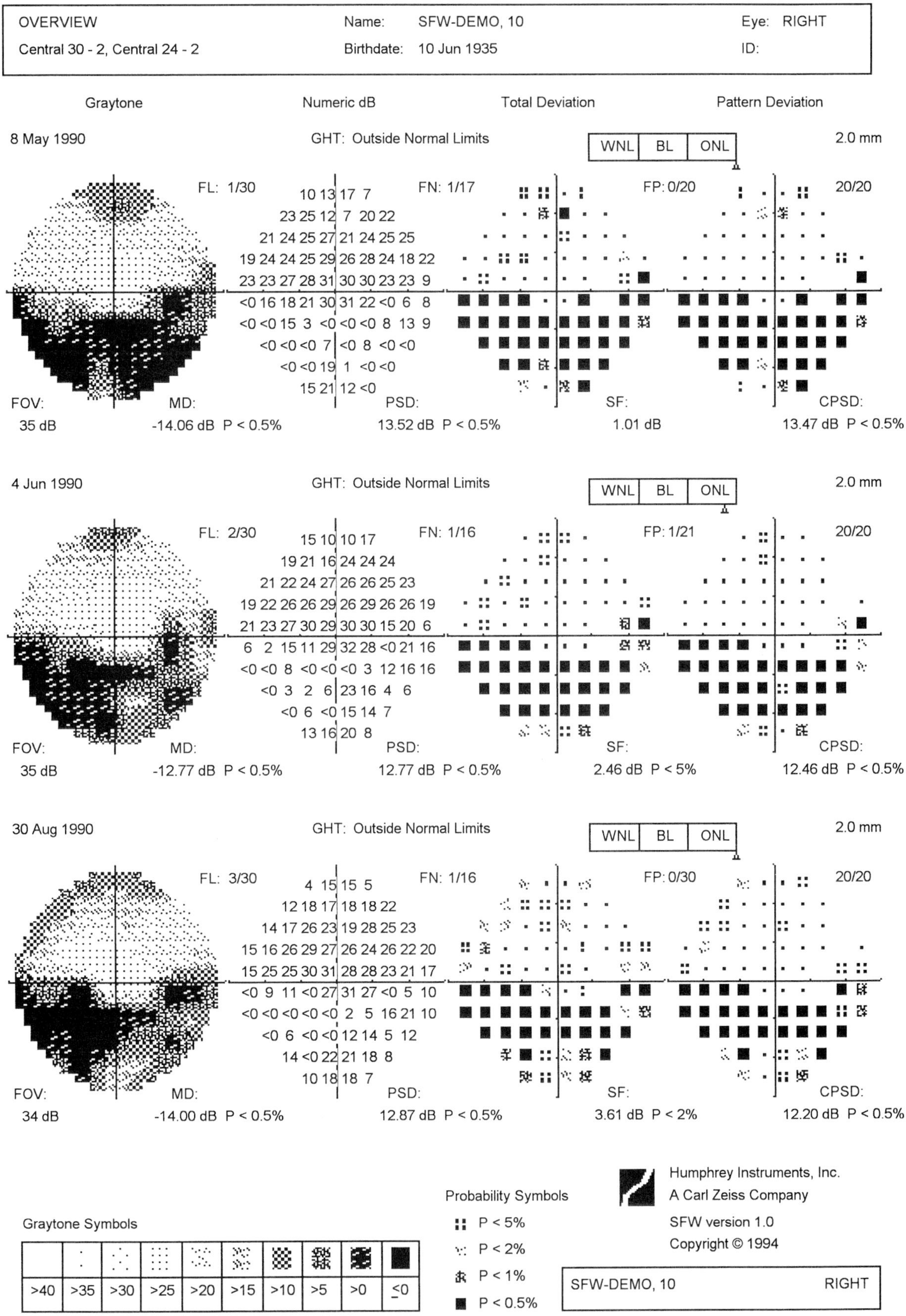
OVERVIEW
Central 30 - 2, Central 24 - 2
Name: SFW-DEMO, 10
Birthdate: 10 Jun 1935
Eye: RIGHT
ID:
Graytone
Numeric dB
Total Deviation
Pattern Deviation
8 May 1990
GHT: Outside Normal Limits
WNL
BL
ONL
2.0 mm
FL: 1/30
FN: 1/17
FP: 0/20
20/20
10 13 17 7
23 25 12 7 20 22
21 24 25 27 21 24 25 25
19 24 24 25 29 26 28 24 18 22
23 23 27 28 31 30 30 23 23 9
<0 16 18 21 30 31 22 <0 6 8
<0 <0 15 3 <0 <0 <0 8 13 9
<0 <0 <0 7 <0 8 <0 <0
<0 <0 19 1 <0 <0
15 21 12 <0
FOV: 35 dB
MD: -14.06 dB P < 0.5%
PSD: 13.52 dB P < 0.5%
SF: 1.01 dB
CPSD: 13.47 dB P < 0.5%
4 Jun 1990
GHT: Outside Normal Limits
WNL
BL
ONL
2.0 mm
FL: 2/30
FN: 1/16
FP: 1/21
20/20
15 10 10 17
19 21 16 24 24 24
21 22 24 27 26 26 25 23
19 22 26 26 29 26 29 26 26 19
21 23 27 30 29 30 30 15 20 6
6 2 15 11 29 32 28 <0 21 16
<0 <0 8 <0 <0 <0 3 12 16 16
<0 3 2 6 23 16 4 6
<0 6 <0 15 14 7
13 16 20 8
FOV: 35 dB
MD: -12.77 dB P < 0.5%
PSD: 12.77 dB P < 0.5%
SF: 2.46 dB P < 5%
CPSD: 12.46 dB P < 0.5%
30 Aug 1990
GHT: Outside Normal Limits
WNL
BL
ONL
2.0 mm
FL: 3/30
FN: 1/16
FP: 0/30
20/20
4 15 15 5
12 18 17 18 18 22
14 17 26 23 19 28 25 23
15 16 26 29 27 26 24 26 22 20
15 25 25 30 31 28 28 23 21 17
<0 9 11 <0 27 31 27 <0 5 10
<0 <0 <0 <0 <0 2 5 16 21 10
<0 6 <0 <0 12 14 5 12
14 <0 22 21 18 8
10 18 18 7
FOV: 34 dB
MD: -14.00 dB P < 0.5%
PSD: 12.87 dB P < 0.5%
SF: 3.61 dB P < 2%
CPSD: 12.20 dB P < 0.5%
Graytone Symbols
>40 >35 >30 >25 >20 >15 >10 >5 >0 ≤0
Probability Symbols
P < 5%
P < 2%
P < 1%
P < 0.5%
Humphrey Instruments, Inc.
A Carl Zeiss Company
SFW version 1.0
Copyright © 1994
SFW-DEMO, 10 RIGHT

5.1B

5.2 DIAGRAMS

Principle

By reducing visual field data to a few numbers or even a single number, it is possible to visualize their temporal course in a diagram or a diagram-like graphic.

Global Mean Defect and Other Standard Indices

The global mean defect (MD) represents the average loss (or gain) of sensitivity compared to that of age-matched normal subjects. Therefore, a diagram of MD versus time shows the average behavior of the entire visual field (Fig. 5.2A). Similarly, other indices, such as those for spatial scatter (PSD, CPSD, LV, CLV), measurement error (SF), and regional mean values (RM), can be plotted versus time.

Box Plot

The box plot represents five values of the cumulative curve: minimum, 15th percentile, median, 85th percentile, and maximum. Contrary to the MD-time plot, the box plot shows not only the average, but also the distribution of values.

Graphical Bar

The graphical bar plot is a stacked histogram of sensitivity classes. Dark areas in the column indicate deep defects, and light areas indicate shallow defects or normal sensitivity. The grayscale or color scale used is identical to the topographical maps. Therefore, it is easy to learn how to interpret these graphics. In contrast to the box plot, the change in a single value may show up if it changes the defect class (Fig. 5.2B).

Combined Representation

The box plot, MD plot, and graphical bar plot can be combined, providing a fairly complete overview of the quantitative behavior of the visual field (Fig. 5.2C).

Figure 5.2A. MD-time-diagram (a portion of the "change analysis" printout, Statpac program, Humphrey Field Analyzer).

Figure 5.2B. Box-plot-time diagram (a portion of the "change analysis" printout, Statpac program, Humphrey Field Analyzer).

Figure 5.2C. Combined representation of the box plot and MD (cross) versus time and the graphical bar plot. For greater readability, the diagram can be viewed in landscape (horizontal) printout mode ("box plot" printout, Peridata program).

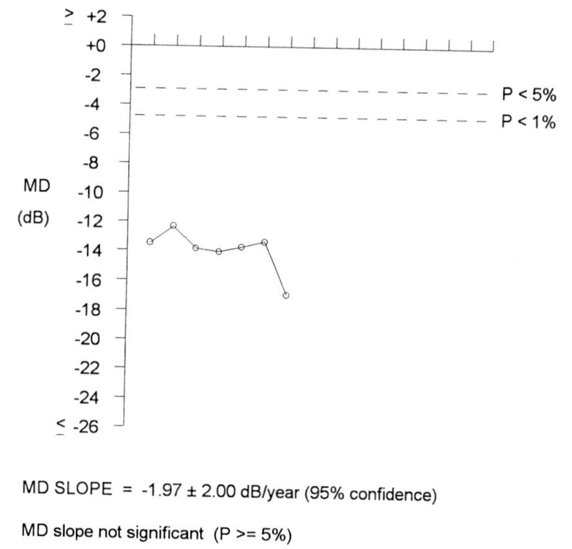
≥ +2
+0
-2
-4
-6
-8
-10
-12
-14
-16
-18
-20
-22
-24
≤ -26
MD
(dB)
P < 5%
P < 1%
MD SLOPE = -1.97 ± 2.00 dB/year (95% confidence)
MD slope not significant (P >= 5%)

5.2A

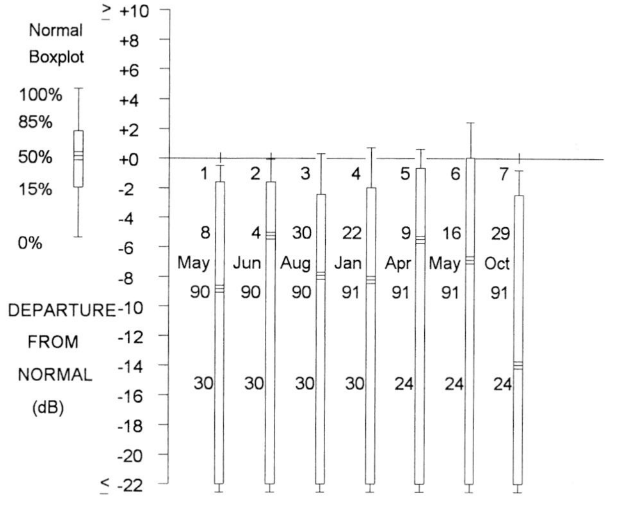
Normal
Boxplot
100%
85%
50%
15%
0%
DEPARTURE
FROM
NORMAL
(dB)
≥ +10
+8
+6
+4
+2
+0
-2
-4
-6
-8
-10
-12
-14
-16
-18
-20
≤ -22
1 2 3 4 5 6 7
8 4 30 22 9 16 29
May Jun Aug Jan Apr May Oct
90 90 90 91 91 91 91
30 30 30 30 24 24 24

5.2B

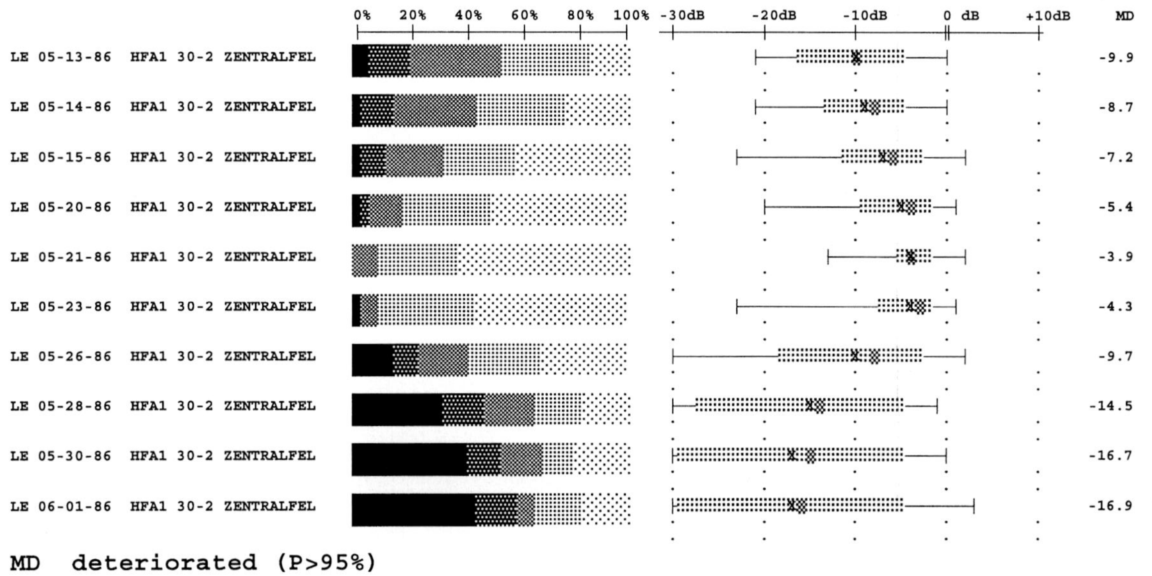
0% 20% 40% 60% 80% 100%
-30dB -20dB -10dB 0 dB +10dB
MD
LE 05-13-86 HFA1 30-2 ZENTRALFEL -9.9
LE 05-14-86 HFA1 30-2 ZENTRALFEL -8.7
LE 05-15-86 HFA1 30-2 ZENTRALFEL -7.2
LE 05-20-86 HFA1 30-2 ZENTRALFEL -5.4
LE 05-21-86 HFA1 30-2 ZENTRALFEL -3.9
LE 05-23-86 HFA1 30-2 ZENTRALFEL -4.3
LE 05-26-86 HFA1 30-2 ZENTRALFEL -9.7
LE 05-28-86 HFA1 30-2 ZENTRALFEL -14.5
LE 05-30-86 HFA1 30-2 ZENTRALFEL -16.7
LE 06-01-86 HFA1 30-2 ZENTRALFEL -16.9
MD deteriorated (P>95%)

5.2C

5.3 POINTWISE TREND ANALYSIS

Principle

Using visual field synopses and diagrams, the examiner must identify changes and evaluate them. With trend analyses, mathematical methods perform the evaluation. The results of such analyses are objective and reproducible. Whether they are more valid than the result of informed subjective human evaluation depends on the concordance between the mathematical model and the field development (e.g., continuous, episodic).

Pointwise trend analysis treats every visual field location separately. The measured data on each location over time are regarded as a time series of a value. Several methods for trend calculation are available.

Linear Regression Analysis

Linear regression assumes that true field change occurs continuously at a constant rate. A line is calculated which falls closest to all measured values (Fig. 5.3A). This line represents the probable true course of the change. The starting point and the endpoint of the line are the most probable starting and ending values of the sensitivity. In case of a large measurement error and a true linear course, these values are closer to the true values than to the measured values themselves. In the Peridata program, these starting and ending values are written under each other (*double numerals,* Fig. 5.3A–B).

The significance of any change is calculated using statistical formulas. The percentage is the probability that the curve has the indicated direction (downward, upward) and is not horizontal or in the alternative direction. Using the Peridata program, the significance is represented by a symbol. On the screen, significance is indicated by colors (green: significant improvement; red: significant deterioration).

Calculation is based on the true time intervals of measurements. For better graphic visualization, Figure 5.3A uses an arbitrary example with constant time intervals.

Figure 5.3A. Principle of pointwise trend analysis with linear regression.

Figure 5.3B. Double numerals representation of the trend analysis of the Peridata program. The two values represent the most probable sensitivity at the beginning and end of the time interval. The symbol represents statistical significance. The numbers are based on the visual field series of Fig. 5.1A–B.

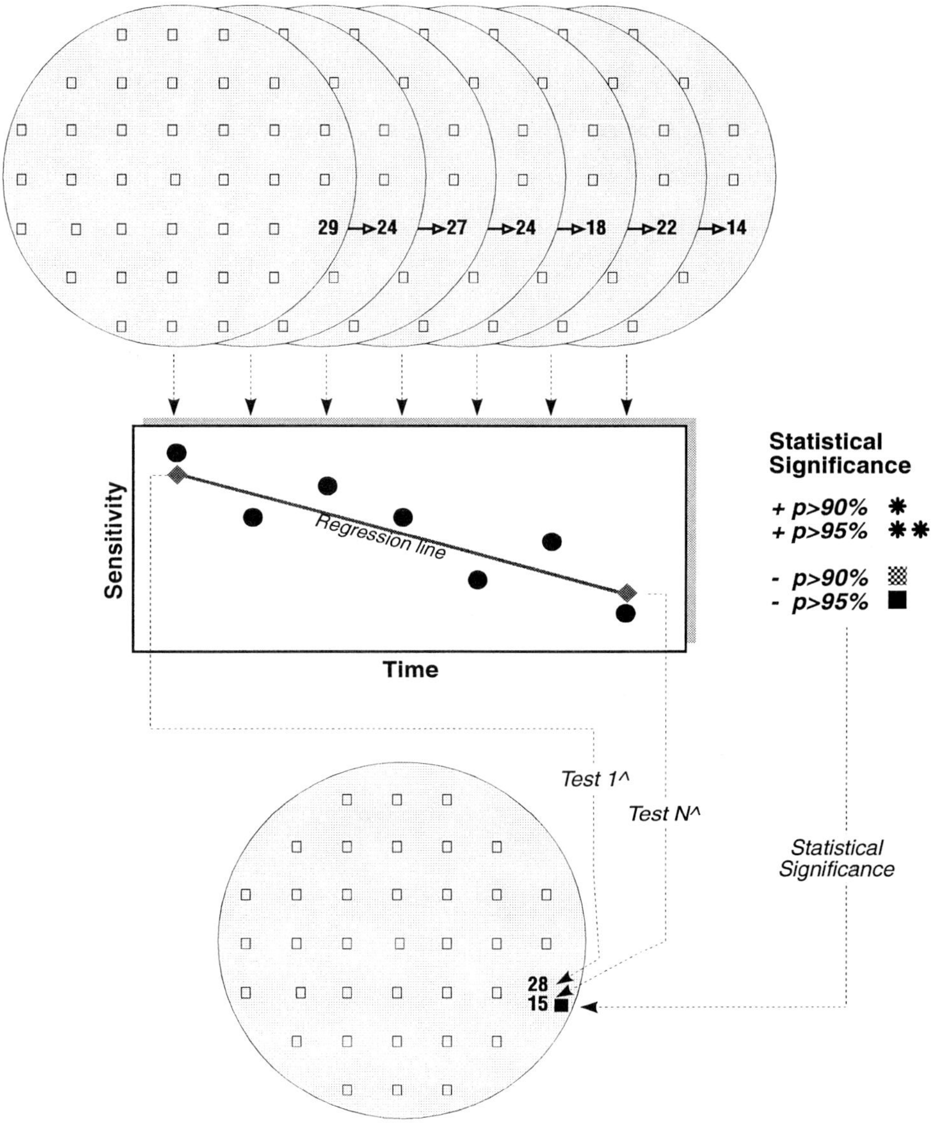
29 24 27 24 18 22 14
Sensitivity
Regression line
Time
Statistical Significance
+ p>90% ✱
+ p>95% ✱✱
- p>90%
- p>95%
Test 1^
Test N^
Statistical Significance
28
15

5.3A

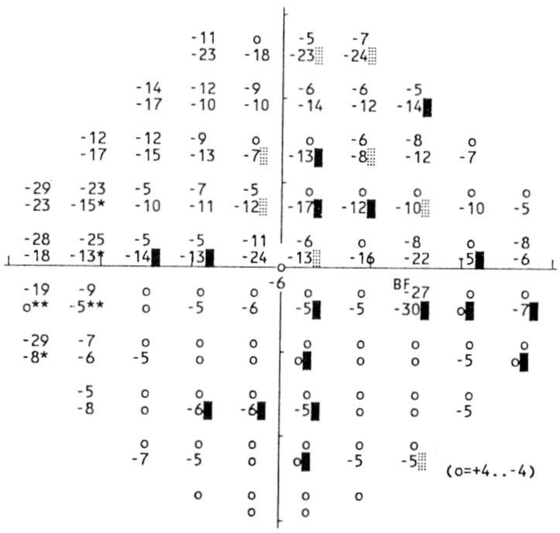
-11 o -5 -7
-23 -18 -23 -24
-14 -12 -9 -6 -6 -5
-17 -10 -10 -14 -12 -14
-12 -12 -9 o o -6 -8 o
-17 -15 -13 -7 -13 -8 -12 -7
-29 -23 -5 -7 -5 o o o o o
-23 -15* -10 -11 -12 -17 -12 -10 -10 -5
-28 -25 -5 -5 -11 -6 o -8 o -8
-18 -13† -14 -13 -24 -13 -16 -22 5 -6
-6
-19 -9 o o o o o BF 27 o o
o** -5** o -5 -6 -5 -5 -30 o -7
-29 -7 o o o o o o o o
-8* -6 -5 o o o o o -5 o
-5 o o o o o o o
-8 o -6 -6 -5 o o -5
o o o o o o
-7 -5 o o -5 -5
(o=+4..-4)
o o o o
o o

5.3B

Empirical Trend Analysis

Empirical trend analysis is based on experimental studies of long-term fluctuation in glaucoma. In a number of glaucoma patients whose condition was stable, follow-up fields were measured several times within a 4-week period. The sensitivity showed a bell-curve distribution around the initial value. The scatter was larger for values of lower sensitivity. Based on these distributions, normal ranges for follow-up fields were developed. They are used in various ways for empirical change analyses.

The Statpac program defines the first two fields as baseline fields and averages them (Fig. 5.3C). For each point, the normal range for successive fields is taken from a look-up table with regard to the baseline sensitivity. Each follow-up field is compared pointwise with these ranges. Values outside the range are considered significantly changed and are indicated by symbols. A series of follow-up fields with change probability symbols is then printed (Fig. 5.3D).

The method of the Peridata program is similar but uses only the last two fields (endpoint) which are most likely to have changed. These last two fields are averaged like the first two to reduce random error. Normal ranges are also smaller. In addition to the change probability symbol, the baseline value and the endpoint value (both averaged) are displayed in a double numerals mode.

Probabilities are valid for the average patient. In patients with widely scattered sensitivities over time (high long-term fluctuation), the probability statements overestimate the true significance. In other patients with very stable values (low long-term fluctuation), the probability statements underestimate the true significance, and continuous visual field decay is detected rather late.

Group Analysis (*t*-Test)

Another statistical procedure divides a series of numbers into two groups and compares them with Student's *t*-test. This method is used in the Delta program. It is suitable if the visual field changed abruptly at one time—for example, after surgery. However, in most diseases (including glaucoma) defects develop slowly and continuously, suggesting that the method of linear regression is more suitable for detecting change.

Overall Evaluation

Pointwise trend analysis is able to recognize and stress regional differences in trends. Overall evaluation based on pointwise analysis is difficult because significant changes in single points do not indicate a trend in the visual field as a whole. Even in stable fields, 5% of all points will lie outside the 95% confidence limit. The number of changed points, the balance between positive and negative trend points, and the concordance with the appropriate anatomy and physiology are not defined.

Figure 5.3C. Principle of pointwise trend analysis using empirical normal ranges for change.

Figure 5.3D. Two follow-up fields using the empirical trend analysis of the Statpac program. Description of maps from left to right: grayscale, norm probability, change in numerals, and change probability symbols.

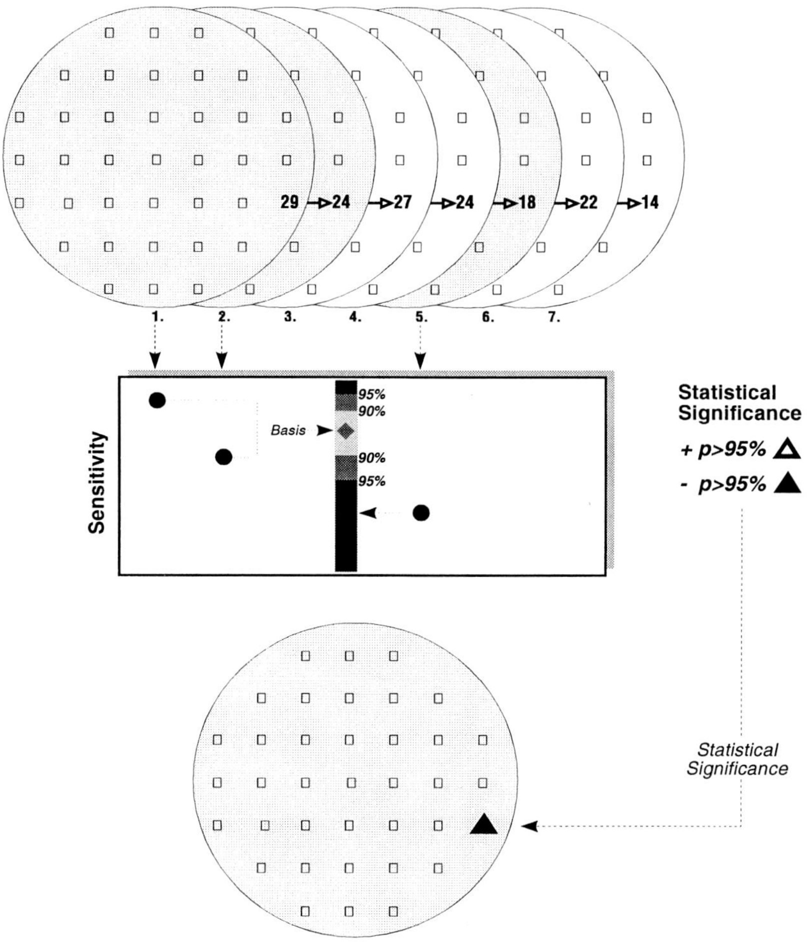
29
24
27
24
18
22
14
1.
2.
3.
4.
5.
6.
7.
Sensitivity
95%
90%
Basis
90%
95%
Statistical Significance
+ p>95%
- p>95%
Statistical Significance

5.3C

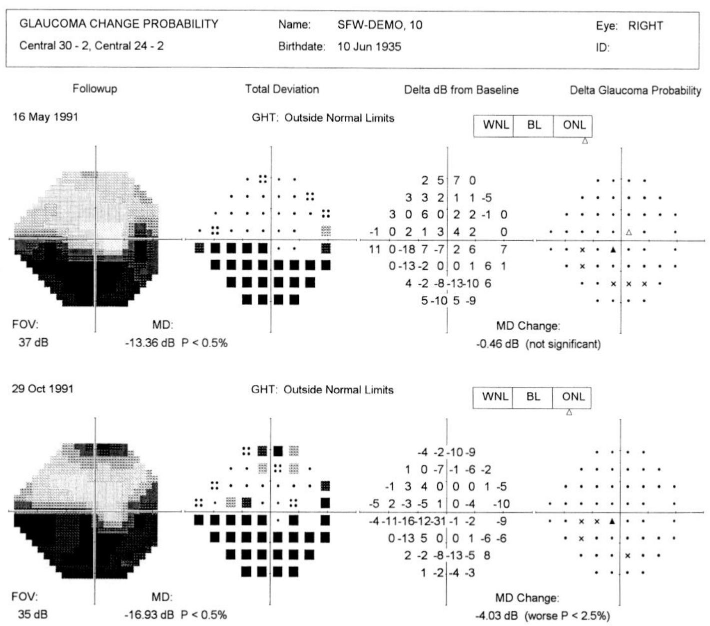
GLAUCOMA CHANGE PROBABILITY
Central 30 - 2, Central 24 - 2
Name: SFW-DEMO, 10
Birthdate: 10 Jun 1935
Eye: RIGHT
ID:
Followup
Total Deviation
Delta dB from Baseline
Delta Glaucoma Probability
16 May 1991
GHT: Outside Normal Limits
WNL
BL
ONL
FOV:
37 dB
MD:
-13.36 dB P < 0.5%
MD Change:
-0.46 dB (not significant)
29 Oct 1991
GHT: Outside Normal Limits
WNL
BL
ONL
FOV:
35 dB
MD:
-16.93 dB P < 0.5%
MD Change:
-4.03 dB (worse P < 2.5%)

5.3D

Choosing a Method

With just a few (two to four) visual fields, empirical trend analysis is the most suitable method. In longer series and with slow, continuous progression, linear regression is superior. In case of a sudden change, Student's *t*-test is the most appropriate choice.

Graphical Analysis of Topographical Trends

Graphical Analysis of Topographical Trends (GATT) is a display which represents both the original field and the change in one graphical image. In can be applied to any type of statistical trend analysis. The image base is the grayscale representation of the initial and final states of the field. Depending on the type of trend analysis used, these may be baseline fields and follow-up fields (empirical analysis), the starting point and ending point of the regression line (regression analysis), or mean values of the first and the second groups (*t*-test). The grayscale images are superimposed. The pattern depends on the amount of change and on statistical significance (Fig. 5.3E).

- In stable regions, both grayscales are equal, and the area is homogenous.
- With statistically significant deterioration, the image is composed of horizontal stripes. The grayscale shows the degree of damage, and the contrast shows the amount of change.
- With statistically significant improvement, the grayscale image is composed of vertical stripes. The contrast shows the amount of improvement.
- In case of nonsignificant change, both images are composed of a checkerboard pattern. The checkerboard has horizontal rectangles in case of deterioration and vertical rectangles in case of improvement.

The information contained in GATT is identical to that of the double numerical map (see Fig. 5.3B). With graphical transformation, the information is more easily visualized and more perceptible. Figure 5.3F shows a typical example. The GATT image contains all the information about progression.

Originally, statistical significance was not shown with GATT. Instead, a graphical trick was used which made significant trends evident. This literal "graphical analysis" was replaced by representations with mathematical significance. Nevertheless, GATT is still partly a graphical analysis. With neighboring points revealing significant trends, a disproportionately large area with stripes is shown, corresponding to the higher importance of trend clusters. Furthermore, larger changes stand out because of the higher contrast of the stripes.

Figure 5.3E. Principle of the grayscale composition of GATT.

Figure 5.3F. Visual field series (top) and GATT (bottom, based on linear regression). A connection developed between the large arcuate scotoma and the blind spot, which is represented by horizontal stripes. This trend is significant. The regression of the shallow upper nasal defect is also significant (representation: Peridata trend analysis).

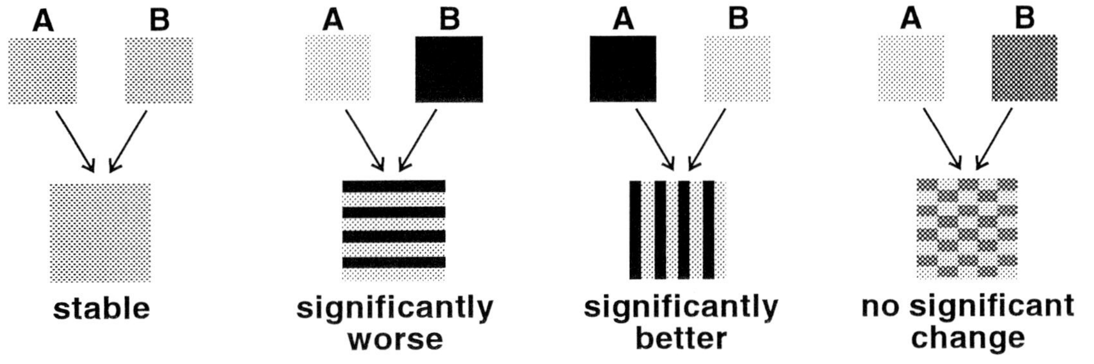
A
B
A
B
A
B
A
B
stable
significantly worse
significantly better
no significant change

5.3E

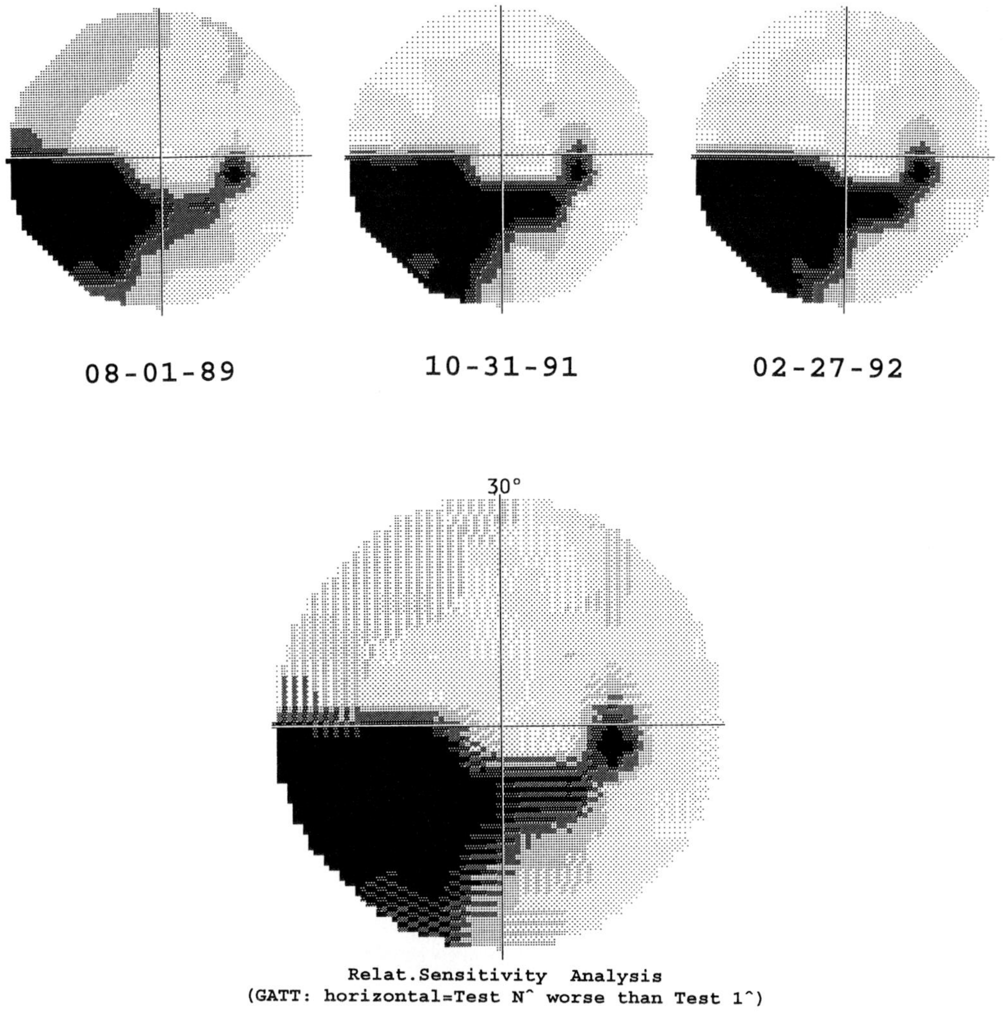
08-01-89
10-31-91
02-27-92
30°
Relat.Sensitivity Analysis
(GATT: horizontal=Test N^ worse than Test 1^)

5.3F

5.4 REGIONAL AND GLOBAL TREND ANALYSIS

Linear Regression Analysis for Regions

Trend analysis in particular regions is based on the regional mean defect (RMD). This mean is analyzed versus time. Linear regression analysis is the preferred statistical approach (see pointwise trend analysis, Fig. 5.3A). Initial and final values of the regression line and the significance of the trend are shown for each region (Fig. 5.4A right). Various regional divisions can be chosen (quadrants, hemifields, sectors, rings, nerve fiber bundles). The active division is printed together with the results (Fig. 5.4A left).

The example is based on the case shown in Figure 5.3F. A quadrant division was chosen. Both upper quadrants improved highly significantly (**), while the lower quadrants deteriorated significantly or highly significantly.

Linear Regression Analysis for Global Indices

Trend analysis of the entire field is based on global field indices, especially the global mean value MD (mean defect). Nearly all programs use linear regression analysis. In addition to the significance level, either the initial and final values of the regression line (Fig. 5.4B left) or the slope (Fig. 5.4B right) are displayed.

The example is based on the case shown in Figure 5.3F and Figure 5.4A. The change in MD from –8.6 dB to –8.1 dB, or +0.2 dB/year, is not significant. The counteracting trends in the upper and lower quadrants have neutralized each other. Heterogeneity (the LV/CLV and PSD/CPSD indices) have increased, which is usually associated with deterioration. The other indices are less important in follow-up.

Graphical Analysis of Numerical Trends

Global trends can be easily detected by changes in the cumulative defect curve. A series of fields may be presented by the cumulative defect curve of the initial field by and the final field or starting point and ending point in regression analysis. These two curves (Fig. 5.4C left), however, do not show which values have changed because the second curve is sorted independently of the first curve. An alternative method is the Graphical Analysis of Numerical Trends (GANT). With this method, changes are indicated by small bars starting at the initial curve (Fig. 5.4C right). Improvement is dotted (screen: green), and deterioration is indicated by solid bars (screen: red).

This example is based on the series shown in Figure 5.3F. The double curve shows that the final field contains higher "good" values (elevation of the left part of the curve) and lower "bad" values (depression of the right part of the curve). GANT shows that this change was caused by an improvement in the originally medium values (middle part with long upward bars) and a decrease in the low values (right part with long downward bars), while the originally good values remained stable (left part without long bars).

Figure 5.4A. Regional trend analysis, quadrant division (Peridata program).

Figure 5.4B. Trend analysis of global indices (Peridata program). Double numerals (left) and change per year (right) are given; both representations contain significance symbols.

Figure 5.4C. Special types of the cumulative curve in the Peridata program indicating global trends: double curve (left) and GANT (right).

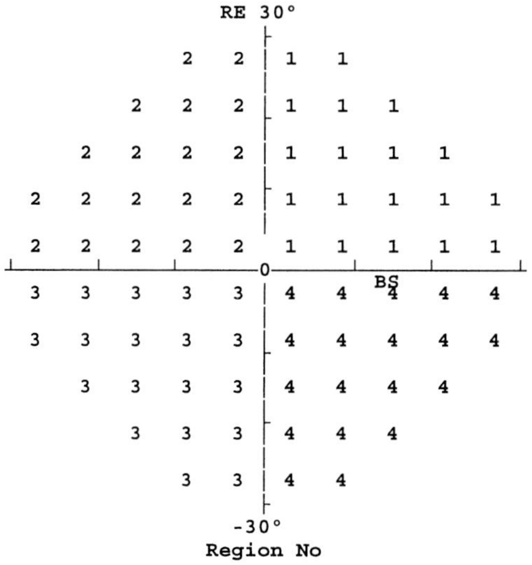

QUADRANTS

R1:	-2.4, -1.2**	(N=18)
R2:	-5.2, +0.2**	(N=19)
R3:	-23.2, -26.1⁞⁞	(N=19)
R4:	-3.9, -5.5█	(N=18)

Relat.Sensitivity Analysis
(Test 1^,Test N^)
(change (neg): ⁞⁞ P>90% █ P>95%)
(change (pos): * P>90% ** P>95%)

5.4A

STANDARD INDICES

* Test 1^,Test N^		
MD	-8.7, -8.2	
LV	107.6,150.2	█
CLV	99.6,143.9	█
PSD	10.4, 12.3	█
CPSD	10.0, 12.0	█
SF	3.4, 2.7	
N	75.0, 75.0	
MS	18.5, 18.8	
FS	55.6, 60.6	**

STANDARD INDICES

* dB/year [±error]		
MD	+0.20 [±0.16]	
LV	+16.60 [±0.08]	█
CLV	+17.22 [±1.69]	█
PSD	+0.74 [±0.00]	█
CPSD	+0.79 [±0.06]	█
SF	-0.28 [±0.34]	
N	0.00 [±0.00]	
MS	+0.11 [±0.18]	
FS	+1.98 [±0.29]	**

5.4B

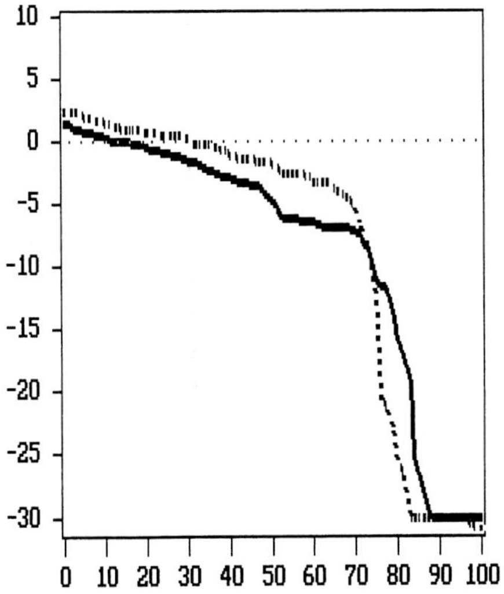

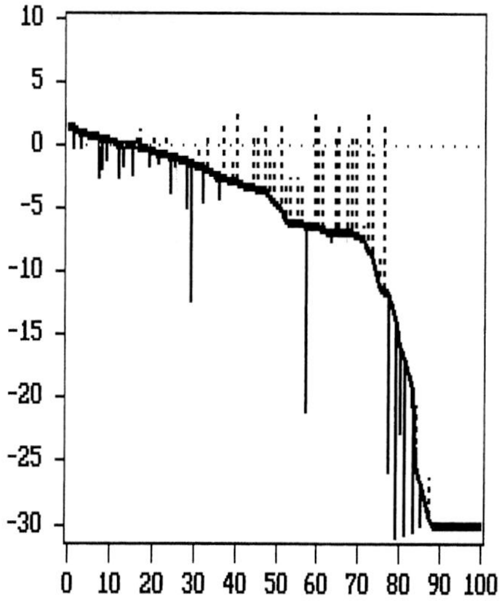

5.4C

5.5 SPECIAL ASPECTS OF FOLLOW-UP EVALUATION

Change in Stimulus Size

In the course of follow-up, it may be necessary to change the stimulus size. Especially when testing badly damaged fields, it may be necessary to change from standard size III (Goldmann notation, visual angle 0.43°) to stimulus size V (visual angle 1.71°) to increase the usable measurement range (Fig. 5.5A). The increase in absolute sensitivity achieved by spatial summation depends on sensitivity, but is about 5 to 10 dB in the lower range. Conversion tables for stimulus size V will soon be incorporated into analysis programs.

Use of Different Perimeters

Since it is possible to store results achieved with different computerized perimeters in the same analytic program and to view them simultaneously, the question of comparability has arisen. Because the examination factors (stimulus duration, background illumination, color, etc.) differ substantially, absolute sensitivities differ. In addition, the definition of decibel scales is different. The use of empirical conversion tables has been attempted, but the wide scatter of converted thresholds makes accurate conversion impossible.

The use of norm-related, relative sensitivity values reduces the differences. The relative sensitivity of normal points is 0 dB for all instruments. Usually the defect depth is similar (Fig. 5.5B). However, larger differences may occur (Fig. 5.5C). In case of suspected change in a visual field, examinations using both instruments on the same day are recommended.

Figure 5.5A. Glaucomatous visual field island, right eye, grayscale representation of absolute sensitivity (Peridata program). The change from stimulus size III to V increases the measured sensitivity. Absolute defects may turn into relative defects if the sensitivity is slightly below the measurement range. Very deep absolute defects remain absolute defects, of course (examination: HFA 30-1 + 30-2; MS = mean absolute sensitivity).

Figure 5.5B. Glaucoma field, examination using the Humphrey Field Analyzer, program 30-2 (left), and Octopus 1-2-3, program G1X (right). Norm-related sensitivity is similar (representation: Peridata norm-related grayscale).

Figure 5.5C. Glaucoma field examination with the Humphrey Field Analyzer, program 30-2 (left), and Octopus 1-2-3, program G1X (right). Norm-related sensitivity is substantially worse in the Octopus examination (representation: Peridata norm-related grayscale).

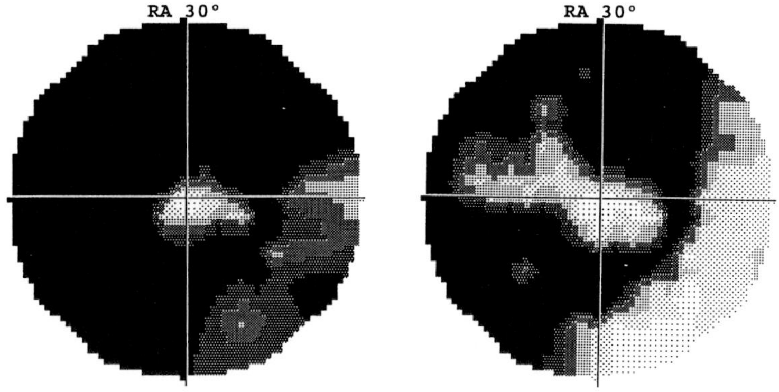

Absolute Sensitivity

Stimulus III
MS = 2.7 dB

Absolute Sensitivity

Stimulus V
MS = 8.3 dB

5.5A

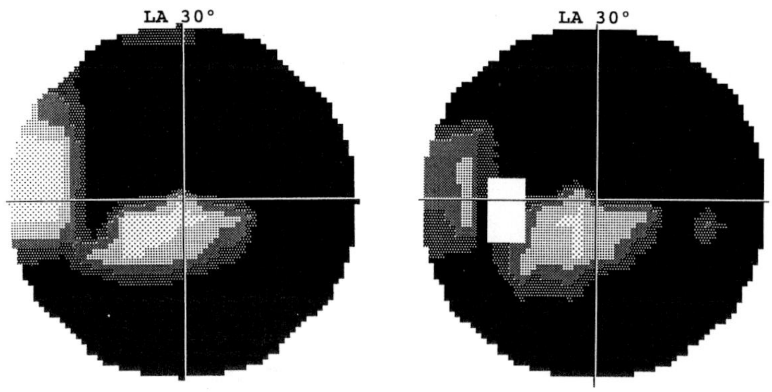

Relative Sensitivity

HFA
MD = -20.2 dB

Relative Sensitivity

Octopus 1-2-3
MD = -22.4 dB

5.5B

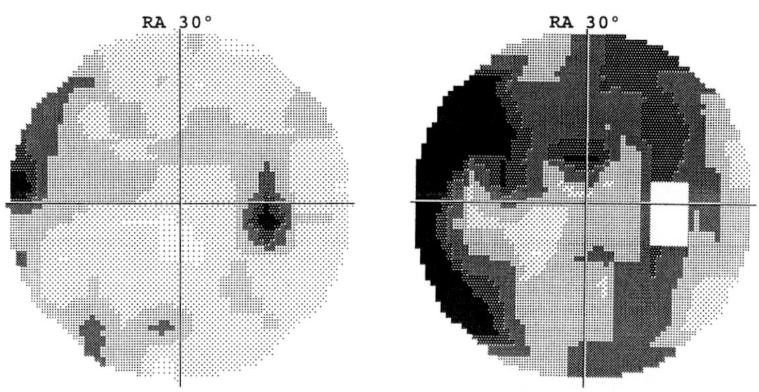

Relative Sensitivity

HFA
MD = -4.0 dB

Relative Sensitivity

Octopus 1-2-3
MD = -10.7 dB

5.5C

Index

ISBN 0-7216-6737-6

90038

9 780721 667379